Viruses and Reproductive

Viruses and Reproductive Injustice

Zika in Brazil

ILANA LÖWY

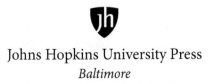

Johns Hopkins University Press

Baltimore

© 2024 Johns Hopkins University Press
All rights reserved. Published 2024
Printed in the United States of America on acid+free paper

2 4 6 8 9 7 5 3 1

Johns Hopkins University Press
2715 North Charles Street
Baltimore, Maryland 21218
www.press.jhu.edu

Cataloging-in-Publication Data is available from the Library of Congress.
A catalog record for this book is available from the British Library.

ISBN: 978-1-4214-4791-9 (paperback)
ISBN: 978-1-4214-4792-6 (ebook)

Special discounts are available for bulk purchases of this book. For more information, please contact Special Sales at specialsales@jh.edu.

CONTENTS

Preface: A Forgotten Virus and Expunged Memories   *vii*

Acknowledgments   *xv*

Introduction. Framing an Epidemic   1

1 Viruses and Mosquitoes: From Yellow Fever to Zika   17

2 Fetuses: Women, Doctors, and the Law   47

3 Surprises: "I've never seen anything like this"   79

4 Zika in Brazil: Producing Partial Knowledge   103

5 Stratified Reproduction: Class, Ethnicity, and Risk   126

6 *Mães de Micro*: Zika and Maternal Care   158

7 After Zika: Open Questions, Complex Legacy   187

Conclusion. Embodied Inequality   203

Further Reading   *215*

Notes   *219*

Index   *269*

A Forgotten Virus and Expunged Memories

Epidemics are often rapidly forgotten. Even the memory of such an immense disaster as the "Spanish flu" pandemic of 1918–20 was suppressed until a revival of interest in this episode in the late twentieth century. In 2016, the rapid transmission of the Zika virus in Brazil and other Latin American countries and its main consequence—the birth of children with severe neurological impairments—were unexpected, frightening, and highly visible developments. With the end of the Zika epidemic in 2017, however, the memory of this event faded quickly, accelerated first by the observation that the main victims of this epidemic had been children of poor, non-white women in northeastern Brazil and then by the advent of the COVID-19 pandemic. When Zika was forgotten, many disturbing aspects of the outbreak of this pathology conveniently disappeared, as did reflections about the relevance of Zika to circumstances in industrialized countries.

In early November 2015, the Brazilian media published alarming reports about a mysterious "epidemic of severe microcephaly" (a phrase that appeared in the Brazilian media in late 2015) among babies in northeastern Brazil. Shortly thereafter, the Brazilian health ministry linked severe birth defects to an infection with the Zika virus (ZIKV). Stories about children born with small heads and severe neurological problems and distressing photographs of the affected babies reached the Western media in early 2016. The accounts underlined the fact that children with severe microcephaly were most often born to women living in poverty but seldom attempted to explain why that was the case. Destitution is often an aggravating factor in an epidemic, but diseases differ greatly in the extent to which they are related to social class: cholera is linked more with poverty than with influenza. Mosquito-borne diseases more frequently affect the poor than they do the affluent, but often the differences are not great. This was decidedly not the case for Zika-induced congenital impairments. The observation that the great majority of the children with microcephaly were born to poor women of color was evident but rarely scrutinized. When this question was discussed, scientists advanced numerous explanations but often avoided the thorny issue of women's reproductive rights.

A *New York Times* article of August 2022, based on interviews with Brazilian specialists, illustrates this trend. The article movingly documents the difficulties of Brazilian families caring for children born with congenital Zika syndrome (CZS) in 2015 and 2016.[1] The challenges of caring for severely neurologically impaired children, it explains, were amplified by their mothers' poverty. A Brazilian researcher quoted in the article reported that 97% of children with congenital Zika syndrome were born to families of lower socioeconomic status and only 3% to relatively affluent families. One obvious explanation for this difference is that women living in poverty are more exposed to mosquitoes. Researchers had shown that about one-third of high-income women in the northeastern city of Recife, one of the epicenters of the Zika epidemic, displayed evidence of ZIKV infection in 2015, while almost two-thirds of low-income women in Recife had come into contact with this virus. This is not a surprising finding: low-income women are less likely to have air conditioning and more likely to live at ground level; most dwell in areas with poor sanitation, which provide breeding territory for mosquitoes. Still, the postulated difference in the rate of infection by the Zika virus cannot by itself explain why only 3% of children with CZS were born to middle-class mothers. Experts interviewed in the *New York Times* article pointed to additional, poverty-related factors that might have increased the likelihood that the Zika virus would cross the placenta and harm the fetus, such as a woman's compromised immune system, the concomitant presence of other infections, or stress during pregnancy. Surprisingly, however, the article did not mention the significant class-based differences in Brazilian women's capacity to control their pregnancies. Affluent women have access to efficient contraception, high-quality prenatal care, and an illegal but safe termination of pregnancy. The article's omission of key factors that allowed middle- and upper-class women to avoid giving birth to children with severe CZS is especially mystifying given the heated public debate over abortion rights in the United States during the summer of 2022. On the other hand, it resonates with Brazilian debates on the Zika epidemic: their focus was nearly exclusively on viruses, mosquitoes, and caring for severely disabled children, not women's sexual and reproductive rights.

Twenty years before the Zika epidemic in Brazil, I became fascinated by another virus propagated by the *Aedes* mosquito, the yellow fever virus. The thread I followed started in 1900, when an epidemic of yellow fever in Senegal, at that time a French colony, killed 45 French soldiers. The colonial authorities isolated the affected areas, a decision that led to riots among local inhabitants and a quarantine on Senegalese merchandise, which hit French traders particularly hard. In 1901, the first results of the US Army expedition that studied yellow fever in Cuba indicated that since the virus was transmitted by mosquitoes, quarantines and sanitary cordons were not efficient approaches to controlling it.[2] French merchants in Senegal asked the Ministry of the Colonies to send a scientific mission to Rio de Janeiro, which was in the midst of a severe outbreak of yellow fever, to verify the "mosquito hypothesis"; they declared their willingness to contribute to the expenses of such a mission. The French parliament voted in July 1901 to create a yellow fever mission under the direction of the Pasteur Institute.[3] The French scientific expedition to Brazil illustrates the role of commerce and colonization in the globalization of health.[4] Its story is also a fascinating one for historians of science interested in the intersections between science, politics, and society.

I stumbled on the story of the French scientific expedition to Brazil partly by chance. Researching other topics in the history of the Pasteur Institute, I found in the institute's archives unpublished reports and correspondence of members of this expedition, Paul Simond, Emile Marchoux, and Alessandro Taurelli Salimbeni. In 1996, I was invited to teach a short course at Fiocruz, Rio de Janeiro, and decided to visit Fiocruz's archives, hoping to find additional information about the Pasteur Institute expedition.[5] Along with information about the expedition, I found an impressive collection of documents about the efforts to control yellow fever in Brazil, especially by the Rockefeller Foundation. Historians thrive on paper trails; I was immediately hooked. The yellow fever story involved multiple areas of interest to me: laboratory and clinical practices, national and international public health campaigns, validation and diffusion of new knowledge, intersections of biomedicine and politics, and North-South relationships. Above all, it allowed me to get in touch with small and bigger aspects of the lives of colorful and fascinating individuals. It was an irresistible mix.

Several years later, in 2001, following an additional sojourn in Rio de Janeiro and several visits to the Rockefeller Institute Archive Center in Sleepy Hollow, New York, and the Wellcome Archive and Manuscript Collection in London, I wrote a book about the efforts to curb yellow fever in Brazil, published in French as *Virus, moustiques et modernité* (Viruses, mosquitoes and modernity).[6] In the same years, Jaime Benchimol, of Casa Oswaldo Cruz, Fiocruz, edited an excellent collection of essays (in Portuguese), *Febre amarela: A doença e a vacina, uma história inacabada* (Yellow fever: The disease and the vaccine, an unfinished history), while in 2016 Rodrigo Magalhães published a detailed history of the efforts to eradicate the mosquito *Aedes aegypti* in Latin America.[7] I was pleased that other scholars were making important contributions to the study of the history of mosquito-borne diseases in Brazil, but I had no plans to return to the topic myself.

The main subject of *Virus, moustiques et modernité* is efforts to control the *Aedes* mosquito in Brazil in the first half of the twentieth century, but the book's last chapter brings this story to 2000. It discusses the eradication of *Aedes* in Brazil in the 1950s, the return of this mosquito in the 1960s and again in the 1970s, and the consequence of this return: outbreaks of dengue fever. It ends with the following statement, "As the 20th century closes, the most urgent problem of control of yellow fever in Latin America is not a too rigid control of this disease . . . but the abandonment of efforts to control Aedes aegypti, justified by economic realism. This abandonment can lead to a very dangerous situation. . . . An epidemic of yellow fever in Latin America, some public health experts believe, is a time bomb waiting to explode; we are here waiting for this to happen."[8]

Predictions are often perceived as prophetic thanks to selective reading. Jules Verne is acclaimed for predicting that flying would be a means of mass transportation, although he foresaw the use of balloons, not machines heavier than air. Science fiction books from the 1950s and 1960s are hailed as prescient because they described a combination of telephone and television that would allow seeing the person to whom one speaks, not chided for their inability to imagine the World Wide Web and radically different ways of transmitting sounds and images. Until now (2023) there have been no new epidemics of urban yellow fever in Brazil, despite numerous outbursts of sylvatic yellow fever (a disease transmitted from jungle animals to humans by mosquitoes other than *Aedes*). The threat of massive urban yellow fever epidemics in Brazil has been averted thanks to the existence of a highly efficient yellow fever vaccine and well-organized vaccination campaigns. Nevertheless, the "time bomb" produced by the reinfestation of Brazil by *Aedes aegypti* did explode, first with increasingly severe outbreaks of dengue fever and then with the arrival of two new viral diseases transmitted by this mosquito: chikungunya and Zika; the latter pathology can also be transmitted through sex.

After the publication of *Virus, moustiques et modernité* I became increasingly interested in intersections between gender and biomedicine. I investigated the history of cancer diagnosis and treatment, with a special focus on female cancers. I then examined the history and present-day practices of prenatal testing. The latter study included observations in a leading Brazilian hospital specializing in the care of pregnant women who had been diagnosed with a fetal anomaly.[9] I was wrapping up the research on the latter topic and starting to plan my next investigation, on the practical consequences of the rapid diffusion of new genomic technologies for clinical medicine and public health. Infection-carrying mosquitoes, or to use the poetic expression of the French philosopher of science Georges Canguilhem, "death with wings," was very far from my preoccupations. But in October 2015 there were alarming reports in the Brazilian media about a mysterious epidemic of microcephaly, abnormally small head size, in newborns in northeastern Brazil. In November 2015 the Brazilian Health Ministry linked the clusters of babies born with small heads to a Zika outbreak several months earlier and declared Zika a Public Health Emergency of National Importance. At first skeptical because an arbovirus (a virus transmitted by mosquitoes) that induced birth defects had not previously been described, I became increasingly intrigued. Not many historians–cum–science studies scholars have studied both inborn anomalies and arboviruses. Zika increasingly looked like a topic I could not avoid, especially when I was asked by colleagues from Fiocruz, Rio de Janeiro, to join a newly created network, Zika and Social Sciences.[10] Zika was a complex, multidimensional phenomenon with a strong gender dimension. I became fascinated again by viruses and mosquitoes.

Zika might have arrived in Brazil as early as 2013, and it induced a large-scale epidemic in northeastern Brazil in early 2015. The awareness that this seemingly benign infection could cause severe fetal anomalies led, in late 2015 and early 2016, to a great fear of the Zika virus. However, from mid-2016 on, the number of children born with congenital Zika syndrome steadily decreased, as did the number of reported cases of Zika in adults. The Brazilian government officially ended the Zika sanitary emergency in May 2017. The virus itself did not disappear from Brazil, and the 2015–16 outbreak left behind thousands of severely affected children. Still, the Zika epidemic came to an end, at least until a possible next outbreak, providing a neat time frame for its study. My research about this epidemic and its consequences, made in close collaboration with Brazilian colleagues and with researchers in France and the United Kingdom, continued in 2018 and 2019. In late 2019 I decided that

I had accumulated sufficient materials to write a monograph on this topic. In early January 2020, when I had just started work on the monograph, Chinese physicians described cases of atypical viral pneumonia in the city of Wuhan, and a few weeks later that city and parts of the province of Hubei were quarantined because of the epidemic risk. It looked at first like a repetition of the SARS (severe acute respiratory syndrome) scare of 2003, an outbreak that, while undoubtedly severe, was restricted to a few countries in Southeast Asia and contained relatively quickly. Two months later, the "Chinese problem" became a pandemic that brought to a halt activities in countries all around the globe, an unprecedented development. France, like almost all of Europe, went into lockdown, while my colleagues and myself, communicating by phone, WhatsApp, email, Skype, and Zoom, scrambled to understand what was going on. When, after several months of a quasi-exclusive focus on COVID-19 fueled by epidemic-related stress, I slowly returned to writing about Zika, the world had changed, and so had I.

COVID-19 is not the main topic of this study—it is discussed only in chapters 6 and 7 and the conclusion—but the new pandemic is omnipresent in the background of this book. It became almost impossible to write about the Zika pandemic without thinking about the much more dramatic pandemic that followed it. In 2014 I had no plans to return to the study of transmissible diseases; in late 2015 I felt compelled to explain why I had decided to abandon my earlier plan to investigate cutting-edge developments in biomedicine and shift to a seemingly more "traditional" topic, an outbreak of a transmissible disease. From 2022 on, there was no need to explain the importance of studying an epidemic. The why became obvious, but in the meantime the how became much more difficult to explain. For two reasons. The first was COVID-19, the numerous questions it raised and the complex ways in which this pandemic, and then its winding down, changed the narrative about the previous one. While this book was written mainly in 2020 and 2021, that is, the period of intensive spread of the SARS-CoV-2 virus, it was revised in late 2022, when the epidemic was perceived as reaching its end and some considered it a topic that should be put to rest, as the Zika epidemic had been.[11] The second reason was a radical change in the perception of the Zika outbreak in Brazil. In 2016 debates on this disease were dominated by fears of a massive epidemic of newborn anomalies. Such fears did not materialize. The Zika outbreak in Brazil was relatively short, concentrated mainly in the northeast, and self-limited. Its principal consequence was the birth of thousands of neurologically impaired children. Between 2016 and 2023 the focus of the discourse about the

Zika epidemic shifted from the multiple aspects of the management of an outbreak by the Brazilian government and international organizations to the plight of children with congenital Zika syndrome and their mothers.[12]

The shift in the perception of the Zika epidemic in Brazil changed the way I understood my task of studying this epidemic. My original intention was to present the chronology of this outbreak, contextualize it, and follow its multiple consequences. I planned to focus on the difficulty of "acting in an uncertain world" and the challenges faced by scientists, clinicians, and public health experts who attempted to reduce the harm produced by the propagation of ZIKV though armed with very partial knowledge. Despite the impressive gains of fundamental research on the Zika virus and the pathologies it induces, scientists did not have an efficient way to halt the propagation of this disease, reliable diagnostic tests, treatments to prevent the induction of fetal anomalies by the Zika virus, or a vaccine against this disease, and human interventions had a limited effect only on the trajectory of Zika in Brazil.[13] My goal to provide a "thick description" of the Zika epidemic in Brazil would be facilitated, I hoped, by this outbreak's short period (two years at most) and its limited geographic area (mainly northeastern Brazil). My initial research goals remain valid, but they were increasingly challenged by the growing identification of the Zika epidemic with the care of children with inborn impairments, or as the title of the *New York Times* article of August 2022 called it, "the forgotten virus."[14] Care of children with CZS is undoubtedly a very important topic, but an exclusive focus on this topic might have meant avoiding other, more disturbing issues. One of the most important jobs of a historian, Peter Burke proposed, is to be a "remembrancer," to remind people of what they would like to forget.[15] Although I initially planned a straightforward narrative of a unique historical event, my research gradually became also an effort to recover elements lost, and sometimes deliberately forgotten, in the new perception of the Zika epidemic in Brazil.

In a public presentation of early results of my research on Zika, I evoked three "Zika ghosts," issues that were absent from the public debate about the new disease: an unwillingness to examine the structural reasons for the persisting failure to control *Aedes* mosquitoes in Brazil; the low visibility of the sexual transmission of the Zika virus; and the difficulty of discussing abortion because of a fetal anomaly or a risk of such an anomaly.[16] As the epidemic receded, also purged from the majority of the narratives about this epidemic were the reasons for the skewed distribution of Zika-induced inborn impairments among social classes in Brazil. Purged elements are seldom truly lost.

In their phantom-like existence, they dwell in a limbo of unresolved issues, ready to come back and haunt us when the time is right.[17] The advent of the COVID-19 pandemic, with its dramatic intensification of disease-linked social injustice, then the undermining of US women's reproductive rights, an especially hurtful development for women from the lower social strata, makes now, I believe, the right time to reexamine Zika phantoms.

A published book is sometimes just a visible part of a much larger endeavor. This is especially true for this book, which relies heavily on studies made by other researchers, especially those on the termination of pregnancy and on the Zika epidemic. I am immensely grateful to the colleagues who conducted these studies and shared their unpublished results and their thoughts with me. I am also grateful to the scientists, health care workers, health administrators, Brazilian officials, and activists who contributed precious information to this book.

The research for this book had two sources. The first was a study of juridical abortion in Brazil, coordinated by Claudia Bonan with the co-participation of Luiz Teixeira (both from the Instituto Fernandez Figueira, Fiocruz), in which I took part. My understanding of prenatal care and abortion in Brazil is largely owing to knowledge acquired during that study. My views on women's reproductive rights in Brazil were also shaped by a long collaboration with Marilena Correa and enriched by exchanges with Cecilia McCallum, Debora Diniz, Wendell Ferrari, Iulia Fernandez, Mariana Lima, Andrea Loyola, Gabriela Victa, and Sylvia de Zordo.

The second source was collective research on Zika through the network Social Sciences and Zika and the project "Acting in an Uncertain World." In late 2015 I was invited to participate in the newly founded Social Sciences and Zika network by the Fiocruz director, Nisia Trindade Lima. Nisia, a social scientist–cum–historian herself, encouraged and sustained all the network's activities. I am greatly indebted to Gustavo Matta, who coordinated the network's activities, and to all its participants. Special thanks to Carolina de Oliveira Nogueira, Elaine Teixeira Rabello, Denise Nacif Pimenta, Lenir Silva, and João Nunes for their generosity in sharing data, experience, and ideas. Together with Ann Kelly, Javier Lezuan, and Gustavo Matta, we conducted the related social sciences project, "Acting in an Uncertain World," financed by the Newton Fund of Great Britain. Our exchanges contributed greatly to my understanding of the Zika outbreak: Ann, Gustavo, and Javier, you know how much I owe you. I am also grateful to two researchers based in France, Koichi Kameda and Helena Prado, who conducted important studies of the Zika epidemic and shared their knowledge with me.

Researchers from my department, CERMES-3 (Centre de recherche, médecine, sciences, santé, santé mentale, société), especially Simone Bateman, Luc Berlivet, Claire Beaudevin, Catherine Bourgain, Maurice Cassier, Jean-Paul Gaudilliere, Myriam Winance, and all the participants in the "café genre" meetings, helped me to clarify my ideas. I am especially grateful to Ann Lovell, who was and is a permanent source of support and inspiration, and to Emilia Sanabria, who greatly improved my understanding of Brazilian society.

Many other colleagues helped me to understand the epidemic, Brazilian medicine and public health, and reproductive injustice. A very incomplete list includes Elisabeth Avad-Porteiro, Nathalie Bajos, Christiana Bastos, Dominique Behague, Jaime Benchimol, Allan Brandt, Carlo Caduff, Maria do Carmo Leal, Marcos Cueto, Claudia Fonseca, Tamara Giles-Vernick, Fay Ginsburg, Cathy Herbrand, David Jones, Simone Kropf, Joanna Latimer, Gabriel Lopes, Laura Mamo, Severine Mathieu, Carlos Henriques Paiva, Diane Paul, Naomi Pfeffer, Camila Pimentel, Scott Podolsky, Rayna Rapp, David Reubi, Marilia Sá Carvalho, Jonathan Sacramento, Alexandra Stern, and Clare Wenham.

Despite the extent of my intellectual debt to colleagues and friends, the standard formula applies for this book, and perhaps especially for this book: all the opinions and interpretations are mine alone, as are any omissions and errors.

I am grateful to the following institutions for their support of studies on social sciences and Zika in which I participated: the British Council/Newton Fund (Institutional Links Programme grant agreement no. 280969145: Acting in an Uncertain World); the Wellcome Trust (ref. 204939/Z/16/Z): the Zika Social Science Network: Sexual and Reproductive Health, Rights, and Justice; the European Commission's Horizon 2020 Research and Innovation Programme (ZIKAlliance grant agreement no.734548); the European Research Council (grant agreement no.715450); and the Oswaldo Cruz Foundation/Vice-Presidency of Research and Biological Collections fund, as well as my home institution, CERMES-3, which partly financed my fieldwork in Brazil but above all provides a highly stimulating environment for scholarly endeavors.

At Johns Hopkins University Press, Matt McAdams strongly supported this project, Adriahna Conway and Charles Dibble followed the manuscript to press, and Joanne Allen provided a careful and thoughtful copyediting. I am especially grateful to the Victoria Miro Gallery and Virginia Sirena for permission to use Paula Rego's painting *The First Mass in Brazil* on the book's cover. Besides being a great work of art, Rego's painting is an inspired visual representation of many of the issues I highlight herein.

My extended family was an infallible source of support—material, intellectual, and emotional. My gratitude goes to Tamara, Rodo, Daniel, Shafak, Naomi, Em, Rachel, Benjamin, Michael, and Eleni. My greatest debt is, as always, to my partner, Woody, for, well, everything. This time his indispensable support included not only a steady supply of physical and intellectual nourishment but also listening to harrowing stories and discussing difficult subjects.

My previous work on prenatal diagnosis made me realize the fragility of fetuses'/ newborns'/children's health and well-being and the role of biological luck in shaping destinies. The present study has made me acutely aware of the importance of luck more broadly defined: the luck of being born and living in the "right" country, having the "right" citizenship, and being reasonably free from major existential worries. We are living now in an increasingly unpredictable world. The Zika pandemic and the much more impactful COVID-19 pandemic occurred in a time of political instability and growing dangers to the planet. My grandchildren may face a more dangerous world than their parents did when they were growing up. In one of my visits to Brazil, in November 2015, I found myself on a flight from Paris to Rio de Janeiro the night following the election of Jair Bolsonaro as Brazil's president. Early the next morning, just before we landed, a flight attendant reported the election's result and then added, "Welcome to Rio de Janeiro, *cidade maravilhosa*—let's hope that it will stay marvelous!" Kyan, Tania, Esteban, Selma, Naama, let's hope that your world will stay a healthy, safe, and wonder-generating place for all children, not just a fraction of children worldwide.

Viruses and Reproductive Injustice

Framing an Epidemic

A Baby in a Bucket

Zika was revealed to the world through images. One of the most striking was a photograph of a dark-skinned baby with a misshapen head sitting in a gray plastic bucket with a red plastic handle while an unidentified woman bathes him. In one photograph the baby gazes at the viewer with a puzzled look; in another he seems frightened, his eyes out of focus. People who saw these photographs often did not know that the baby was seated in a bucket of cold water to calm his convulsions, but they instinctively felt that something was very wrong.[1] The baby, José Wesley Campos, photographed by Brazilian Associated Press photographer Felipe Dana, became one of the first faces of a microcephaly epidemic in Brazil, especially after the broadcast of a BBC program that documented the harsh conditions in which José and his family were living.[2] When José was born, his mother, Solange Ferreira, from a small town in the state of Pernambuco, had never heard the reports of an unusual incidence of babies born with abnormally small heads in northeastern Brazil. She only learned of the diagnosis of microcephaly when he was two months old. At that time Ferreira, like many lower-income women in Pernambuco, especially those living outside major cities, had limited access to services provided by the Brazilian National Health Service, the Sistema Único de Saúde, or SUS.

Felipe Dana first visited Solange Ferreira in December 2015. He met the 38-year-old Ferreira when she was waiting with her son for a doctor's appointment. At that point, Ferreira hoped that José's problems were not severe. Dana didn't contradict her, because he didn't want to be the one to dash her hopes. After Ferreira heard from the doctor that José had severe microcephaly, she seemed to be in shock, but she agreed to be interviewed and photographed by Dana the next day.[3] Visiting her in her house in the small town of Poço Fundo, Dana photographed a baby who would scream uncontrollably for long stretches, turning red in the face and contracting his already stiff limbs; he thrashed when being fed. Putting José into a bucket of cold water, a method Ferreira had learned from a hospital nurse, calmed him for a while. Dana visited Ferreira and José again three months later, in February 2016. By then, they had moved to the town of Bonito, closer to the state's capital, Recife, so that they had easier access to the health care professionals who treated José.[4] José's health problems, Dana reported, became more severe. While his mother was saddened by the downturn in her son's symptoms, she better understood the scope of his condition and realized that he would need a high level of care for the rest of his life.[5]

Epidemics Are Messy

The Zika-induced microcephaly epidemic in Brazil was a short, intense, and frightening episode. The Zika virus arrived in the country in either 2013 or 2014. In April 2015, Brazilian researchers in northeastern Brazil noticed a cascade of cases of a febrile disease accompanied by a rash. At first, they suspected that this was a mild variant of dengue fever, but they later ascertained that the agent was another arbovirus (a virus transmitted by mosquitoes): the Zika virus (ZIKV). ZIKV belongs to the same family of RNA viruses, called flaviviruses, as the dengue virus and the yellow fever virus. Like these viruses, ZIKV is transmitted by the *Aedes aegypti* mosquito. However, unlike other arboviruses, the Zika virus can also be transmitted through sexual contact. Beginning in August 2015, clinicians in northeastern Brazil observed clusters of children born with small heads (microcephaly) and other severe brain anomalies. Later these anomalies were diagnosed as congenital Zika syndrome (CZS). The linking of brain anomalies with the Zika virus produced a wave of fear among women of reproductive age. Some epidemiologists predicted, on the basis of an earlier occurrence of Zika in the Pacific Islands, that the outbreak in northeastern Brazil would be relatively short-lived. On the other hand, they feared that ZIKV might move to other regions of Brazil and other Latin American countries and produce an epidemic of microcephaly. These fears never materialized. Cases of CZS in Brazil were mainly concentrated in northeastern Brazil, while the intensive phase of the epidemic in Brazil lasted less than a year. The Zika virus continued to produce sporadic fetal anomalies, but from mid-2016 the number of children with CZS decreased considerably. This was true in other Latin American countries as well. Infection with the Zika virus remains a risk for pregnant women, but this pathology is no longer perceived as a global threat.[6]

The story of the Zika outbreak in Brazil might seem straightforward. It has a central thread, is limited to one country, and apparently, at least, has a well-defined beginning and end. But studies of diseases are rarely simple. In 1927 Ludwik Fleck, a pioneering scholar of the social history of science, explained that diseases are complex events that cannot be grasped from a single point of view.[7] This is particularly so when dealing with a multidimensional event such as an epidemic. Nevertheless, scholars who write about epidemics, the historian of medicine Charles Rosenberg proposed, often produce linear narratives focused on moments of acute calamity. Such narratives start at a given moment in time, describe an event limited in space and duration, follow a plotline of increasing and revelatory tension, move to a crisis of individual and collective character, then drift toward closure—often a successful halt of the disease's spread.[8] The popularity of such linear narratives of epidemics is not surprising: people like stories with a definite beginning and a happy ending, or at least an ending of some sort. When the story is about an outbreak of a transmissible disease, they also yearn for a progress narrative that presents developments in modern medicine as a promise of salvation.[9]

The desire for reassuring stories of salvation through scientific progress has a long tradition. In 1919 the Brazilian writer and activist Monteiro Lobato predicted that science would end the country's backwardness: "The veil has been lifted. The microscope has spoken."[10] But a microscope's light beam also produces shadows, and the study of such shadows may be no less important than the investigation of brightly illuminated areas. Promoters of a faith in the unstoppable advance of science aspire to replace fears generated by an epidemic with the promise of a secure and predictable future. Real-life epidemics, however, are often untidy and complicated, and they rarely fit into neat narratives.[11] Existential threats like epidemics awaken people's sense of contingency, feelings of vulnerability, fears of disintegration, and awareness of the existence of uncontrollable events, unresolved issues, and vast zones of darkness.[12] The investigation of epidemic outbreaks can thus be enriched by paying more attention to what is subdued, hidden, and repressed in social life and examining the specific ways that power links individual bodies to the collective body politic.[13]

Biology Matters

Social scientists recognize that diseases are indissociably biological and social events, but they often concentrate on their social aspects and pay less attention to their biological ones. They investigate topics such as patients' experience of disease, ethical dilemmas of professionals, or the organization of health services and tend to neglect the biological aspects of pathologies. They may thus overlook important differences between diseases, the distinct ways they can be prevented, contained, and treated, and their dissimilar consequences for individuals' lives and developments in society.[14] The observation that the main harm produced by the Zika outbreak in Brazil—the birth of severely impaired children—was concentrated among poor, non-white women may seem to be a statement of the obvious.[15] Lower socioeconomic status is nearly always linked with a higher vulnerability to transmissible diseases. Still, not all transmissible diseases are identical. Their biological traits influence their pattern of spread and distribution in the population. Airborne infections tend to be more "democratic" than those directly linked to poor sanitation, some diseases occur more frequently among specific occupation groups, and others among people who live in specific places, and in some cases middle-class individuals who are protected from an encounter with a given pathogen as children are more vulnerable to this pathogen as adults.

Pathologies disseminated in Brazil by the *Aedes aegypti* mosquito, responsible for the dissemination of Zika, dengue fever, and chikungunya, are more prevalent among people from lower social strata, who are more often exposed to these mosquitoes. On the other hand, the association between social class and infection by an arbovirus is not as straightforward as, for example, the association between childhood diarrhea and lack of access to clean water. Dengue and chikungunya, while more frequent among the poor, can strike anybody.[16] Anecdotal evidence from northeastern Brazil indicates that in 2015, when the prevalence of Zika in the region was very high, this disease affected people from all social strata. Moreover, some epidemiologists maintained that the majority of the inhabitants of this region had been infected with ZIKV.[17] This was decidedly not true for the distribution of cases of congenital Zika, which were much more frequent among poor women.

Infections that induce fetal anomalies—gathered under the acronyms TORCH (toxoplasmosis, other diseases, rubella, cytomegalovirus, herpes simplex) and, in countries with a high prevalence of congenital syphilis, STORCH—are also perceived as relatively "democratic." This is not entirely accurate. Babies with congenital syphilis are born to women who, because of inadequate prenatal surveillance, were not treated for this condition when pregnant. In industrialized and intermediary countries such women usually belong to marginalized social groups. Similarly, babies with congenital rubella are born to women who were not vaccinated against the disease as children or teenagers; such women too often belong to marginalized segments of the population. But in the case of pathologies for which there is no vaccine or efficient treatment, infection of a pregnant woman by a pathogen that induces fetal anomalies is seen mainly as bad luck, not as related to her socioeconomic status.[18]

There is no vaccine or treatment for Zika. Infection with ZIKV is akin to infection by pathogens, such as *Toxoplasma gondii*, cytomegalovirus, herpes simplex, or parvovirus B19, which can affect pregnant women from all social classes. Therefore, the socioeconomic status of women infected with the Zika virus during pregnancy does not explain the strongly skewed class distribution of CZS, which was both put to the fore and concealed.[19] The media and progressive social scientists accurately described the typical mother of a microcephalic child as poor and Black or "Brown" (*parda*). However, they rarely dwelled on the specific reasons for the concentration of children born with CZS in lower social strata. This topic became marginalized through two district approaches: a quasi-exclusive focus on the care of children with CZS and a reluctance to discuss the absence of interventions that might have reduced the number of infants with CZS among poor women—from efficient contraception to reliable prenatal diagnosis and decriminalization of abortion for a fetal indication.

History Matters

Recently, sociologists, anthropologists, and historians have become interested in traces of past events. The past, the anthropologist Ann Stoler points out, creatively reconfigures the present.[20] Traces of efforts to control transmissible diseases, argue Paul Wenzel Geissler, Guillaume Lachenal, John Manton, and Naomi Tousignant, are not confined to vestiges of the past. They are an integral part of the present and actively participate in the construction of the future.[21] History matters, but in complex, nonlinear ways. The Zika epidemic in Brazil was shaped by efforts to control the mosquito *Aedes aegypti*, the main vector of the yellow fever virus and the dengue virus.[22] Early efforts to get rid of *Aedes* mosquitoes, such as Oswaldo Cruz's highly publicized campaign against yellow fever in Rio de Janeiro (1903–7), relied mainly on fumigation.[23] In the 1920s, 1930s, and 1940s the control of *Aedes* mosquitoes was the responsibility of the Brazilian Yellow Fever Service, organized and directed in the interwar era by Rockefeller Foundation (RF) experts and after World War II by Brazilian specialists. The guiding principle of the Yellow Fever Service was the elimination of *Aedes aegypti* larvae.[24] This approach was initially successful. Brazil was declared free of *Aedes* by the Pan American Health Organization in 1958. The elimination of *Aedes* put an end to urban outbreaks of yellow fever. This impressive achievement was eroded later, however. In the 1970s and 1980s Brazil was reinfested by *Aedes aegypti*, and the government gradually abandoned its hopes not only of eradicating this insect but of even significantly reducing its prevalence.[25] The omnipresence of *Aedes* made it impossible to contain the spread of diseases carried by this mosquito, above all dengue fever.[26] Dengue, absent from Brazil for fifty years, reappeared in the 1980s. Between 1997 and 2002 the country reported more than 2 million cases of dengue, 70% of the cases recorded in Latin America in that period. In the twenty-first century dengue fever has become hyperendemic in the majority of Brazilian states.[27] Zika reached Brazil in 2013 or 2014. At the same time another viral disease diffused by the *Aedes* mosquito, chikungunya, had arrived in Brazil. Reactions to these diseases were shaped by the country's long history of trying, with limited success, to control *Aedes aegypti*.[28]

All Politics Are Reproductive Politics

The German physician, scientist, and politician Rudolf Virchow explained in 1848 that medicine is a social science and politics is but medicine writ large.[29] The US anthropologist Laura Briggs proposed 170 years later that all politics becomes reproductive politics.[30] Politics is indeed concerned with the reproduction of individuals and societies, an element, one may argue, already implicitly contained in Virchow's original statement. During the Zika epidemic in Brazil, Briggs's proposal was accurate in a very concrete sense. Since the main harm of an infection by ZIKV is the induction of inborn anomalies, reproduction and "maternal politics" were at the very center of the Zika crisis.

The veneration of maternity, including the suffering linked with being a mother, occupies an important place in Brazilian social imagery. It is displayed by the popular expression "To be a mother is suffering in paradise."[31] All the social classes glorify maternity as inseparably linking joy and suffering, but it is especially associated with poor women, admired as devoted and self-sacrificing mothers. This social imagery, I propose, shaped attitudes about prenatal diagnosis and termination of pregnancy. It favored the widespread perception of abortion, described as "getting rid of the baby" (*tirar o bebê*) as a morally repugnant act, or at least a shady one. Many Brazilian women might have agreed, at least at a discursive level, with the statement made by Pope Francis, who explained in February 2016 that the Zika epidemic was not a sufficient reason to suspend the interdiction of abortion: "Abortion is not a theological problem. It is a human problem, it is a medical problem. You kill one person to save another, in the best-case scenario. Or to live comfortably, no?"[32] The widespread social imagery that glorifies maternal suffering and condemns women's supposed wish "to live comfortably" favored the relegation of the debates on the material aspects of abortion, especially an abortion for a fetal indication, to the domain of "public secrets," things that are often done but are rarely discussed openly. A negative image of abortion has concrete consequences, such as an insufficient training of physicians to perform legally permitted abortions. It also hampers the development of an accurate prenatal diagnosis of fetal anomalies in the public sector, especially outside highly specialized medical centers.[33] Abortion is also a politically explosive topic in Brazil. Only Far Left politicians openly defend woman's right to end a pregnancy. Others, including socially progressive ones, implicitly support the criminalization of abortion. Thus during the presidential campaign in the fall of 2022 the supporters of the left-leaning Luiz Inácio Lula da Silva, in order to discredit Lula's adversary, the Far Right sitting president, Jair Bolsonaro, called attention to an old interview in which Bolsonaro had declared that abortion was a private matter that should be decided by families.[34]

From 2018 on, studies of the Zika epidemic in Brazil focused on the care of children with CZS and their mothers. This was certainly not the case in early 2016, when I became part of a collective effort to understand the epidemic. At that time, my colleagues and I sought to follow in real time reactions to an outbreak of a new disease. We aspired to understand how the knowledge about such an outbreak is produced and diffused, how individuals and institutions react to unexpected and dramatic developments, how the politics of Zika in Brazil was influenced by developments in the international arena, and how the management of the Zika epidemic had changed with time. Some of the questions we asked were specific to mosquito-borne diseases, others to pathologies that affect the fetus; some were focused on events that took place in Brazil, while others were about developments in global health. We did not predict the shortness of the Zika epidemic in Brazil or its consequence, a drastic decrease in the research on the disease. Nor did we predict that the rapid waning of the Zika outbreak, coupled with its public image as an epidemic of microcephaly, would rapidly lead to a redefinition of Zika as the problem of caring for several thousand severely impaired children and their mothers' struggle to provide such care.

The redefinition of Zika as a problem of children with multiple inborn disabilities had important positive consequences. Thanks to a rich corpus of studies in pediatrics, neurology, psychiatry, social medicine, social work, psychology, sociology, and anthropology, the immense effort invested in the daily care of children with CZS was made evident and recognized in all its complexity. These studies exposed important differences between approaches to disability in industrialized and developing countries, examined shifting meanings of motherhood and religious faith, and provided detailed analyses of patterns of self-organization and empowerment of mothers of children with multiple impairments. On the other hand, when Zika became identified with suffering, militant, self-sacrificing, or heroic mothers, other important questions linked with the pandemic gradually disappeared from the public debate. The redefinition of Zika as a problem of care diminished the interest in national and international reactions to the Zika outbreak. An emphasis on individual mothers' sacrifice and courage drew attention away from the role of care in promoting radical social and political change.[35] A focus on the material and emotional difficulties of mothers of children with CZS also detracted attention from developments that led to children being born with congenital Zika and the reasons for the concentration of such births among poor, nonwhite women.

During the Zika epidemic, women's sexual and reproductive rights were, following the words of the philosopher Jutta Schikore, a "wicked problem." When dealing with such problems, Schikore explains, the scientist's agency is limited by stakeholders outside the laboratory as well as by other agents who conceptualize and frame the problem differently and who have a different understanding of the problem's overall significance.[36] Once the Zika epidemic passed its peak, and the main issue was not how to prevent births of children with CZS but how to provide adequate care for children born with this condition, Zika became a less fraught issue. A "wicked problem" became a part of a mundane political debate over the allocation and distribution of resources.

Stratified Risks and Targeted Interventions

Brazil is proud of its national health service, the SUS. The Brazilian constitution of 1988 grants a universal right to health. In practice, the services provided by the SUS are highly variable. The health service is very efficient in some areas of health care and much less so in others; it provides reasonably good care in some parts of Brazil, less so in other parts. Brazil's transition to democracy has been marked by a constant struggle to effectively satisfy citizens' "right to health" and to extend health care to areas where it is limited. This is particularly true for approximately three-quarters of the Brazilian population, who rely exclusively on SUS services.[37] Middle-class citizens with private health insurance, especially those who have high-end health plans, have access to quality medical care, while low-income citizens have much more limited access to such care. The gap in access to health services between the middle and lower classes is especially evident in women's reproductive health. Middle- and upper-class women seldom if ever use SUS gynecology and obstetrics services, while lower-class women are entirely dependent on public services in this area.

Brazilian progressive physicians and social scientists framed the Zika epidemic as a political and social issue. In March 2016, one of the leading experts of the Brazilian Association for Collective Health (Associação Brasileira de Saúde Coletiva, ABRASCO), Leo Heller, declared that the right response to the Zika outbreak was to improve sanitation and the water supply.[38] In April 2016, an official declaration issued by ABRASCO's epidemiology commission similarly emphasized the key role of control of the *Aedes* mosquito in containing the Zika epidemic. It also stressed the need to intensify scientific research on Zika and CZS and strengthen the SUS.[39] The Brazilian government put the onus of preventing CZS on individual women, encouraging them to keep their houses free from mosquitoes, postpone pregnancies during the epidemic's peak, and avoiding mosquitoes when pregnant. Progressive public health professionals and feminist organizations strongly criticized this approach and insisted on the social dimension of the Zika epidemic, above all the government's responsibility for flawed sanitary and social policies, which had resulted in an uncontrolled spread of *Aedes* mosquitoes.[40] To state a distinction made by Charles Rosenberg, Brazilian authorities saw the Zika outbreak through the prism of the reductionist "contamination" model, which focuses on the role of circulation of pathogens and their vectors, while progressive public health specialists saw it through the prism of the holistic "configuration" model, which perceives contagious diseases in a wider ecological, socioeconomic, political, and cultural context.[41]

The "configuration" framework, which pointed out that the Brazilian government had produced the conditions that made possible the Zika epidemic, was, however, very broad and did not address the biological specificity of this pathology. Zika's main threat was not to Brazil's population as a whole but to a specific group: pregnant women. Thus it might have been important to act quickly to reduce the immediate risk to this group, above all through targeted interventions in the area of women's reproductive health to reduce the frequency of severe CZS. Only a handful of feminist groups promoted such targeted interventions. Progressive political and professional organizations openly debated women's reproductive rights, among them the right to terminate a pregnancy, but they did not press the government to rapidly implement measures to protect lower-class women from the consequences of Zika. Such measures might have included the distribution of effective contraceptives and information about the risk of sexual transmission of ZIKV, first-rate prenatal diagnoses in public facilities, and the decriminalization of abortion, including for a fetal indication. However, Brazil is a society that extols maternity and in which conservative religions wield considerable political power. In such a society, to venture beyond a general discourse on women's rights and actively promote specific interventions in the reproductive domain was to walk into a political minefield. Few groups and organizations, including those sincerely committed to the ideal of collective health, risked such a step.[42]

The Brazilian journalist Mino Carta explained in March 2021 that "in Brazil, health, like education, is nearly exclusively a privilege of the affluent class."[43] The Zika story was at first one of a localized disaster and scared women, then became one of a global threat, and ended as a story about the care of severely disabled children. But it is also a narrative about the consequences of entrenched social injustice. It exposed not only the impressive gap in Brazil that separates the ultra-rich ("Brazilionaires") from the rest of the population but also the gap that separates the members of the middle class, who have access to services provided by the private health sector, from lower-class people, who rely exclusively on the SUS.[44] The gap between the rights and privileges of the haves and the have-nots is especially evident in the area of women's reproductive rights.

Zika in Context: The Organization of This Book

The history of the Zika epidemic is inseparable from one of the insect vectors of this disease, the mosquito *Aedes aegypti*. The first chapter of this book, "Viruses and Mosquitoes: From Yellow Fever to Zika," tells the complex story of Brazil's effort to control mosquito-borne diseases, yellow fever and then dengue fever. Until the early 1930s, scientists believed that the only natural hosts of the yellow fever virus were humans, and the only way to control this disease was to eliminate its vector, *Aedes aegypti*. They believed that eliminating the mosquito would rid Brazil of yellow fever. In the 1930s they had learned, however, that the yellow fever virus was present in jungle animals and could be transmitted by jungle mosquitoes. It was therefore not possible to eradicate this virus. It *was* possible to control its spread through the elimination of *Aedes*, an intervention that prevented urban yellow fever, and vaccination, which protected people at risk of contracting the sylvatic variant of this disease. Both efforts were initially successful. In the late 1930s, Brazil was the first site of mass production and testing of an efficient anti–yellow fever vaccine, and in the late 1950s Brazil eradicated the *Aedes* mosquito. Alas, this was only a temporary achievement. *Aedes* reinfected Brazil, and Brazilian health authorities gradually abandoned hope of controlling its spread. No Brazilian government, right, center, or left, was willing to make the massive investments in sanitation and infrastructures necessary to efficiently contain this insect. As a result, it became nearly impossible to control the diseases propagated by Aedes—dengue fever, then chikungunya and Zika.

One of the key factors shaping reproductive politics in Brazil was the criminalization of abortion. Chapter 2, "Fetuses: Women, Doctors, and the Law," examines the consequences of criminalizing abortion in Brazil, especially for poor women. Criminalization of abortion increased the gap between the experiences of lower- and middle-class women, since only the latter have access to a safe, although illegal, termination of pregnancy. There are nevertheless a few exceptions to the criminalization of abortion. A woman who learns about a severe, potentially lethal anomaly of the fetus can petition a court for permission to legally terminate the pregnancy. "Juridical abortions" are, however, rare and difficult to obtain. Women who submit a request to legally end a pregnancy face a true obstacle course with an uncertain outcome. The criminalization of abortion in Brazil not only increased the suffering of poor women but made it more difficult for all women to receive an accurate prenatal diagnosis. In the great majority of cases, accurate detection of a fetal anomaly does not improve the pregnancy's outcome, since only a few therapeutic interventions are possible before birth. With no legal possibility of terminating a pregnancy for a fetal indication, Brazilian physicians who work in the public sector do not have a strong incentive to promote an accurate diagnosis of fetal anomalies—including those induced by the Zika virus.

The Zika outbreak was an unforeseen event. Chapter 3, "Surprises: 'I never saw something like this,'" discusses the Brazilian reaction to the surprising finding that the epidemic of microcephaly had been caused by an arbovirus, ZIKV. This virus, long considered a relatively harmless pathogen, induced in the twenty-first century massive outbreaks, first on the small Pacific island of Yap in 2007, then in French Polynesia in 2013–14. During the latter outbreak, scientists discovered that ZIKV could be transmitted through sexual contact. In early 2015, Brazilian epidemiologists identified a massive outbreak of Zika in northeastern Brazil. In August and September 2015, Brazilian gynecologists and pediatricians observed a cluster of cases of unusual, very severe microcephaly in newborns. The Brazilian researchers rapidly linked these cases and other cases of severe brain anomalies in newborns with Zika infection during pregnancy. In November 2015, the Brazilian Health Ministry declared a Public Health Emergency of National Importance (Emergência em Saúde Pública de Importância Nacional, or ESPIN) and established a special registry to closely follow cases of microcephaly in newborns. At first, the postulated link between Zika and microcephaly was not contested by international experts; in early 2016, however, this link was questioned by some, mainly because of suspicions that Brazilian data on the prevalence of microcephaly were unreliable. One of the main goals of the declaration of Zika as a Public Health Emergency of International Concern (PHEIC) by the WHO in February 2016 was to clarify the nature of links between Zika and fetal anomalies.

The intensive efforts to learn more about the new disease and to contain it had mixed results. Chapter 4, "Zika in Brazil: Producing Partial Knowledge," follows the trajectory of the Zika epidemic in Brazil to its rather abrupt end and examines questions that remained unanswered in the aftermath of the Zika outbreak. The declaration of Zika as a PHEIC by the WHO, and fears of the spread of the Brazilian epidemic of microcephaly to other Latin American countries and possibly other parts of the world led in 2016 and 2017 massive investments in research on Zika. These investments made possible a better understanding of the molecular structure of ZIKV, its mutations, and the mechanisms by which it harms the fetal brain. They did not lead, however, to the elaboration of reliable and inexpensive diagnostic tests for Zika. In the absence of such tests much about this epidemic, including the reasons for the high prevalence of children with congenital Zika syndrome in northeastern Brazil, remains unknown. Extensive investment in studies of ZIKV did not lead to the development of an efficient treatment for Zika and CZS or an anti-Zika vaccine. Moreover, international funds mobilized in response to the Zika pandemic were not channeled to reducing sexual transmission of Zika, curbing ZIKV infections in pregnant women, or alleviating the plight of children with CZS, their mothers, or their families. Thus the conclusion of some experts that the international answer to the Zika crisis had failed Latin American women.

Mosquito-borne diseases affect people from all social strata, while CZS cases occurred largely among the poor. Chapter 5, "Stratified Reproduction: Class, Ethnicity, and Risk," examines the reasons for the almost exclusive concentration of congenital Zika syndrome among poor, frequently non-white women. Since the Brazilian government was reluctant to intervene in the area of women's sexual and reproductive health, women who relied exclusively on SUS services often had no protection against the Zika threat. This was decidedly not the case for middle-class women in Brazil. Not only were people living in affluent neighborhoods less exposed to *Aedes* mosquitoes than those living in poor areas but, crucially, during the Zika epidemic middle-class women of reproductive age were able to take several additional steps to minimalize their risk of giving birth to a child with CZS. They took extra care to avoid contact with mosquitoes, employed effective insect repellents, delayed pregnancy, and negotiated safe sex with their partners. Moreover, when pregnant, they had access to an accurate diagnosis of Zika and fetal malformation induced by ZIKV and then, if applicable, to safe abortion. Taken in isolation, each of the risk-limiting steps was imperfect, but—following the "Swiss cheese model," popularized by efforts to limit COVID-19 risk (a single slice of Swiss cheese has many holes, but layering several slices with differently distributed holes produces a near-perfect seal)—their combination strongly reduced the probability of giving birth to a child with congenital Zika syndrome. It also reduced the psychological consequences of living in fear and feeling helpless.[45]

The perception of the Zika outbreak in Brazil radically changed over time. Chapter 6, "*Mães de Micro*: Zika and Maternal Care," investigates the transformation of the narrative about the Zika epidemic in Brazil into a story focused on care of severely disabled children. Debora Diniz's important book on Zika in Brazil, published in 2016, is subtitled *From the Brazilian Backlands to Global Threat*, but Zika actually followed an opposite trajectory: from a global threat, Zika became a story about Brazilian backlands, or rather of about a specific segment of the backlands population.[46] The chapter follows the unfolding of stories about children with CZS and their mothers, referred to as *mães de micro*. (Fathers often left after the birth of an impaired child, and those who stayed are rarely present in narratives about the care of children with CZS.) It starts with the definition of legally confirmed CZS, a condition that gives access to specific privileges, and the problem of numerous children with severe inborn anomalies who failed to be recognized as affected by CZS and were denied access to the advantages linked with such recognition. It then examines the trajectories of mães de micro: their organization as groups and their struggle to obtain better care for their children but also their problematic interactions with researchers who studied children with CZS. Mães de micro suspected that because Zika had become an important research topic, scientists were more interested in using their children as research material than in promoting their well-being. A 2019 parliamentary debate on providing a life-long pension to children with CZS exposed the political tensions surrounding the topic, while in a 2021 exhibition about Zika in Brazil Zika was identified with the care of severely disabled children.

The disease does not end when an epidemic stops. Chapter 7, "After Zika: Open Questions, Complex Legacy," looks at the aftermath of the Zika outbreak. It examines the role of international organizations in the management of Zika in Brazil. The Zika outbreak highlighted the important scientific contributions of Brazilian researchers and offered them highly interesting research opportunities. On the other hand, these opportunities were mainly restricted to fundamental research, seldom focused on the specific problems of Brazil, and became much more limited after the Zika epidemic ended in 2017. Zika is still present in Brazil and other Latin American countries, but it has been "normalized" as one of the several endemic diseases transmitted by mosquitoes, and one among the many transmissible pathologies that induce fetal impairments. In all probability endemic Zika too selectively harms fetuses of women from lower social strata. But while at its height the Zika epidemic made visible the concrete consequences of stratified reproduction in Brazil, reproductive injustice became much less visible when narratives about the Zika epidemic shifted from general considerations about disease-related risks to problems of care of children with CZS, above all their mothers' hardship and sacrifice. Such a focus, the psychologist Jorge Lyra, of the Federal University of Pernambuco, explains, forced the mothers to maintain an image of saintly women instead of talking about their rights.[47] At the same time, the emotional power of stories of mães de micro, whether disheartening or uplifting, stifled interest in the developments that led to a highly uneven distribution of CZS cases. It also curbed the readiness to engage with complex subjects and ask unsettling questions.

Many aspects of the Zika epidemic in Brazil prefigured developments during the "next plague," the COVID-19 pandemic. The conclusion, "Embodied Inequality," examines reproductive injustice in Zika times. Progressive Brazilian health professionals and social scientists, deeply concerned about Zika's aggravation of inequalities between poor and middle-class women and families, proposed expanding social justice by improving the living conditions, sanitation, and health care of lower-class people and reinforcing the SUS. These important long-term goals are not, however, specific to Zika. One may argue, along with thinkers such as Nancy Fraser and Avishai Margalit, that in the face of a health emergency it might have been more fruitful to focus on the elimination of reproductive injustice.[48] Expanded social justice may have multiple meanings, from a truly egalitarian society to moderate improvement of the well-being of people at the lower rungs of the social ladder. A rebellion against social injustice is different. It is frequently directed against phenomena that cannot be tolerated at all because they undermine human dignity and the foundations of a decent society. Reproductive injustice, this study argues, is such a phenomenon. There is no halfway solution for a woman faced with a brutally violent male partner, a scary illegal abortion, or continuing a pregnancy against her will. Middle-class women whose social status protects them from such traumatic experiences inhabit a different world from that of women who have already faced such experiences or live in apprehension of the moment they may face them.[49] The advent of the COVID-19 pandemic underscored the specificity of the Zika epidemic but also its important resonances with COVID-19. The two outbreaks were very different in their magnitude, the biological properties of the pathogen, and their consequences, but in both, embodied injustice had a key role.

Sidelined Stories

I observed the Zika epidemic in Brazil from a privileged perspective. First, I was able to observe it from its earliest stages, and second, I benefited from the collective experience and generous help of members of two closely related research groups: Social Sciences and Zika (Rede Zika Ciências Sociais) and the program "Acting in an Uncertain World: Mapping Public Health Responses to the Zika Epidemic in Brazil," financed by the Newton Foundation. These groups conducted formal interviews (more than 25) with leading scientists, clinicians, and government officials directly involved in the management of the Zika epidemic and had numerous exchanges with other actors.[50] In parallel, I had numerous semiformal and informal talks with professionals and activists, made direct observations in the laboratory and the clinics, and participated in workshops, meetings, and conferences on Zika. My study was greatly facilitated by the fact that the professionals who had helped me in my previous work on prenatal diagnosis in Brazil were willing to do so again, shared with me unpublished materials and preprints, directed my attention to the relevant governmental documents, and introduced me to other health professionals. Much of the material in this study was acquired by a process akin to osmosis: an imperfect, idiosyncratic, but I hope efficient adsorption of information from a milieu in which I was immersed.

Despite my privileged access to many sources, analyzing all the aspects of the Zika epidemic was well beyond my capabilities. This work does not pretend to be a definitive history of the Zika outbreak in Brazil, a complex, multilevel event, but is closer to a collection of imperfectly fitting fragments. Moreover, it is a decidedly subjective interpretation of the observed events. Nevertheless, I hope that it can suggest new ways of thinking about this epidemic.

Discussing in the spring of 2021 the "pharmaceuticalization" and "judicialization" of health in Brazil, the anthropologist João Biehl explained that during the Zika epidemic "a mundane disease of the tropics proved to be a source of tremendous distress for women. The key protagonists were not physicians and scientists, but mothers-to-be."[51] Biehl's statement that the main protagonists of the Zika epidemic were the mothers-to-be is intriguing. At some level at least, people directly affected by a given disease are by definition the key protagonists of a story about this disease. Biehl might have been referring to a different, indeed unique feature of the Zika epidemic: the emphasis on the plight of women who gave birth to children with congenital Zika syndrome. Such an emphasis may reflect the difficulty of constructing a narrative about an epidemic whose trajectory was only minimally affected by a successful human intervention. The Zika epidemic did not end because of the development of a vaccine, an efficient treatment, or a better way to control the *Aedes* mosquito. Since human ingenuity did not play a significant role in the course of the Zika outbreak, a focus on the experience and struggles of mães de micro could provide a framework for an alternative story about an epidemic, with its dramatic moments, room for interpretation, and lessons for the future. The prominent place given to that story led, however, to the sidelining of nearly everything else about the Zika epidemic in Brazil. What was sidelined, including embodied reproductive injustice, is at the center of this study.

CHAPTER ONE

Viruses and Mosquitoes

From Yellow Fever to Zika

Necrotorium: Hunting for Viruses in Cemeteries

In the 1930s local authorities constructed in many Brazilian cemeteries a small, windowless building with a large stone or concrete table in the center. Some of these buildings resembled a garden shed or a storage room, others a small funerary chapel, still others a tiny house. Many had no inscription on their facade, but a few were designed as the property of the Brazilian Yellow Fever Service.[1] These buildings had a very specific use: a rapid sampling of the cadaver's liver, visceroctomy, with a specially designed instrument, the visceroctome. In each case of sudden death from a suspicious fever, public health authorities were obliged by the law to provide a sample of the liver tissue of the dead person before delivering a burial permit. The sample was sent to a specialized laboratory in Rio de Janeiro or Salvador, Bahia, and examined for the presence of typical changes induced by the yellow fever virus. At that time there were no simple diagnostic methods to detect the presence of the yellow fever virus. Searching for characteristic pathological lesions in the liver was an efficient way to spot yellow fever deaths. Decree no. 21434, of May 23, 1932, which defined the parameters of intervention by the Rockefeller Foundation–directed Brazilian Yellow Fever Service, instituted the legal obligation of burial in authorized cemeteries and stated that a burial permit in these cemeteries would be granted only after the family received approval from the local representative of the visceroctomy service.[2]

Not infrequently the deceased individual's family saw visceroctomy as a desecration of the body and strongly resisted it. The reaction was especially extreme when the sample was taken from the body of a young child. Vis-ceroctomy might have been seen as an especially brutal intervention, differ-ent from a regular autopsy. Autopsies took place in the sterile atmosphere of a hospital's pathology department and were conducted by professionals, whereas visceroctomies were conducted furtively, often not by a physician but by a person named the local visceroctomist, who was sometimes a doctor but often a pharmacist, a male nurse, or a trained worker from the funeral services. An autopsy was for a long time forbidden even to doctors; with visceroctomy, a routine violation of the integrity of dead bodies became trivialized in the name of public health. At the same time, the 1937 instructions for the estab-lishment of visceroctomy posts insisted on the secrecy of this endeavor. The instrument itself should not be shown to people outside the visceroctomy service. The puncture should never be made in the presence of outsiders. If the sampling of liver tissue was conducted at home, it should be made in an isolated room with closed curtains and shades; if it was performed in a cem-etery, only the visceroctomist and in some cases the patient's doctor should have access to the necrotorium.[3] The precautions and the secrecy were seen as necessary to prevent violent incidents. The Rockefeller Foundation's ex-perts' attitude toward visceroctomy was often ambivalent. They recognized the scientific value of this practice but also its messiness, and they were aware of the ethical dilemmas linked with its use. Such dilemmas were not new. From its early days, research on yellow fever was linked with ethically doubt-ful practices, among them risky experiments on human beings.

Mosquito-Borne Diseases and Human Experiments in the Early Twentieth Century

Pioneering studies of transmissible diseases often were done in colonial and postcolonial settings.[4] Tropical diseases that threatened colonial armies and white settlers were seen as a major obstacle to colonization. Before the advent of microbiology and immunology, the tropical climate and environment were seen as intrinsically hostile to white people. The solution was either slow ac-climatization, especially through raising a second and third generation born in colonialized countries, or intermarriage with the presumably "racially re-sistant" natives. In the late nineteenth and early twentieth centuries, the prob-lem of the "hostile environment" of the tropics was redefined as the presence of parasites that attacked people coming from abroad: worms, microscopic parasites, bacteria, filterable viruses. It then became possible to propose tech-nical solutions, such as a physical separation of settlers from "contaminating" native populations, the protection of the colonists through vaccination, and the development of efficient cures. At the same time, infectious diseases that originated in the Global South, such as cholera or yellow fever, were increasingly perceived as a threat to populations of Europe and North America. It was important to find ways to contain them.[5] Colonies and semicolonized countries became in the late nineteenth and early twentieth centuries a vast laboratory for studying transmissible diseases, their prevention, and their management. In some locations, such studies were conducted exclusively by European and North American scientists, who employed the native population as a research material. In other cases, especially in "intermediary" countries with an already existing scientific tradition, scientists from Europe and North America collaborated with local researchers and doctors. They were sincerely persuaded to be engaged in a true exchange with the local researchers and believed that such an exchange would benefit not only both groups of professionals but above all their experimental subjects, populations affected by the studied pathologies. Scientists from industrialized countries overlooked, however, important asymmetries of power and differences in goals.[6] Moreover, scientific collaborations led occasionally to problematic experiments on humans, such as those conducted by the Reed mission, which studied yellow fever in Cuba, and the Pasteur mission, which studied yellow fever in Brazil.

Yellow fever is a disease of tropical regions, with occasional outbreaks in temperate climates as well, especially in ports where mosquitoes carrying yellow fever were brought by ships returning from the tropics and in centers of slave trade. The first epidemics of yellow fever in the Americas were observed in the seventeenth century. In the eighteenth and nineteenth centuries there were significant yellow fever epidemics in the United States (Philadelphia, New York, Saint Louis, New Orleans, Savannah) but also in Central and South America and in Europe (Gibraltar, Barcelona, Saint-Nazaire). Yellow fever was an especially dreaded pathology, with dramatic symptoms (delirium, black "fomites") and very high mortality. Since it was especially dangerous for newcomers to the tropics, it was viewed as a major obstacle to colonization and military expeditions. In the absence of an animal model of yellow fever or a possibility of cultivating its etiologic agent in a test tube, it was also a disease that was especially difficult to study in the laboratory.

The Reed mission (1900–1902) was sent by the US Army to Cuba to test the hypothesis that yellow fever was transmitted by the mosquito *Stegomya facilities*, later renamed *Aedes aegypti*.[7] To confirm this hypothesis, Walter Reed and his colleagues conducted experiments on humans. Volunteers—North Americans, mainly US soldiers, who, one may assume, acted mostly from altruistic motives, and Spanish new immigrants to Cuba, who were promised a significant monetary compensation—were deliberately infected with yellow fever through bites of contaminated mosquitoes. Since yellow fever was often fatal, these experiments have raised important ethical issues. Reed's biographer William Beam claimed that the North American researchers in Cuba maintained very high ethical standards.[8] The claim that all the volunteers in Reed's mission experiments on humans freely respected a contract they had signed, is, however, at odds with the description of Reed's experiments produced by General William Gorgas. According to Gorgas, the experimental subjects were placed in an isolated camp under military control and were physically prevented from leaving it.[9] A key element in the success of Reed's experiments was the presence of armed guards around the compound where these experiments were conducted. There were no reported deaths among the volunteers inoculated with yellow fever by Reed and his colleagues in 1901. The same year, the Cuban physician Juan Guiteras, who collaborated with Gorgas, attempted to immunize people against yellow fever by exposing them to bites of mosquitoes infected by feeding on mild cases of this disease. Three of the eight participants in these experiments died from yellow fever.[10]

In 1901 the Pasteur Institute, in Paris, sent a scientific mission to Rio de Janeiro to study Reed's hypothesis of transmission of yellow fever by mosquitoes. A proof that this disease was mosquito-borne could put end to expensive and bothersome quarantines on people and merchandise coming from countries affected by yellow fever outbreaks. The French parliament voted in July 1901 to create a yellow fever mission under the scientific direction of the Pasteur Institute to investigate the transmission of yellow fever by mosquitoes. The mission was funded by the French Ministry of Colonies and the Association of French Merchants in Senegal.[11] The mission members, Paul Luis Simond, Émile Marchoux, and Alessandro Taurelli Salimbeni, arrived in Rio de Janeiro in November 1901. They established a laboratory in the São Sebastião Isolation Hospital, the main yellow fever hospital in Rio de Janeiro, and started to study yellow fever patients.[12] These investigations were limited in scope. In September 1902, Simond complained that the results they had obtained so far were very modest given their efforts.[13] The main obstacle to progress was the absence of an animal model of yellow fever. The Pasteur experts decided, therefore, with the encouragement of the Pasteur Institute vice director, Émile Roux, to start experiments on human beings.[14] They recruited paid volunteers from among new immigrants to Brazil, isolated them in an experimental camp in the mountains, a zone free of mosquitoes able to transfer this disease, and in early 1903 started their efforts to produce yellow fever in the volunteers under controlled conditions. This was a complicated task, and at first their progress was very slow.

Nothing in the abundant paper trail left by the Pasteur Institute mission— official publications, report to the institute directors, correspondence—hinted that their experiments had had fatal outcomes.[15] However, in the 1990s Louis Simond's grandson donated to the Pasteur Institute Archives additional papers of his grandfather, among them his laboratory notebooks from the yellow fever studies.[16] These notebooks revealed that the mission's official report, which presented a well-organized and systematic study, masked chaotic and hurried experiments on humans. The main reason for the precipitation was a fear that the French Ministry of Colonies, disappointed by the mission's slow progress, would cut the funding.[17] The mission's members felt pressured to produce rapidly concrete results. They also wanted to exploit a lucky break: a successful production of a case of severe yellow fever in one of their experimental subjects. They employed the blood of this subject to infect several other volunteers. As a consequence, in June 1903 two men died from yellow fever, while another was killed during a brawl in the isolation camp where the volunteers were held.[18] In fine, the Pasteur mission did confirm that yellow fever was transmitted by mosquitoes, as did several other groups at the time, but the mission's experiments on humans did not produce original observations, while the dramatic events that occurred during these experiments remained hidden. In 1905 Simond and Marchoux received the Legion d'honneur for their "outstanding contribution to the yellow fever commission's work and the impressive intelligence they brought to this extremely difficult and dangerous endeavor."[19]

Aedes aegypti Mosquitoes in Brazil: Geographies of Risk

From 1901 on, efforts to control yellow fever were identified with the efforts to control its vector, the mosquito *Aedes aegypti*. *Aedes* is a "domesticated" insect. It lives near human habitations and is a day mosquito; it bites mainly at dawn and dusk. In heavily infested zones, swarms of mosquitoes are found in and around houses, as are their eggs, larvae, and pupae. Photographs from the 1920s and 1930s show the inspectors of the Brazilian Yellow Fever Service shining a flashlight into a domestic water reservoir (*caixa d'água*), a big jar, or a dark corner. Indeed, the distribution of more powerful flashlights increased the inspections' efficacy. Nevertheless, the main instrument for discovering *Aedes*'s breeding locations was and is the trained eye. Although *Aedes* breeds in public and semipublic spaces—gardens, cemeteries, construction sites, waste disposal grounds, or neglected urban areas—the majority of its breeding sites are in and around private habitations. Sanitary agents responsible for mosquito control, who until the 1970s were practically all men, had to negotiate with the individuals responsible for the management of domestic spaces, that is, mainly women, to gain access to houses and yards, to communicate to them the results of their inspections, and, if applicable, to punish them for failing to implement sanitary rules.

The first campaign against *Aedes* mosquitoes in Brazil was conducted in the early twentieth century by Oswaldo Cruz (1872–1917), one of the founders of biomedical research in Brazil. In 1902 President Rodrigues Alvez named Cruz, a young doctor trained at the Pasteur Institute in Paris, head of the General Directorate of Public Health (DGSP) of the capital, Rio de Janeiro. His main task was to control infectious diseases in the city.[20] These diseases, especially yellow fever, projected an image of Brazil as a backward country, dangerous for foreigners and unsafe for trade, and hindered its aspiration to be included among the advanced nations. Moreover, the effort to control yellow fever in Brazil in the early twentieth century was complicated by racial considerations: the high priority given to efforts to control yellow fever, a disease especially dangerous for European migrants, revealed the importance given to the task of "whitening Brazil."[21] Between 1903 and 1906 Oswaldo Cruz conducted an energetic campaign in Rio against smallpox, plague, and yellow fever. Some aspects of this campaign were strongly resisted by Rio's population. Many people opposed the vaccination campaign against smallpox because of its authoritarian character. They also opposed the forced sanitation of Rio: the banning of street vendors from the center of the city and the destruction of "unhealthy" neighborhoods, an intervention that pushed Rio's poor to the hills surrounding the city's center.[22] Oswaldo Cruz's measures led in 1904 to a popular rebellion, the Vaccine Revolt. This rebellion was led by a heteroclite coalition of the Positivist Church (an organization inspired by the writing of Auguste Comte and popular among Rio de Janeiro's middle class), cadets from the Military School of Praia Vermelha, and the poor.[23] The urban rioting was partly successful. President Alves suspended the smallpox vaccination requirement. He did not halt, however, the destruction of popular neighborhoods in the center of Rio, seen as an essential part of his project of modernization of Brazil's capital.[24] By 1907 the transmission of the targeted pathogens had decreased greatly and the majority of Rio de Janeiro's inhabitants had become reconciled to Cruz's sanitary measures. From a vilified overzealous health promoter, Cruz became a national hero, celebrated as the person who had brought progress to Brazil.

Oswaldo Cruz created a specialized unit to fight mosquito infestation, the Yellow Fever Prophylaxis Service. Its sanitary workers were dubbed mosquito slayers (*mata mosquitos*). The main anti-mosquito measure instituted by Cruz was massive fumigation of buildings with sulfuric acid, which was regarded at the time as an advanced, science-based approach. Fumigation machines became a visible symbol of the use of modern technology to promote public health.[25] To limit the risks of propagation of yellow fever agents, poor yellow fever patients were sent to isolation hospitals, while affluent patients were allowed to isolate in their homes in rooms equipped with mosquito nets. Cruz's anti–yellow fever measures were effective. In 1903 there was 584 yellow fever deaths in Rio de Janeiro; in 1907, 37 deaths; in 1908, 4; and in 1909, none.[26] Yellow fever remained endemic in many parts of Brazil, especially in port cities. In the second decade of the century outbreaks of this pathology were fought by applying Cruz's approach, above all the pulverization of insecticides. At that time yellow fever was dangerous mainly for newcomers to the country and was not perceived as a major public health problem. Brazilian experts were much more preoccupied with the poor health of many Brazilians, especially in rural areas. Early in the decade, a group of Brazilian physicians affiliated with the Serological Institute of Manguinhos, founded by Oswaldo Cruz (renamed the Oswaldo Cruz Institute after Cruz's death in 1917) conducted a series of sanitary expeditions to remote regions of Brazil, attempting to overcome the traditional division between the culturally and economically advanced littoral and the undeveloped interior. They described the extreme poverty and the catastrophic health status of inhabitants of the visited areas. Their reports, reproduced in national newspapers, stimulated the rise of the Brazilian Sanitary Movement, active between 1916 and 1920 and dedicated to the improvement of health in the interior of Brazil.[27]

One of the founders of the Sanitary Movement, the president of the Brazilian National Academy of Medicine, Miguel Pereira, declared in an oft-quoted discourse of October 1916, that "except for the capital Rio de Janeiro, where there is now a reasonably efficient sanitary surveillance, and a handful of other cities, Brazil is an immense hospital." The inhabitants of the country's interior, Pereira explained, were weakened by hookworm and malaria, degraded by syphilis and leprosy, devastated by alcoholism and diminished by hunger, ignorant, and abandoned. It is not surprising that they fail to identify with a state that was willing to put a rifle in their hands but denied them access to literacy.[28] Pereira's list of diseases that afflicted the inhabitants of Brazil's interior did not include yellow fever. This disease was also not listed among the main pathologies targeted by the institutions developed as a result of the Sanitary Movement activism, the Rural Prophylaxis Service (Serviço de Profilaxia Rural), founded in 1919, then the National Department of Public Health (Departamento Nacional de Saúde Pública, DNSP), founded in 1920.[29] In the second decade of the twentieth century, the control of *Aedes* mosquitoes was not seen as a major problem by Brazilian public health activists. It became an important target of public health campaigns, however, following the arrival of the Rockefeller Foundation (RF) experts.

Yellow Fever as a Demonstrative Disease: The Rockefeller Foundation in Brazil

Experts of the international division of the Rockefeller Foundation selected yellow fever as one of the main targets of their intervention in Brazil because they thought it could be an especially effective "demonstrative disease." Its elimination, they believed, would show the importance of using scientific methods to control disease. In 1923, an agreement between the international division of the foundation and the Brazilian government gave RF experts the right to organize a nationwide yellow fever service in Brazil. The main goal of this service was to prevent the proliferation of *Aedes* mosquitoes. Fumigations, RF specialists argued, are dramatic but not very effective because they provide only short-term relief. Control of mosquitoes has to be grounded in the systematic elimination of their breeding places. Since *Aedes* lives in and near houses and can breed in even very small containers filled with water, it is crucial to ascertain that no such containers are available. Yellow Fever Service inspectors visited houses and examined their exterior and interior for the presence of potential breeding sites. RF experts also introduced larvae-eating fish in ponds, fountains, and other larger sites with stagnant water, sponsored the diffusion of domestic water reservoirs with tight covers, and where it was possible, promoted a central distribution of water to houses.

The goal of carefully eliminating *Aedes* breeding sites was established during RF experts' first period of activity in Brazil, 1923–29. The goal of the Yellow Fever Service was not the elimination of all such sites, only the majority. At that time, the RF epidemiologists adhered to the "key focus" theory. They believed that (*a*) humans were the only hosts of the yellow fever virus; (*b*) the

Aedes aegypti mosquito was the only vector; (*c*) the disease existed only in Brazil's littoral cities, where the density of infected humans and mosquitoes secured uninterrupted chains of transmission; and (*d*) to break the chains of transmission it was sufficient to reduce the "mosquito index," the number of houses infected by *Aedes* (i.e., houses in which a careful inspection found either breeding sites of this mosquito or adult insects), to less than 5%.[30] Such a reduction, RF experts were persuaded, would put an end to the transmission of yellow fever in a given locality. Consequently, it was not necessary to impose very stringent measures to eliminate all the mosquito larvae. Soft control, based on persuasion and education, was sufficient, especially when coupled with additional measures such as the distribution of larvae-eating fish and control of sources of stagnant water in public spaces.[31] Brazilian doctors familiar with yellow fever had serious doubts about the validity of the key focus theory. They believed that yellow fever was endemic in the country's interior and that eliminating this pathology from littoral cities would not be sufficient to eradicate it from Brazil. However, in the first years of the RF's intervention its approach seemed to work well. Between 1923 and 1926 there was a drastic reduction in the number of cases of yellow fever, and no new cases were recorded in 1927. The RF gradually closed its Yellow Fever Service branches and planned to end to its yellow fever campaign in Brazil.[32] These plans were cut short in 1928 by a dramatic outbreak of the disease in Rio de Janeiro. The outbreak lasted more than a year. Clementino Fraga, who at that time headed Rio de Janeiro's health services, fought the outbreak with massive fumigations, a method that regained its status as the visible face of "war against mosquitoes."[33]

The Rio de Janeiro outbreak started with cases imported from Brazil's interior, from sites that according to the key focus theory should have been free of yellow fever. It became increasingly clear to RF experts that their theoretical assumptions were erroneous. In 1930 Fred Lowe Soper was named head of the RF's Brazilian bureau, a post he held until 1942. In the 1940s Soper directed campaigns of elimination in insect vectors of diseases in North Africa, Italy, and the Middle East, and from 1947 to 1959 he directed the Pan American Sanitary Bureau (PASB), which in 1958 was renamed the Pan American Health Organization (PAHO).[34]

From the beginning of his tenure Soper was persuaded that the foundation's main mistake was failing to pay attention to the presence of hidden cases of yellow fever in Brazil's rural areas, and, one might add, to the opinions of Brazilian physicians.[35] The final demise of the key focus theory came from the observation, made in 1932 during a yellow fever epidemic in the state of Espírito Santo, that the yellow fever virus could be transmitted by mosquitoes other than *Aedes aegypti* and that it also infected jungle animals.[36] The description of sylvatic (or jungle) yellow fever put an end to hopes of eradicating this disease from Brazil. It was not possible to eliminate the yellow fever virus or to prevent sporadic cases of this disease in people who had close contact with the jungle. The goal of eliminating yellow fever shifted to one of eliminating *Aedes aegypti*, which was responsible for massive urban outbreaks of the disease.[37] During the second phase of the RF campaign to control yellow fever in Brazil (1930–39), conducted under the leadership of Fred Soper, the campaign's goal was to drastically reduce Aedes's density.

The second phase of RF intervention was shaped by two events: the abandonment of the key focus theory and the arrival to power of Getulio Vargas. Vargas, who became president in 1930, would probably be described today as a populist, and his regime, especially after its turn to the right in 1937, as an illiberal democracy. Until today, historians' evaluations of the Vargas regime have varied. Some have stressed the positive aspects, such as the striving to modernize Brazil and reduce the gap between the littoral and the interior, or the promotion of labor legislation that protected workers. Others have emphasized the repressive aspects, such as the brutal elimination of left-wing opposition and, especially in the late 1930s, the regime's close links with European fascist regimes.[38] In the early years of his presidency, Vargas was especially interested in modernizing Brazil and fascinated by the United States. His close collaboration with RF experts was prompted by his aspiration to imitate the North American model of development.

In 1932 Varga's government provided a legal framework for the intervention of the Yellow Fever Service, the decree of May 23, 1932. This law, elaborated in close collaboration with Soper and his colleagues, greatly increased the power of the Yellow Fever Service. The service's inspectors were given authorization to inspect all private and public buildings, all ships in Brazilian ports, and all the public spaces; to conduct an autopsy in any case of "unexplained death"; to order inhabitants to eliminate larvae in their houses, yards, and gardens; and to fine those who resisted inspections or failed to eliminate the larvae from their premises.[39] Since the new goal of the Yellow Fever Service was to eliminate *Aedes* mosquitoes, not merely reduce their number— Soper's slogan was "Any is too many"—it was important to make the inspections highly efficient. The Yellow Fever Service shifted accordingly from a model of "soft control" to one of "rigid control" of larvae, inhabitants of infested areas, and work of the service's inspectors. The inspectors, uniformed and with distinctive insignia according to their rank, were expected to follow a strict routine of rounds of inspections and to provide accurate reports of these rounds. They were also permanently supervised by their hierarchical superiors, who made control inspections in the targeted areas. Soper considered efficient supervision of the work of service inspectors key to success; 20–25% of the budget of the service was dedicated to such supervision. Another important element of the success of the service's work was the homogenization and centralization of the collection of data. The service's inspectors employed standardized forms and made several copies of each report, making possible the compilation of data on the regional and the state level and better-organized anti-larvae campaigns.[40]

In the 1930s, anti-*Aedes* campaigns were grounded in a complex system of surveillance of areas targeted for the elimination of mosquitoes. Inspectors of the Yellow Fever Service made weekly visits to every house in a targeted area, inspected it carefully, and eliminated all the containers holding stagnant water, which might become breeding places for *Aedes*. Repeat offenders were fined. Domestic water reservoirs, an important item in modest-income households, had to be carefully covered to prevent the breeding of *Aedes* larvae. Inspectors poured kerosene into reservoirs or containers that were not covered, making their future use for the storage of drinking water impossible. Alternatively, if the uncovered container was made of clay, the inspectors broke them, severe punishment for poor people, for whom the purchase of a water container was an important expense. This punitive measure was seen as especially drastic in northeastern Brazil, a region often plagued by severe droughts.[41] The work of rank-and-file sanitary inspectors was systematically controlled by their superiors through verification of their written records, spot checks of inspected houses to check whether lower-level inspectors had failed to notice mosquito foci, and "adult mosquito capture," an independent measure of the progress of the anti-mosquito campaigns.[42]

Reports of RF experts who coordinated Yellow Fever Service activities rarely mention women and do not discuss the inclusion of women in efforts to control *Aedes*. This is somewhat puzzling since women were responsible for cleaning the house and keeping it in order, and one of the goals of RF intervention in Brazil was to modernize the country, including through teaching women the principles of domestic hygiene. This was one of the main activities of the RF-sponsored Hygiene Institute of São Paolo, founded in 1918. The institute offered women courses in domestic economy, dietetics, puericulture, and science-based housecleaning. Every area of daily life, students were told, could be greatly improved through scientific management.[43] While the Rockefeller experts energetically promoted the teaching of science-based home economy to middle-class women, I did not find evidence of attempts to educate lower-class women about mosquito control. The uniformed male agents of the National Yellow Fever Service, seen as soldiers of an anti-mosquito army, were very different from the (nearly always female) teachers of domestic hygiene.

Only rarely do field diaries of RF experts explicitly mention women. In one case Porter Crawford, who directed the Yellow Fever Service in the state of Paraíba in the 1930s, noted that while the general rule was to destroy water containers in which the inspectors had found *Aedes* larvae, they allowed one old woman to keep hers because she could use it to keep coal for cooking.[44] In another case, reported by Soper to illustrate the necessity of thoroughly examining the interior of a house, an inspector asked a housewife whether there were water containers in her house, to which she replied that there were none. Doubting this statement, Soper made a careful inspection of the house and found a vase with live flowers and an old conserve tin filled with water.[45] A woman could be an object of compassion or a person who could not be trusted but not a potential partner in the effort to control *Aedes* mosquitoes.

Since the control of mosquitoes was mainly grounded in repressive actions such as the destruction of water recipients and imposition of fines, it is not surprising that occasionally people rebelled against the interventions of Yellow Fever Service inspectors, sometimes violently. Several inspectors were killed by angry homeowners who resisted inspections and fines. Soper and his colleagues regretted these incidents but argued that such incidents, like the killing of a few visceroctomy agents, were an acceptable price for ridding Brazil of yellow fever. They added that the system of eliminating mosquitoes developed by the Yellow Fever Service worked well. In the great majority of the sites controlled by the service, the mosquito index fell below 1%. This was an important achievement, especially when compared with the 1920s goal of a 5% index. Moreover, in the spring of 1933 service inspectors observed in some areas a total absence of *Aedes* mosquitoes and decided to halt control measures in those areas. The size of the *Aedes*-free zones had increased gradually. Complete eradication of *Aedes* was initially an unintended effect of carefully planned and meticulously organized mosquito control programs. It inspired Soper to develop his approach of "eradication of disease vectors" through short, intensive campaigns that gradually enlarged the size of *Aedes*-free zones.[46]

Yellow Fever Agent in the 1920s and 1930s: Laboratory Studies and Epidemiological Surveys

Until 1926 scientists failed to reproduce yellow fever in a laboratory animal. In the absence of an animal model of a transmissible disease or the possibility of cultivating its agent in the laboratory, the only means of discovering its presence was an accurate identification of its symptoms. Typical clinical symptoms of yellow fever were easily observed during an epidemic, but when the disease was relatively rare its manifestations could be easily confused with those of other pathologies, such as severe malaria. In 1912 the Brazilian physician Henrique da Rocha Lima described the typical changes produced by severe yellow fever in the liver. This led to the practice of examining the liver for evidence of such changes, which became the basis of the visceroctomy service.[47] Rocha Lima's method was very useful for uncovering hidden cases of yellow fever that ended in death. It was less useful for discovering mild to moderate cases. However, as early as the early twentieth century Cuban and Brazilian doctors proposed that in endemic areas yellow fever was usually a mild childhood disease. This view was adopted by the Pasteur Institute researchers who study yellow fever in Rio de Janeiro.[48] Children, they proposed, were immunized through an early encounter with the yellow fever virus. In areas with a high density of *Aedes* mosquitoes, young children were a permanent reservoir of yellow fever, yet only rarely did a child—or an adult with insufficient immunity—develop severe, easily diagnosed form of yellow fever. In areas devoid of non-immunized foreigners, the disease might be endemic and occur very frequently, but in the absence of suspicious deaths it would be invisible to researchers.

The difficulty of visualizing the "filterable virus" that induced yellow fever led some scientists to doubt its existence. In the second and third decades of the twentieth century, a well-known RF expert, Hideo Noguchi, proposed that yellow fever was induced by a bacterium, *Leptospira icteroides*.[49] Because of Noguchi's prestige as a leading Rockefeller Foundation bacteriologist, his hypothesis was seriously considered in the 1920s by the RF experts who worked in Brazil. It was reinforced by Noguchi's visit to Brazil in 1923. During this visit, Noguchi claimed that he had identified two strains of *Leptospira*, specific to Brazil, that were responsible for yellow fever outbreaks there.[50] Other specialists failed, however, to reproduce Noguchi's results. In 1926 Andrew Sellards and Max Theiler, of Harvard University's School of Tropical Medicine, contested Noguchi's findings. They claimed that the putative agent of yellow fever, *Leptospira icteroides*, was identical to a known bacterium, *Leptospira icterohemmorhagiae*, that induced jaundice known as Weil's disease, clinically quite different from yellow fever. A year later they showed that a *Leptospira* could not be transmitted by the *Aedes* mosquito, disqualifying definitively this microorganism as a possible agent of yellow fever.[51] The same year, three North American researchers, Adrian Stokes, Johannes Bauer, and Paul Hudson, induced for the first time yellow fever in a laboratory animal, the rhesus monkey. They were successful, after numerous failed attempts by other scientists to infect monkeys with yellow fever, because they counterintuitively employed an Asian rather than an African or Latin American monkey, thus an animal from a continent free of yellow fever.[52]

The infection of rhesus monkeys with yellow fever virus was the first step in the development of laboratory studies of this pathogen, elaboration of accurate diagnostic tests, and the manufacture of a vaccine. It became possible to test whether a given individual had antibodies against yellow fever by checking whether their blood protected a rhesus monkey from an experimental infection. Monkeys were expensive, however. The next decisive development was in 1930, when the virologist Max Theiller, who joined the RF virology laboratory that year, successfully adapted the yellow fever virus to grow in a mouse brain, a less onerous method of maintaining this pathogen in the laboratory. Testing whether a serum protected mice from yellow fever infection was a much less expensive way to detect anti–yellow fever antibodies. The mouse protection test detected both ongoing and past infections, including mild ones. It thus made possible direct visualization of the presence of yellow fever in Brazil. One of the main innovations of the RF-piloted Brazilian Yellow Fever Service was the construction of networks that linked the laboratory and the field and favored the circulation of biological samples such as sera or liver tissue. While such networks existed already, mainly thanks to scientific expeditions that collected biological samples and took them for further analysis to major scientific centers, the Brazilian Yellow Fever Service transformed a whole country into a vast area of sample collection.

The mouse protection test was used to confirm a suspected diagnosis of yellow fever, especially in patients who survived the disease. The main application of this approach was, however, to conduct epidemiological surveys. Widespread collection of sera made it possible not only to determine whether yellow fever had been present in a given area but also to provide an idea of when. Through the collection of sera from people of all ages, including children, it became possible to determine whether the disease was endemic (in which case anti–yellow fever antibodies were found in the sera of all the people living in the area) or had been present in an earlier period, then disappeared (in which case only older people would have anti–yellow fever antibodies). Collection of sera for research purposes is never simple. It is particularly complicated in populations that lack access to basic education and sanitation. The RF experts recorded encounters with "superstitious natives" who feared to give their blood and took the experts for emissaries of the devil. In practice, the RF experts often secured the collaboration of local elites—physicians, pharmacists, politicians, and teachers, sometimes also priests. They also occasionally bribed people with presents to allow them to draw their blood and, an especially challenging task, the blood of their children. Yellow fever laboratories in Salvador, Bahia, and Rio de Janeiro centralized the mouse protection tests. The final result was the construction of detailed maps that indicated the presence of yellow fever and guided anti-*Aedes* campaigns.

The collection of sera was a frequent but not systematic endeavor. Visceroctomy—the systematic collection of liver samples from people who died from a suspicious "fever"—was, by contrast, an obligatory method of surveilling the Brazilian population. Since according to the decree of May 23, 1932, obtaining a burial permit required the permission of the local representative of the visceroctomy service, in principle at least, all cases of death from yellow fever were recorded by the Yellow Fever Service. Visceroctomy was performed in cases of death from a nondefined "fever"; in cases of a strong presumption of death from yellow fever a complete autopsy was performed. The use of the visceroctome, an instrument specially devised to produce a small sample of liver tissue, streamlined the collection of samples from a cadaver's liver. A trained visceroctomist was expected to perform this procedure in a minute or less, which was an advantage when it was important not to attract attention to this activity. The procedure was, however, brutal, and the instrument crude. Unsurprisingly, families of the deceased often attempted to prevent it. One frequent method of escaping the obligation of visceroctomy was a clandestine burial. Another, less frequent, was preventing visceroctomy by force. There were numerous reports of fights between the visceroctomist, who sometimes was protected by soldiers or policemen, and family members of the deceased person armed with knives and in some cases riffles. The violence occasionally led to the death of the visceroctomist, either when he attempted to collect the liver sample or later, as an act of vengeance for profanation of the body.

In 1937, Wilbur Sawyer, then the director of the RF's international division, heard that six visceroctomists had been killed in fights with people who opposed visceroctomy and many others had been wounded in such fights; some of their opponents also had been killed or wounded. Appalled, he wrote to Soper asking him to consider suspending this practice or at least limiting it to cases in which a partial biopsy was essential. Soper strongly disagreed. He believed that visceroctomy was indispensable for the control of yellow fever in Brazil, and he noted that considering the number of visceroctomies performed—more than 100,000 a year, often in regions known for their religious fanaticism—the violence that accompanied visceroctomy could be described as very mild. Sawyer was not persuaded, but Soper refused to reduce the use of the procedure. Nevertheless, in his 1977 autobiography, while he defended the practice as a very useful public health tool, Soper did recognize that sampling of a cadaver's liver was a "somewhat gruesome business at best."[53]

Yellow Fever Vaccine in Brazil: Virology and Public Health

With the identification of sylvatic yellow fever it became clear that while urban populations could be protected from yellow fever through the control of *Aedes*, the only way to protect people in contact with jungle mosquitoes was vaccination. At first, scientists attempted to produce a vaccine that contained inactivated viruses, or rather heat-inactivated tissues of infected animals, but they discovered that such vaccines did not work. Efficient vaccination was possible only using a live, attenuated virus. In 1932 the director of the yellow fever laboratory at the Rockefeller Foundation, Wilbur Sawyer, together with his colleagues S. F. Kitchen and Wray Lloyd, developed the first live vaccine with an attenuated yellow fever virus, 17E, grown in fertilized eggs. However, this virus was not sufficiently stable and could be safely used only when mixed with immune serum from people who had recovered from yellow fever.[54] In 1936, the virology laboratory of the Brazilian Yellow Fever Service, at the Oswaldo Cruz Institute, Rio de Janeiro, founded by the experts in the RF's international division, started a culture of the 17E strain. In 1937, an important epidemic of sylvatic yellow fever in the state of Parana led to the first large-scale field trial of the 17E vaccine in Brazil. Scientists conducting the trial noted that some of the recipients of the virus mixed with an immune serum developed jaundice.[55] Similar findings were reported in vaccination campaigns in Africa. Researchers aspired, therefore, to develop a vaccine that could be administered without immune serum.[56]

Also in 1937, Max Theiler and his colleague Hugh Smith developed another attenuated strain of yellow fever, 17D, that could be administered without immune human serum.[57] That same year, Smith traveled from New York to Rio de Janeiro, where, together with a Brazilian colleague, Henrique de Azevedo Penna, he perfected the culture of 17D in fertilized eggs, enabling rapid production of the new vaccine. The 17D vaccine was first employed in Brazil during an outburst of sylvatic yellow fever in Minas Gerais in December 1937.[58] In 1938, more than a million Brazilians were vaccinated with the 17D virus.[59] Because of unknown risks linked with a distribution of a live vaccine for a dangerous disease, the Brazilian Yellow Fever Service staff outlined a strict protocol of postvaccination surveillance. Each vaccination site had two tables: one for preparing the vaccine, diluted from a lyophilized (dried at a low temperature) stock, and the other for paperwork. Personal data on each vaccinated person—name, age, sex, occupation, address—were recorded in a vaccination book. One copy of this book was kept locally, and another in Rio de Janeiro. After each vaccination campaign physicians designated by the Yellow Fever Service visited the vaccinated locality twice, first after a few weeks and then after a few months, to assess the efficacy of the vaccination campaign and possible secondary effects of the vaccine. Detailed data recorded in the vaccination book facilitated their task.[60]

The protocol elaborated in Brazil for the early 17D vaccination campaigns was maintained during the impressive scaling up of the vaccination: in 1939 alone more than a million Brazilians received the 17D vaccine.[61] In 1939–41 there were several incidents of iatrogenic effects of the vaccine. These incidents led a researcher of the Oswaldo Cruz Institute, Angelo Moreira de Costa Lima, to accuse the Rockefeller Foundation experts of using Brazilians as guinea pigs.[62] This was, however, a minority opinion. The yellow fever vaccination campaigns were generally well received, probably because of fear of this disease but also because the campaign organizers successfully mobilized the support of local authorities and elites. Moreover, while vaccination-related incidents were far from negligible, the efficient surveillance of the consequences of vaccination campaigns favored their rapid detection. As the RF experts in Brazil explained, "The best protection against future accidents is the careful surveillance of vaccinated individuals."[63]

The main pitfalls of using a live, neurotropic vaccine, maintained through multiple passages in fertilized eggs, were that the virus might be too weak (excessive attenuation) or too strong (insufficient attenuation) and that the vaccine might be contaminated by an external infectious agent. All three possibilities did occur during the mass production of the 17D yellow fever vaccine in Brazil. In 1939 a vaccination campaign in the state of Espírito Santo was followed by epidemics of yellow fever. The cause, researchers in the Rio laboratory discovered, was that the virus used in the vaccine had been weakened through too many passages in fertilized eggs; accordingly, they limited the number of such passages.[64] In June 1941, doctors observed a rise in the incidence of encephalitis after a vaccination campaign in the state of Minas Gerais. An investigation concluded that the outbreak had been induced by vaccination with an insufficiently attenuated virus. This incident led to a tightening of controls of attenuation of the virus.[65]

The most serious accident with the 17D vaccine in Brazil was, however, its contamination by a "jaundice agent," later identified as hepatitis B virus. During a vaccination campaign in the state of Espírito Santo in late 1939 and early 1940, postvaccine follow-up identified more than 1,000 cases of jaundice, with 22 deaths. The Rockefeller Foundation experts and their Brazilian colleagues decided to halt immunization with 17D until they discovered the jaundice's source. First, they excluded the possibility that it had been produced by a mutation of the yellow fever virus itself: there was no correlation whatsoever between the presence of jaundice and the level of antibodies against yellow fever. They then carefully examined all the components of the production chain and through an elimination process concluded that the culprit was normal human serum employed as a suspension fluid to protect the fragile yellow fever virus.[66] Virologists who produced yellow fever vaccine in Rio de Janeiro decided to discard all the old batches of vaccine, imported a new strain of 17D from New York, and started the production of a vaccine in which human serum was replaced by liquid from fertilized eggs. There were no more cases of vaccine-related hepatitis in Brazil.[67]

The conclusion that a serum, even when inactivated by heating it to 56°C, could induce jaundice was not surprising. There had been numerous earlier reports of this phenomenon, among them the finding by the South African professor of veterinary medicine Arnold Theiler of jaundice in horses vaccinated against the African horse sickness with a combination of a live virus and horse immune serum.[68] Moreover, George Marshall Findlay and his colleagues in the Wellcome Foundation's virology laboratory in London described jaundice in people vaccinated against yellow fever and attributed it to the presence of a contaminated human serum in the vaccine.[69] It is reasonable to assume that these studies were known to the virologists confronted with an outbreak of postvaccination jaundice in Brazil, as well as to the scientists who produced the 17D vaccine in New York, especially because Max Theiler was Arnold Theiler's son, while Findlay and his colleagues at the Wellcome had frequent exchanges with RF experts. Virologists from the New York laboratory were also aware of the decision made by their Brazilian colleagues in 1940 to produce a serum-free vaccine. Nevertheless, in early 1941, when New York began massive production of yellow fever vaccine for the US Army, the vaccine contained normal human serum.

The New York virologists, led by Sawyer, confident in the technical superiority of their vaccine production process, believed that postvaccination jaundice in Brazil was the result of contamination of their yellow fever virus cultures by another virus owing to a failure to adequately supervise virus cultures in a technically "inferior" setting.[70] They were confident that such problems would not arise in the cutting-edge virology laboratory in New York, with its rigorous control of all the steps of manufacture of yellow fever vaccine, and therefore did not see any reason to change their production protocol. When, in 1941, the yellow fever laboratory was asked by the US Army to drastically scale up the vaccine production to vaccinate the soldiers sent to the Pacific arena, Sawyer and his colleagues saw no reason to change their production protocol. Between January 1, 1941, and April 9, 1942, the New York laboratory supplied the US Army with 7.7 million doses of yellow fever vaccine.[71] In March 1942 the army reported massive outbreaks of jaundice, in all probability linked to the vaccination against yellow fever. The number of cases rose very quickly. The New York laboratory halted the manufacture of yellow fever vaccine in early April 1942 and started production of serum-free vaccine a few weeks later.

The report of an internal investigation of the Rockefeller Foundation published in 1944 estimated that more than 26,000 soldiers developed postvaccination hepatitis.[72] Later, epidemiologists estimated that at least 40,000 soldiers were hospitalized for this indication, of a total of 300,000 soldiers immunized with contaminated batches of the vaccine, the largest known iatrogenic incident of vaccination in US history.[73] Nevertheless, the commission that investigated the massive contamination of yellow fever vaccine by hepatitis virus absolved the RF laboratory of responsibility for the incident.[74] The report also did not mention that the same problem had been successfully solved two years earlier in Brazil thanks to an efficient combination of high-tech virologic knowledge with a low-tech public health approach: a careful postvaccination surveillance of the vaccinated population.[75]

Control of Yellow Fever in Brazil in the 1950s, 1960s, and 1970s: The SNFA's Insufficient Forms

In 1940, the Yellow Fever Service (Serviço de Febre Amarela, or SFA), led by Rockefeller Foundation experts, was replaced by the Brazilian-led National Yellow Fever Service (Serviço Nacional de Febre Amarela, or SNFA). The SNFA was expected to faithfully reproduce the SFA patterns of intervention codified by Soper and his collaborators.[76] Instruments such as the standardized epidemiological forms, the backbone of Soper's SFA were, however, increasingly perceived as inadequate. One of the key reasons was a slow erosion of the rigid guidelines for describing suspicious cases of "fever" and sudden deaths from such "fevers." Without the coaching of RF experts, Brazilian workers in the Yellow Fever Service found it difficult to describe the drama of sudden death, frequently of a young child, in preprinted epidemiological survey forms. The forms used by sanitary workers in the 1950s were inherited from the 1930s and 1940s SFA, but by the 1950s the mind-set of the employees who filled them out had gradually shifted. One difference was the inclusion of doubts about diagnoses in the epidemiological record. For example, in the case of Feliciano Vaz de Goias, who died on December 11, 1944, the family rejected the laboratory's diagnosis of yellow fever. The family's doctor at first took the family's side, then six months later changed his mind. In the case of Ruffino da Silva Matos, who died on August 22, 1944, the pathologist found nonspecified "suspicious lesions"; the laboratory result was negative for yellow fever, but the case was reclassified on January 5, 1951, as yellow fever, with no supplementary explanations in the file. Many files carried the expressions "suspicious, possibly negative," "insufficient quantity adequate material," or "suspicious lesions." Some of the cases were never elucidated: the "suspicious" cases remained suspicious, at least in the epidemiology files.[77]

Another difficulty was a growing desire to integrate a different kind of information into the standard forms, above all details about the lives of the people who carried the viruses. Since the forms were printed, SFA employees increasingly added information in the margins or at the bottom of the page. Sometimes the form contained marginal notations in several different colors of ink. Thus one physician found it difficult to establish the precise cause of death in children who suffered from several parasite diseases and other conditions linked with poverty. He refused to complete the standard epidemiological survey form and wrote instead that "the information we have is not sufficient to provide an adequate classification of the patient's symptoms. Despite my efforts, I am unable to follow this model." Other doctors added question marks in their reports, noted that they were not sure that the answers they proposed were correct, stressed that the deceased person suffered from multiple pathologies, or added in small, cramped writing in the margins of the printed forms numerous details about the deceased person's family and life conditions. Such remarks were especially abundant when the deceased was a child.[78] The administrative methods elaborated by the RF experts were, at least until the 1960s, an efficient way to control mosquitoes and viruses. They may have been less efficient when dealing with people.

The Yellow Fever Service files from the 1940s and 1950s provide a rich description of the routine functioning of a public health service in Brazil. They also indicate that at that time cases of yellow fever were rare. The majority of suspected yellow fever cases and unexplained deaths were finally identified as cases of different conditions, in some cases other infectious diseases, in others intoxication, including with medication, that produced severe jaundice. The few cases of confirmed yellow fever were of a sylvatic variant. Since 1942 there have been no identified cases of *Aedes*-transmitted urban yellow fever in Brazil. Moreover, until 2015, the annual number of cases of sylvatic yellow fever was usually under 100 and often under 50 (one exception was 1954, with more than 200 cases).[79] Selective vaccination of vulnerable populations became an efficient way of containing this pathology. Containing the *Aedes* mosquito was much more complicated.

Eradication of *Aedes* in Latin America: Success and Failure

From the 1930s to the 1970s experts believed that the only efficient way to control diseases propagated by the *Aedes* mosquito was to eradicate this mosquito. Soper's goal of extending the anti-*Aedes* campaign to all of Latin and Central America became more feasible after World War II with the development of a highly efficient anti-mosquito compound, DDT. In 1947 the Pan American Health Organization, inspired by Fred Soper, officially adopted the goal of eradicating *Aedes aegypti* from the Americas.[80] Soper was aware of the difficulty of scaling up anti-*Aedes* campaigns. Continentwide eradication of the *Aedes* mosquito was more difficult than organizing local or national campaigns. It required efficient cooperation of sanitary authorities in all the infested countries and reliable monitoring of the progress of the eradication work.[81] Moreover, efforts to eradicate *Aedes* from the Americas were also hampered by US sanitary authorities' reluctance to join eradication programs. The United States formally supported the 1947 program for the continental eradication of *Aedes*. In 1957 the US Public Health Service created a pilot pro-gram to test the feasibility of *Aedes* eradication in Pensacola, Florida. The program was successful, and in 1962–63 it served as the basis for the proposal of a countrywide eradication program. The program was never implemented, and the United States officially abandoned its *Aedes*-eradication efforts in 1969. Soper believed that there were multiple reasons for the low enthusiasm for eliminating *Aedes* in the United States: the absence of a direct yellow fever threat, the high cost of anti-mosquito campaigns, US citizens' resistance to these campaigns, the lack of a reliable system for monitoring the progress of *Aedes* elimination, and the low credence US sanitary authorities gave to the risk of contamination of other countries by mosquitoes originated in the United States.[82] An additional obstacle was the rise of DDT-resistant strains of *Aedes*, a problem that became especially acute in the Caribbean region.[83] Soper ac-knowledged in 1968 that the eradication of *Aedes* in the Americas was slower than expected, but he had no doubts about its eventual success.[84]

In the mid-1970s the continental eradication of *Aedes* could have been presented as a partial success. The last colonies of *Aedes* mosquitoes in Brazil had been detected in 1955, and in 1958 Brazil had officially been declared an *Aedes aegypti*–free country. Several other countries—Argentina, Belize, Ber-muda, Bolivia, Chile, Equator, the Panama Canal Zone, Paraguay, Peru, and Uruguay—were also declared free of *Aedes*. On the other hand, the United States, Colombia, Cuba, the Dominican Republic, Guyana, the Caribbean is-lands, and Venezuela never eliminated this mosquito. The continued presence of *Aedes* in these countries contributed in the late 1960s to the infestation of countries previously certified *Aedes*-free.[85] Their reinfestation was attributed to the increasingly dense population, the degradation of sanitary conditions in the cities, the increase in migration and tourism, the existence of zones of intensive illegal trafficking, the uncontrolled circulation of small planes, the continental trade in old automobile tires, and a gradual abandonment of mos-quito control efforts by public authorities.[86] The difficulty of controlling *Aedes* in the Americas may have been aggravated by the inaccuracy of reports about the progress of eradication work. In the early 1960s many PAHO experts were unaware of the extent of infestation of the Caribbean region by *Aedes aegypti* and of the growing risks of propagation of dengue by this insect.[87]

The Rockefeller Foundation officially left Brazil in 1939, although some RF experts—virologists, entomologists, and epidemiologists—continued to work with their Brazilian colleagues from the Yellow Fever Service. In the 1950s and 1960s, the elimination of *Aedes* from Brazil was conducted by organizations affiliated with the Health Ministry, first the DNSP, later the Departamento Nacional de Endemias Rurais, or DNERu (National Department of Rural Endemic Diseases), created in 1953. In 1967 the control of yellow fever became the responsibility of the newly created Superintendência de Campanhas de Saúde Pública, or SUCAM (Superintendence of Public Health Campaigns), born from a fusion of DNERu with campaigns to eradicate smallpox and malaria.[88] SUCAM was active until 1991, when it was officially replaced by the Fundação Nacional de Saúde, or FUNASA (National Foundation of Health). The foundation of SUCAM accelerated the mutation of the original SFA into a very different kind of organization. The RF experts viewed inhabitants of "controlled" areas mainly as vehicles for the proliferation of *Aedes* larvae and trained SFA workers to strictly respect rules and maintain a rigorous, US-style work discipline.[89] SUCAM workers were not expected to adhere to such a strict discipline, and many became sincerely interested in helping the communities they served. In the 1980s SUCAM opened an internal competition for memoirs of its sanitary workers, who at that time were still almost exclusively men. Authors of the best memoirs received a prize, and their essays were published. These essays provide a vivid image of fighting mosquitoes in the 1960s, 1970s, and 1980s in remote regions of Brazil. SUCAM agents were often poorly paid and worked under difficult conditions. Their essays reveal their adherence to an ideal of public service but also the role of their Catholic faith in support of this ideal. They were often struck by the extreme poverty of some of the people they visited, their poor health, and the stark contrast between the needs of vulnerable populations and the paucity of the means dedicated to sanitary and public health work.[90]

The declaration of Brazil as an *Aedes*-free country in 1958 was perceived as a triumph of the patient efforts of sanitary agents. Dedicated sanitary workers were, however, unable to prevent the return of *Aedes* to Brazil. In July 1967 a physician in Belem (Pará) captured a mosquito identified as *Aedes aegypti*. When sanitary agents arrived in Belem the next month, they found a significant *Aedes* presence in the city and in several inland localities. DNERu inspectors immediately started an energetic eradication campaign. At first, this campaign was hampered by a reduction in the number of agency technicians and difficulties in obtaining sufficient quantities of insecticides, but later it was presented as a success.[91] In 1973 PAHO again declared Brazil *Aedes*-free. The second official eradication period did not last long. In 1976 and 1977 *Aedes aegypti* was found in Rio de Janeiro and Salvador, Bahia, and then in nearly all the Brazilian states.[92]

New Configuration: *Aedes* and Dengue Fever

The reappearance of *Aedes aegypti* in Brazil in the 1970s was followed by outbreaks of dengue fever, a disease absent from Brazil for 50 years.[93] Dengue
was first spotted in 1981–82 in the northern state of Roraima, but the first
important outbreak of this was the 1986 outbreak in the state of Rio de Janeiro.
This outbreak coincided with the end of twenty years of military dictatorship
in Brazil and the rise of civil movements that promoted the engagement of
citizens in the democratic process.[94] The dengue outbreak started in April
1986 in the region Baixada Fluminense. Epidemiologists feared that it would
spread to other areas and soon reach the city of Rio de Janeiro.[95] According
to *O Globo*, one of the main Brazilian newspapers, that would be a sad rever-
sal of Oswaldo Cruz's campaign to "civilize Rio." With the arrival of dengue
fever, Rio would "uncivilize itself."[96]

Public health authorities tried at first to convey that the risk of dengue was
not very high. Local activists strongly disagreed. At that time, civil organizations in Baixada Fluminense such as the Movimento de Amigo de Bairros, or
MAB (Friends of Neighborhoods), the Federação das Associações de Mora-
dores do Estado do Rio de Janeiro, or FAMERJ (Federation of Associations of
Residents of the State of Rio de Janeiro), and the progressive Catholic association Caritas Diocesana (Diocesian Charity Association) were engaged in a
struggle for the extension of democratic rights, especially at the local level.[97]
Women played a key role in these popular movements. They were also directly
involved in protests in favor of aggressive anti-mosquito measures. MAB's
leader, the physician Lucia Souto, stressed the importance of intensifying such
actions and of the involvement of inhabitants of infested areas in mosquito
control.[98] The state of Rio de Janeiro's sanitary authorities recognized in April
1986 that SUCAM, responsible for mosquito control, could not deal with the
high density of *Aedes* mosquitoes in the Baixada Fluminense region: they
had only 500 agents and 15 fumigation machines for a population of 7 million
people.[99] The detection of cases of dengue in Rio de Janeiro prompted the State
Department of Health to strengthen its anti-mosquito interventions, above
all fumigations with the insecticide malathion. The Department of Health
purchased 32 powerful fumigation machines in the United States. It also
declared May 25, 1986 the "Day of a fight against dengue" and mobilized high
school students to educate the inhabitants about the importance of eliminating breeding sites of *Aedes* larvae.[100]

The combination of education and fumigation, claimed Claudio Amaral, secretary of health for the state of Rio de Janeiro, would lead to the elimination of dengue.[101] MAB activists were more skeptical. Fumigations and sporadic removal of some of the *Aedes* breeding places, Lucia Souto explained, would not solve the severe structural problems that had led to the proliferation of *Aedes* mosquitoes, such as ineffective garbage collection, poor sanitation, or the failure to act against vendors who left piles of used tires outdoors. To protest against the shortcomings of the state investment in public health, representatives of inhabitants of five cities of Baixada Fluminense blocked the Via Doutra, one of the main access roads to Rio de Janeiro, on May 27, 1986. The demonstration was organized by MAB and neighborhood committees and was supported by progressive Catholic groups. Photographs of this demonstration show that the majority of the participants were women. A carnival car carried demonstrators in mosquito costumes. Some posters called for the return of Oswaldo Cruz, others proposed that the name of the mosquito *Aedes aegypti* be changed to *Aedes brasiliensis*.[102]

In June, the state of Rio de Janeiro health department purchased additional fumigation machines and mobilized soldiers to conduct fumigations.[103] Journalists, as well as external experts, regarded these efforts as insufficient and strongly criticized years of severe neglect of sanitary interventions.[104] The prevalence of dengue decreased however in late June, a development that the sanitary authorities attributed to the efficacy of their anti-Aedes measures, above all fumigations, presented as an improved version of Oswaldo Cruz's campaign.[105] In retrospect, the sanitary authorities recognized that the efforts to control *Aedes* in the state of Rio had yielded only modest results.[106] The dengue epidemic of Baixada Fluminense was the first in a long series of such outbreaks. It also marked the beginning of the transformation of dengue fever, earlier seen as a rare pathology, into a major public health problem in Brazil.[107] The widespread presence of dengue fever was seen as an indicator of the increasing severity of social problems. A survey in the late 1980s found that 33.8% of Brazilian homes lacked a clean water supply and 39.8% had no garbage collection. The catastrophic sanitary situation in the rapidly and chaotically growing poor urban and peri-urban neighborhoods, coupled with the degradation of security conditions in these neighborhoods, facilitated the increased density of *Aedes*.[108]

In the mid-twentieth century, favelas were seen as relatively safe places, less plagued by crime than the more affluent neighborhoods. The security situation in the favelas deteriorated dramatically, however, in the last quarter of the century, with the rise of favela-based drug trafficking, controlled by increasingly aggressive crime gangs, sometimes in collaboration with the police.[109] In the 1990s Brazilian public health experts believed that the spread of dengue could be halted through intensive education about the importance of anti-*Aedes* measures and the enrollment of leaders of affected communities in these efforts. At the same time, public health specialists recognized that targeted campaigns to reduce the density of mosquitoes in a given locality provided only short-term solutions. Lasting prevention of dengue fever implied a radical improvement of sanitation in poor neighborhoods, a long-term and costly endeavor. In 1996 the Brazilian Health Ministry elaborated an ambitious project of nationwide eradication of *Aedes aegypti*, but this project was never implemented. In fact, just the opposite occurred. At that time, Brazilian sanitary services that dealt with mosquito control became increasingly perceived as too expensive and not sufficiently cost-effective; their size was drastically reduced in the 1990s, as part of an overall reduction of public spending under the neoliberal presidents Fernando Collor, Itamar Franco, and Fernando Henrique Cardoso. In the absence of systematic and sustained efforts to eliminate *Aedes* mosquitoes, their density continued to increase, as did the threat of the diseases they transmitted. In 1999 Rio de Janeiro fired approximately two-thirds of the sanitary agents responsible for mosquito control in the city. In 2002 the city suffered a massive dengue epidemic.[110]

In the early twenty-first century the eradication of *Aedes* disappeared from Brazil's public health agenda, while the proliferation of these insects was further favored by an increase in the volume of air travel, the mosquitoes' growing resistance to insecticides, and the consequences of global warming. The mosquito has won. In 2001 the Brazilian government officially abandoned the 1996 project to eradicate *Aedes* and proposed instead a Plan of Intensification of Actions to Control Dengue. In 2002, this plan was replaced by a new plan, the National Plan to Control Dengue. Its goals, supported by the left-wing government of Luiz Inácio Lula da Silva, were to develop permanent programs of mosquito control, to elaborate large-scale information and education campaigns to stimulate community-based anti-mosquito measures, to integrate the control of mosquitoes with other programs of basic public health such as the popular Program of Family Health (Bolsa Familia), and to perfect tools of epidemiological surveillance. This plan did not promote, however, large investments in sanitation in poor neighborhoods. Mosquito control was not seen as a high priority in a country struggling with severe social problems and plagued by high inequality. In the late twentieth and early twenty-first centuries, Brazil made important advances in the reduction of extreme misery and improved the access of the poor to primary health care and education. It did not make similar advances in providing clean water, sewage, and trash collection to destitute neighborhoods. Hopes that new scientific developments would halt the proliferation of mosquitoes did not materialize either.[111]

Between 1997 and 2002 Brazil reported more than 2 million cases of dengue, 70% of the cases of this disease recorded in Latin America.[112] Dengue fever was no longer confined to specific Brazilian states but was distributed across the nation. The broad diffusion of dengue fever was accompanied by an increase in the number of cases of a more severe form of this disease, hemorrhagic dengue fever, and deaths attributed to this pathology. In the first years of the twenty-first century, effective control of *Aedes* mosquitoes in Brazil was increasingly presented as an impossible task. In 2010 Rio de Janeiro suffered the worst dengue epidemic in the city's history, and the disease has become hyperendemic in the majority of Brazilian states. Brazil could be described again, as it was in the early 1920s, as a land filled with mosquitoes.[113] The distribution of mosquitoes, especially of the most dangerous among them, *Aedes aegypti*, is, however, uneven. Brazilian social scientists describe the unequal distribution of environmental risks among different segments of the population as "environmental racism." The absence of even rudimentary sanitation in many poor areas increased the exposure of the inhabitants of these areas to toxic substances, pathogenic microorganisms, and disease-carrying insects.[114] Dengue fever became one of the "normal" hurdles of life. It is perceived as annoying and sometimes severely handicapping, but less dangerous than the endemic violence deeply embedded in daily life in many poor neighborhoods.

In the twenty-first century, it has become increasingly difficult to imagine a complete elimination of the *Aedes aegypti* mosquito from Brazil. Experts expect at best to achieve a moderate reduction in its density in urban and peri-urban areas.[115] Their main hope is that technical solutions such as the sterilization of mosquitoes, their genetic modification, or their infection with the bacterium *Wolbachia* will limit the capacity of *Aedes* mosquitoes to disseminate diseases.[116] Some Brazilian experts have maintained that only high-tech solutions will contain the spread of *Aedes* mosquitoes in Brazil.[117] Others continued to situate the efforts to eliminate these insects in a broader social context.[118] In the meantime, while some localities did achieve better control of mosquitoes, there were no tangible signs of improvement for the country as a whole. A 2011 assessment of the control of infectious diseases in Brazil stated that the Brazilian government had invested 900 million reais a year (at that time equivalent to more than half a billion US dollars) in vector control campaigns, but these campaigns had failed to halt the spread of dengue fever. The prospects for the future, the authors of the survey concluded, were not encouraging.[119] They were right. The economic crisis in Brazil, which had started in 2013, led to further degradation of urban and peri-urban environments and the reduction of public health budgets. The prevalence of dengue fever in Brazil has not diminished, and new mosquito-borne diseases, chikungunya and Zika, appeared in 2013 and 2014. Unsurprisingly, inhabitants of poor areas, especially those infested by mosquitoes, were at increased danger of contracting these new diseases.[120]

The Return of Sylvatic Yellow Fever: The Epidemics of 2016–18

Studies of the yellow fever virus in the 1930s and 1940s and the mass production of the yellow fever vaccine favored the development of virology in Brazil. With the sharp decrease in the incidence of this pathology, Brazilian virologists focused on other viral diseases, such as influenza and polio. One of the main sites of development of Brazilian virology was the virology laboratory of the Oswaldo Cruz Institute, Rio de Janeiro, originally a key site of studies on the yellow fever virus and the 17D vaccine. In the 1970s, this laboratory, headed by the virologist Hermann Schatzmayr, was transformed into an independent research center, the Centro de Virologia Médica (CVM). The CVM introduced innovative methods of virologic research, among them the use of monoclonal antibodies; it also perfected diagnostic tests for viral diseases. In the early 1980s, with the reappearance of dengue in Brazil and disquieting news about the epidemics of hemorrhagic dengue in Cuba in 1981, the CVM turned to studies of the dengue virus and, following the 1986 epidemic of dengue in Rio de Janeiro, opened a laboratory dedicated to the studies of flaviviruses; a group of pathogens was named after its most deadly member, the yellow fever virus. This laboratory became an internationally recognized center for study of this group of pathogens. In 2015–16 it played an important role in studies of the Zika virus. It also continued studies of the yellow fever virus [121]

Although for more than 70 years the prevalence of yellow fever in Brazil was low, experts were aware that the number of cases might explode and feared that the failure to control the *Aedes* mosquitoes might lead to an outbreak of the urban form of this disease as well. In 2016 there was a significant increase in the incidence of sylvatic yellow fever, especially in southeastern Brazil, in the states of Rio de Janeiro, Minas Gerais, Espírito Santo, and São Paolo. The outbreak continued in 2017 and 2018 and led to at least 2,251 human cases and 772 deaths. It was contained through mass vaccination. The possible reason for this outbreak was a combination of ecological variables and the low frequency of anti–yellow fever vaccination. Uncontrolled deforestation and consequences of climate change led to the degradation of natural habitats of jungle monkeys, the main carriers of the yellow fever virus, and the *Hemagogus* mosquitoes, which transferred this virus to humans. Another important element was the unvaccinated populations in the affected regions. These regions were not considered to be at high risk of yellow fever and therefore had not been included in previous vaccination campaigns. The spread of yellow fever might have been facilitated by the presence of asymptomatic cases of this disease, which scientists had discovered to be much more frequent than previously suspected. Ideally, some public health experts argued, all Brazilians should be immunized with the highly effective 17D vaccine. Ideally, vaccination should be combined with the reduction of the density of infestation of *Aedes aegypti*, which would reduce the risk of the "urbanization" of yellow fever.[122]

With the increased frequency of yellow fever, people in the affected regions erroneously blamed monkeys for the outbreak, and some started to kill these animals. However, not only did killing monkeys not halt the spread of yellow fever—there was a very large reservoir of yellow fever in jungle animals—but it hampered the detection of new sites of the yellow fever virus. Dead monkeys were an early warning sign of the presence of this virus in a given area.[123] In response to the yellow fever outbreak, the Brazilian government started an intensive vaccination campaign in all the affected regions. This campaign was at first hindered by a shortage of vaccines. The production of the 17D vaccine in Brazil was sufficient to deal with endemic yellow fever, but it was difficult to scale it up rapidly. In order to vaccinate all the adults in targeted states, the government injected people with one-fifth of the usual dose, an emergency vaccination that, although imperfect, could protect for at least one year.[124] Another initial problem was an uneven geographic distribution of the vaccine. Some vaccination centers did not receive enough vaccine doses, so that people had to wait many hours in line. They became discouraged and failed to return when more vaccines became available.[125] Later, however, the Brazilian manufacturer of yellow fever vaccine, Biomanguinhos (Fiocruz), successfully accelerated its production, while the Brazilian National Health Service greatly improved the distribution of this vaccine, thanks, among others things, to the development of mobile vaccination units, sent to areas with low vaccination rates.[126] The yellow fever outbreak ended in 2019. To everybody's relief, despite the high density of *Aedes* mosquitoes in Brazilian cities, there was no outbreak of the urban form of this disease.

The management of yellow fever epidemics in Brazil in 2015–19 was described as an overall success but also a partial failure. The successful control of a yellow fever outbreak and the prevention of the most feared outcome, epidemics of *Aedes*-transmitted urban yellow fever, reflected the important achievements of the biomedical sciences and public health in Brazil: excellent research on mosquito-borne viruses, efficient and rapid local production of the vaccine despite some initial problems, a competently organized mass-vaccination campaign. On the other hand, this episode also exposed failings in Brazil's epidemic preparedness: delays in the detection and reporting of the rise of cases of yellow fever, especially in nonendemic areas; insufficient vaccine coverage in rural and peri-urban areas; incomplete immunization for rural workers who live close to forest areas; and the persistence of poor sanitation that facilitated the proliferation of mosquitoes.[127]

The outbreak of sylvatic yellow fever in Brazil coincided with the Zika epidemic. Even though these two outbreaks were produced by closely related flaviviruses, they were rarely discussed together. One reason might be the important differences between these two diseases. Yellow fever is a severe, often lethal infection, while Zika is nearly always a benign pathology. The main harm induced by ZIKV is infection of the fetus. The other reason might be differences between affected populations. Yellow fever was found mainly in young men exposed to jungle mosquitoes because of their work as loggers, hunters, or farmers. Although they were mainly working-class men, sylvatic yellow fever is usually seen as a professional rather than a class-related pathology. Zika was especially dangerous for pregnant women and affected mainly those from lower social strata. A third reason might be the difference in vectors that spread these diseases: the jungle mosquitoes that diffuse sylvatic yellow fever do not behave in the same way as the *Aedes* mosquito. Finally, an efficient solution made possible the containment of the yellow fever outbreak: vaccination. The main problem was how to organize a mass vaccination campaign. There was no similar solution to the Zika outbreak. Nevertheless, these outbreaks shared two important traits: a lack of attention to the gradual degradation of sanitary conditions in Brazil and a low level of preparedness for a health crisis. As Weverton Rodrigues, a Rio de Janeiro public health expert, explained: "Unfortunately I see the culture of our country as very short-sighted. You work according to demand. You put out fires. A problem comes up and let's deal with it."[128]

CHAPTER TWO

Fetuses

Women, Doctors, and the Law

Operation Herod

In October 2014, an article in a major Brazilian newspaper, *O Globo*, reported that 57 people, among them 6 physicians, 7 nurses, 2 lawyers, 6 plainclothesmen, 1 firefighter, and 2 politicians, were arrested as part of Operação Herodes (Operation Herod, the saving of innocent babies from murder), a crackdown on clandestine abortion clinics in Rio de Janeiro. All were accused of the "crime of abortion" and described as a "criminal band," a term usually reserved for drug traffickers.[1] The article reported that an 88-year-old gynecologist, Dr. Aloisio Soares Guimarães, previously condemned several times for illegal abortions, headed a vast and exceptionally lucrative network of clandestine abortion clinics. He operated in a high-end clinic in the center of Copacabana and supervised the activities of six additional clinics in various parts of Rio de Janeiro. Several of the arrested physicians also had previous condemnations for illegal abortions. The average price of an abortion was 7,500 reais (at that time about US$2,000). The article was accompanied by a photograph of an elderly man (presumably Guimarães), his face covered with his vest, being led to a police car. The caption read "Shame."

According to *O Globo*, the clandestine clinics had agreements with policemen, who protected them from raids. The police declared that Operation Herod put an end to 30 years of impunity in Rio de Janeiro. Gynecologists in Rio reported soon after Operation Herod that middle- and upper-class women who wished to end an unwanted pregnancy were obliged to travel to São Paolo; the most affluent among them often elected to travel abroad. Less than two years later, a prominent Rio de Janeiro gynecologist, Antônio José Farias de Andrade, and his collaborator, the anesthetist Juvenal Siqueira Azevedo Filho, were arrested for performing an abortion in a high-end clinic in Copacabana, not far from one of the clinics of Dr. Aloisio Soares Guimarães. This time the police also arrested a woman who was in the middle of surgical termination of pregnancy; they took her to prison despite her state. In all probability the arrest was prompted by a report made by a member of the clinic's staff.[2]

Abortion Is a Crime

Abortion is illegal in Brazil, as it is (in 2023) in the majority of Central and Latin American countries. Article 2 of the Brazilian Civil Code states that life starts at conception. Abortion is punishable by one to four years of imprisonment for the person performing the abortion. The inclusion of abortion as a crime in Brazil's criminal code of 1830 was confirmed in the criminal code of 1890 and consolidated in the penal code of 1940, still valid today. From the 1970s on, Brazilian feminists have fought to liberalize abortion, but the only important change has been the decriminalization of abortion for anencephaly (absence of a brain in the fetus) in 2012.[3] Abortion performed by a pregnant woman on herself is considered a criminal act too, but in practice Brazilian women have seldom been punished for a self-induced termination of pregnancy.[4] Until 2012, abortion was only legal in cases of immediate risk to the mother's life and rape. A woman who declares that her pregnancy is the result of rape is automatically entitled to an abortion in a public facility, although it may not be easy to find a hospital willing to perform the act.[5] Abortion for a risk to a mother's life has to be approved by a judge on the basis of a declaration from the woman's physician. This indication allows, in principle at least, some interpretive freedom for the judge. In 2012, mainly as a result of campaigns made by human rights and women's rights advocates, such as the Institute of Bioethics, Human Rights, and Gender (ANIS) at the University of Brasília, abortion for confirmed anencephaly was legalized.[6] This modification of the law was justified by the fact that all anencephalic babies died shortly after birth. Decriminalizing abortion for this indication was thus presented as a consequence of a decision that had been already taken by God or Nature, not as allowing a woman to decide what the fate of her pregnancy will be.[7]

Abortion was first criminalized in Brazil in 1830. The passage of the 1890 penal code expanded the 1830 characterization of criminal responsibility in infanticide and abortion laws. The code incorporated more technical legal and medical definitions of fetal and infant life and implemented harsher sentencing practices for abortion and infanticide. While the 1830 code only criminalized the abortion provider, the 1890 code punished both the provider and the woman. However, the law took the woman's intention into account. If she had an abortion or committed infanticide to maintain her honor, her punishment was reduced.[8] Main provisions of the 1890 law were incorporated reformulations of laws regulating abortion in Brazil. They were not changed by the left-leaning government of the Workers' Party (PT, 2002 to mid-2016), and since 2016 they have been reinforced by the turn to the right in Brazilian politics.[9]

The usual argument in favor of voluntary termination of pregnancy is women's right to control their bodies and their fertility, or as in the United States, their right to privacy. During the Brazilian debates on the termination of pregnancy in the case of an anencephalic fetus, and then on the decriminalization of abortion in the context of the Zika epidemic, the main claim was different: the intolerable mental suffering of a woman obliged to continue a pregnancy with a nonviable fetus or uncertain what the fate of her pregnancy would be. Such suffering, activists that supported the decriminalization of abortion argued, was akin to torture. Since international law opposed torture, to force pregnant women to suffer its equivalent violated her basic human rights. Still, if every fetus is regarded as a living person and every abortion is perceived as murder, a woman's suffering, however great, may not be seen as a sufficient reason to justify this act. This may be especially true in countries such as Brazil, where religious opposition to abortion is combined with a strong valorization of the maternal role. In Brazil, even women who have had an abortion—or several abortions—sometimes severely condemn other women who elected to terminate a pregnancy. Thus young women from a Rio de Janeiro favela hospitalized in the 1990s for complications from induced abortion made declarations such as "I think that it is a crime for a woman to go to a hospital to take out a child" (*tirar o bebê*, a popular term for an induced abortion); "Once she is with child, she has to accept him"; or "Some favela women get rid of their children because they are shameless, they refuse to take care of these children."[10]

It is not easy to oppose an amalgam of religion, macho culture, and glorification of maternity. In a society that combines a long tradition of rejecting abortion with a high occurrence of (illegal) abortions, an argument in favor of voluntary termination of pregnancy may be based on a plurality of opinions. "Abortion wars," the US legal scholar Katie Watson argued, cannot be won, because of innumerable interpretations of the nature of the fetus and the role of women in society. What can be won, is the acceptance of the principle that members of a given society can agree to strongly disagree on specific issues, and still live harmoniously together, or as Watson put it, "I am not asking you to like abortion. I am asking you to like pluralism. I am asking you to acknowledge that your feeling, opinions, belief, or convictions about the moral status of embryos and fetuses cannot be proven to the level required to force them on others through the force of law."[11] On the other hand, this argument relies on the strength of a democratic tradition, absence of polarization, and willingness to compromise, a combination that in 2023 seemed increasingly challenging to attain.

Another powerful argument against the criminalization of abortion, especially in highly stratified societies, is social injustice. Many years ago, at an international bioethics conference, I met a Belgian bioethicist who was also a Jesuit priest. He explained that although as a Catholic priest he strongly opposed abortion, he was against its criminalization. When he met a woman who wanted to end an unwanted pregnancy, he did everything in his power to persuade her to change her mind. However, he knew from experience that in the majority of cases the woman could not be persuaded. If she had a legal and safe abortion, she would sin against her unborn child. If she went to a backstreet abortionist, she would put her life at risk and therefore also sin against herself and against her family, who might need her. One sin was better than three. The Belgian priest might have added that when abortion is criminalized, affluent women usually find a way to safely end an unwanted pregnancy. The risk of harming herself and her family is much greater for a poor, vulnerable woman. As the celebrated Brazilian physician and TV personality Drauzio Varella put it, "Abortion is already free in Brazil; to prohibit it is to punish those who do not have money."[12]

Real-Life Abortions: "I am afraid of dying"

A young psychologist, Wendell Ferrari, was engaged by a nongovernmental organization to work in a clinic in a favela in the southern zone (Zona Sul) of Rio de Janeiro. This relatively small favela is situated in close proximity to an affluent part of the city, and its inhabitants have easy access to the beach, as well as to high-end shops, the metro, and numerous bus lines. It is therefore perceived as somewhat atypical and privileged. It is still a favela, chaotically constructed, with no solid infrastructure, inhabited by people from lower social classes, and dominated by drug dealers. Ferrari elected as a theme of his study the sexuality of teenage girls in the favela and their experience of abortion. At the center of his dissertation, later published as a book, are ten interviews with young women who had an abortion before they turned 18. Only one among these young women defined herself as "white."[13] The interviewees included only young women who agreed to share their abortion experience with a researcher. While probably nonrepresentative, the narratives collected by Ferrari provide a rare opportunity to learn how young, poor women aborted in Brazil in the second decade of the twenty-first century.[14]

Four of the young women interviewed had had a surgical abortion in a clandestine clinic in the favela, three had had a surgical abortion in a more upscale clinic outside the favela, and three had used the abortive drug misoprostol (Cytotec). In the moral economy of this favela, misoprostol was distributed by the same networks that distributed illegal drugs, and only men were allowed to purchase it. A woman who wanted to buy this drug has to ask a man to do it for her, an extreme expression of male control of female fertility.[15] The three favela women who used misoprostol reported more harrowing experiences than those who underwent a surgical termination of a pregnancy, probably because they did not know what to expect and were not prepared for the side effects of this abortifacient—severe cramps, pain, bleeding, and gastrointestinal symptoms. All three were alone when these symptoms occurred. One took the drug in the house of her male partner, who supplied it, but then he left her alone and went to work. One was able to end the abortion without additional medical intervention; nevertheless, she reported that she was in severe pain for many hours and very scared—she described her experience as "horrible." She was also shocked to see the expulsed "product of abortion," a bloodied sac with fetal remains. Thankfully, a friend who had already aborted with misoprostol reassured her later that this was normal, just as it was normal to experience heavy bleeding several days after a drug-induced abortion. The friend also advised her to undergo a control ultrasound examination in one of the inexpensive ultrasound clinics in the city. The result was negative. Learning that "there was nothing there," she felt greatly relieved.[16]

Two other young women who used misoprostol had to end their pregnancies with a curettage (surgical abortion). One of the women started an abortion with misoprostol, then suffered pain and severe cramps. She panicked, and upon the advice of her sister she went to a public hospital. This was, she reported, the worse part of her abortion. The nurse who received her first put her in a room with two women with advanced pregnancies; she believes this was done deliberately to shame her. The doctor who talked with her disbelieved her story of undergoing a spontaneous miscarriage and treated her with contempt. He performed a curettage, then told her to come back "only if you are at the point of dying." In that case, the hospital staff's suspicion that she had taken a drug to end the pregnancy was justified, but their disparaging treatment of a patient who was scared and in severe pain was not. The second young woman told Ferrari that her first pregnancy had ended in a spontaneous miscarriage and that when she and her mother had gone to a public (SUS) hospital, nobody believed that she had not taken an abortive drug.[17] The second time she got pregnant, she took misoprostol to end the pregnancy. She suffered severe pain and hemorrhaging, but because of her previous traumatic experience she categorically refused to visit a public hospital. She ended by going to one of the clandestine abortion clinics in the favela, dubbed the "witch's house," where the woman who administered abortions provided her a curettage for a reduced price of 300 instead of 500 reais.[18] All three women who took misoprostol affirmed that the process was very painful, frightening, and messy, but all were reluctant to provide more details about their experience because they wanted to forget their trauma. As one of them put it, "Nobody deserves to go through such a thing."[19]

Four young women elected to have an abortion in the "witch's house."[20] While restricting the purchase of misoprostol to men was a way for men to control women, the "witch's house" was an exclusively female domain. Men were not allowed to enter it, and all the negotiations with the abortionist were conducted by the woman who wanted to end her pregnancy and her female friends. The "witch" herself was described as an elderly woman, solitary, and "strange," while the "witch's house" was presented as a scary place: a small house, dirty, and repulsive (*imonda*). "It looked like a dog house, it was horrible. . . . There was blood on the sheets, the place was very dark, it was like being inside a horror movie."[21] On the other hand, the surgical abortion itself was performed under general anesthesia, and the lay abortionist was described as being "serious" and "professional." Some women mentioned pain and bleeding for a few days after the abortion, others refused to speak about the physical effects. Nevertheless, none among the five women who aborted in the favela's clandestine clinics had serious postabortion complications, and none mentioned hearing about such complications from other young women. It is possible that the abortionist either was a trained health professional or had learned from competent professionals and her own experience how to perform surgical abortions under general anesthesia.[22]

Two women had abortions in a private clinic in a more affluent part of the city, and one in the private apartment of a health provider (probably a physician, but this is not specified). In the latter case, and also in the case of one of the women who aborted in a "better" clinic, the man who got the woman pregnant paid for the abortion. In both cases, the man was older and married. The women who aborted in professional surroundings described their experience as "good": they were treated correctly and received instructions on what to do in case of postabortion complications. The third woman who had an abortion in a clinic outside the favela found herself pregnant after a casual sexual encounter. She did not want to risk her life in the favela's "witch's house" because she had heard frightening stories about the clinic: "Nobody died there as for now, but it is a very scary place and I did not want to die or to go to prison." Encouraged by a friend, a nurse in a high-end gynecology clinic, she decided to have a safe abortion in that clinic. Because the price of an abortion in the high-end clinic was more than five times the price in the favela clinics, she borrowed money from drug dealers. They lent her the money at high interest, and to pay off her debt she worked for six months after school and on weekends in a bookstore. Despite the abortion's high cost and the stress of paying off her debt—at one point the drug dealers threatened her because she was not paying them back fast enough—she was persuaded that she had made the right choice. She was treated by competent and sympathetic professionals who told her what to expect and reassured her that the abortion itself was a "super-safe" operation.

The work in a bookstore had an unexpected benefit: it introduced this young woman to feminism. She mentioned especially a book called *How to Be a Woman*, by Katie something (in all probability Caitlin Moran's book).[23] "It's about everyday feminism. . . . This book helped me a lot, I adore this book, I want to give it to all my friends to read. And I understood what feminism is, because nobody speaks to us about feminism, at home or in school. . . . When I finished this book I cried, and I became sure that I am a feminist. I also read Simone something's book *The Second Sex*. It is very difficult, in two volumes, full of biology and science. I did not understand many things. But in the second volume, she speaks about the experience of being a woman— I loved this book! I read it in a week and it really changed my life. I mega-identified with it, you see? I lived it in my life too, the humiliation to be another sex, not to be a man. Why don't women get it? [*Nossa, como as mulheres nao percebem isso?*] I really loved these two volumes; when I have more money, I'll buy them."[24]

Two young women interviewed by Ferrari told him that they had been strongly opposed to abortion until they faced the decision whether to end a pregnancy themselves. None among the interviewed women was supported by her parents. Their mothers, described by the majority of the women as "mega-religious," Catholic or evangelist, were never consulted. Six received some help, mainly material, from the men who had gotten them pregnant, but their main source of moral and sometimes material support was their female friends, especially those who had had an abortion. Despite their peers' support, the experience of abortion was a solitary one, stressful and often scary. Their main fear was that they would die as a consequence of the abortion. The woman who elected to contract a heavy debt to have a safe abortion did it mainly out of fear. The young women also were afraid of late complications from interrupting a pregnancy and of being denounced to the police for an illegal act. Probably, the language used by the three women who took misoprostol to terminate their pregnancies—all three said "I believed that I am dying"—was linked to a deep-seated fear of dying as a result of an unsafe abortion, as was the reluctance of many of the interviewed women to provide details about the abortion itself. At the same time, women from this self-selected sample reported being greatly relieved once the abortion was over: they had survived, were physically unharmed, and had not gone to jail. Several young women said that their abortion had led them to think about why they had been forced to undergo such a stressful and frightening experience. They had learned to be more careful and to avoid risky situations by using contraception or insisting that their partners use a condom. Some women also expressed anger toward the men who had gotten them pregnant and then refused to take responsibility for it or, at most, limited their support to paying for an abortion or purchasing abortive drugs.

Humanizing Abortion: The Atenas Project

A pregnant woman who takes the abortifacient drug misoprostol and then goes to a public hospital with drug-induced bleeding, as a rule hides as well as she can the fact that she has taken the drug, pretending that she is undergoing a spontaneous miscarriage. Such women, as well as women truly undergoing a spontaneous miscarriage—a very common event in early pregnancy—are often treated in a cold and impersonal way and, not infrequently, with the disrespect that verges on mistreatment. The declared aim of the Atenas Project, developed in a public hospital in Salvador, Bahia, was to humanize abortion and promote a dignified and respectful treatment of women having an abortion in a public hospital. The health professionals who started this program hoped that its principles would be adopted elsewhere, although this ambition seems to have been thwarted by obstacles to the integration of this program into a big public maternity hospital. Beyond the specific problems encountered by the Atenas Project, the project's fate illustrates the structural difficulties of dealing with the thorny issue of abortion in Brazil. Such difficulties became more evident during the Zika crisis.

The concept of the humanization of abortion was not invented in Salvador. It first appeared in official texts of the Brazilian Health Ministry. The document "Humanized Care of Abortion" was first issued in 2005 and then revised in 2011. It frames the treatment of women in the "situation of abortion." It is a rather surprising text. While it reaffirms that "abortion is a crime," it can be read as a disguised plea for the legalization of abortion. The long theoretical preamble of this document explicitly states that in countries in which abortion is legal it is a very safe medical procedure: its rate of mortality is lower than 1in 100,000 interventions. By contrast, in Brazil illegal abortion is one of the principal causes of maternal mortality. Moreover, it is the origin of numerous health problems. The introduction also clearly states that the criminalization of abortion does not reduce the number of women who terminate their pregnancy; just the opposite is probably true. Finally, the document declares that its goal is to ascertain that all the Brazilian health professionals, independently of their religious and moral convictions, will provide competent and respectful treatment to women who abort and respect their dignity and rights.[25]

The generous principles proclaimed in the document are, however, rarely applied in real life. As numerous studies by anthropologists and sociologists attest, the publication of this document did not seem to modify practices and did not end the frequent mistreatment of women arriving at a public hospital with symptoms of a miscarriage.[26] In 2015, two physicians at the maternity hospital in Salvador, Bahia, created an initiative to implement the "humanization of abortion," with a double goal: first, to provide nonjudgmental medical and psychological help to women in a situation of abortion, and second—and this was the innovation of the project—to offer them an opportunity of a "watchful waiting," that is, an opportunity to go back home and wait for a natural termination of the abortion process. The background for this project was studies that documented mistreatment of women in situations of abortion in public hospitals in Bahia and frequent obstetrical violence in these situations. Such violence was rooted in moral condemnation of women who abort, labeled "bad mothers" and not considered deserving of respect or compassion on the part of hospital staff.[27]

The project, formalized in 2017 and located in the maternity Climéterio de Oliveira, in Salvador, was named Atenas after a well-known song of the singer and poet Chico Buarque, "Mulheres de Atenas" (Women of Athens), which expresses sympathy for the invisible and silenced wives of heroes of ancient Athens.[28] The program was aimed at women in a situation of abortion, less than 12 weeks pregnant, and without comorbidities. Its goals were defined as (a) reestablishment of the patient's autonomy by giving her the choice between a surgical termination of pregnancy, a medical one, and a physiological one; (b) reduction of the number of hospitalizations related to abortion; (c) promotion of women's sexual and reproductive rights and family planning; (d) reduction of psychological, physical, social, and moral violence directed toward women in a situation of abortion; and (e) sensitization of health professionals to this problem.

During its first, introductory phase (2015–17) the Atenas Project provided extra-hospital assistance to 564 women. These women received care from a multidisciplinary team that included health professionals, psychologists, and social workers. Women qualified for inclusion in the project after an ultrasound that determined how far along the pregnancy was and a medical examination that excluded comorbidities. They were then given a choice between a surgical abortion, a drug-induced abortion, and an expectative (physiological) approach. The surgical abortion was performed by curettage or, more frequently, a manual aspiration of the uterine content. The drug-induced abortion was performed through an intravaginal administration of misoprostol (the document states that this drug could be legally administered only in a hospital). The woman was then sent home to wait for the expulsion of the fetus. If this did not happen within a week of the initial administration of misoprostol, she could return to the hospital and receive an additional dose of this drug. An abortion employing misoprostol alone is usually slower and less efficient than abortion with a combination of mifepristone (RU-486) and misoprostol; this combination is employed to induce abortions in the majority of Western countries. The use of mifepristone is, however, illegal in Brazil. If a woman chose an expectative approach, she was told to wait for a "natural" end of the pregnancy, which could take a very long time.

Health professionals who participated in the Atenas Project were instructed not to ask women whether their abortion was spontaneous or induced. In practice, when they spoke with their patients, they often maintained the fiction that the pregnancy loss was spontaneous. Although the declared goal of the project was to be nonjudgmental, health professionals' implicit attitude obliged women who took misoprostol to end their pregnancy to show grief over their pregnancy loss. Those who failed to display signs of grief might be labeled "anti-*mãe*" (hostile to motherhood), a derogatory description in the context of the glorification of maternity in Brazilian culture.[29]

Women who elected the physiological solution and were sent home to wait for their pregnancy to end were told what to expect and given phone numbers of health professionals they could call if they had a problem or felt anxious. In addition, an Atenas Project worker (either a nurse or a social worker) regularly contacted them to ask how they were doing. After the expulsion of the fetus, women were offered a control ultrasound to confirm the end of the pregnancy. Although in principle women were free to choose a surgical, medical, or physiological solution, in practice the program strongly encouraged the latter approach, which was presented as especially safe and one that would not imperil the woman's reproductive future. A table presenting the three choices offered to women in a situation of abortion explained that the physiological solution was less painful (++) than a medical abortion with misoprostol (+++) or a surgical abortion by aspiration (+++); did not have a higher likelihood of infection than the two other solutions; and above all was free of the risk of uterine perforation, a risk that did exist for medical abortion (+) and surgical abortion (++).[30]

An ethnographic study of the Atenas Project indicated that 56% of the women initially included in this project elected the physiological solution and had an abortion during the waiting period; 20% received misoprostol, and 24% elected a surgical abortion. Women who chose the physiological approach appreciated the personalized attention they received, perhaps because they were not used to receiving such attention in their other interactions with SUS and because they initially feared being mistreated because of their situation of abortion. Health professionals also hailed the opportunity of a more personal interaction with patients.[31]

The professionals engaged in the Atenas Project listed safety as the main advantage of the physiological approach. Another advantage of this approach was the avoidance of hospitalization. Women who underwent a surgical termination of their pregnancy spent two or three days in the hospital. Many among the women who took part in the Atenas Project wished to avoid such a disruption in their lives and perceived a slow process of pregnancy loss as more "natural." The absence of hospitalization, some of the health professionals who participated in the project explained, also saved public money.[32] The disadvantages of the physiological approach were a long waiting period, which could last up to two months, pain and bleeding, the need to cope with expulsion and disposal of the "abortion product," that is, the fetus, which in pregnancy beyond ten weeks might have a "humanoid" form, and the need to abstain from sexual relations or to ask their partner to use a condom until the abortion process ended.[33]

The motto of the Atenas Project, "If one can humanize childbirth, why not an abortion," refers to the widely publicized program of humanization of childbirth in public maternity services in Brazil. Nearly all middle-class Brazilian women give birth in private clinics, where a C-section has become the norm. For them, childbirth is an elective surgery, with its rites, including in some clinics organized festivities.[34] The choice of a "natural" (i.e., vaginal) birth is available only in selected upper-end hospitals and clinics, and often middle-class women who make this choice have to pay more for it. By contrast, lower-class women who give birth in public hospitals are encouraged to have a vaginal birth but often are passive recipients of forms of overmedication, such as practically automatic episiotomies and the widespread use of oxytocin to accelerate birth. As the sociologists Simone Diniz and Alexandra Chacham put it, Brazilian women, according to their social class, are submitted either to a "cut above" or a "cut below."[35]

The important research project "Nascer no Brasil" (Birth in Brazil) displayed the multiple problems, physical and psychological, linked with birth in the public sector in Brazil.[36] The project coordinators strongly advocated a humanization of childbirth in SUS facilities: respectful treatment of the birthing woman, the right to be accompanied by a person of her choice, elimination of unnecessary interventions such as systematic episiotomies and the use of oxytocin or forceps to accelerate birth, the right to be mobile when in labor, and access to nonmedical interventions designed to reduce pain, such as massage and psychological support. The recommendations did not include, however, women's right to pharmacological alleviation of pain, above all epidural anesthesia.[37] The implicit subtext of the Nascer no Brasil project is that since childbirth is a natural process, healthy women do not need any medical intervention.[38] Leaders of this project agreed in principle that epidural anesthesia should not be put in the same category as excessive episiotomies or pressure on women to undergo an elective C-section, but at the same time they reaffirmed their strong support of medication-free birth.[39] In practice, epidural anesthesia is available to women who have a vaginal birth in high-end private clinics but is rarely available to women who give birth in SUS hospitals. A definition of "natural birth" that does not include pain relief for women who may feel they need it matches the Atenas Project's definition of "natural abortion."

Three strophes of Chico Buarque's poem "Mulheres de Atenas," reproduced on the title page of the document introducing the Atenas Project, describe women who produce for their husbands the new children of Athens; young widows and abandoned pregnant women; women who keep quiet, dress in black, conform, dry up, and shrink serving their husbands, the heroic men of Athens. Buarque's powerful poem focuses on women's suffering, self-effacement, and sacrifice. Professionals involved in the Atenas Project sincerely aspire to empower "silent women" and make them more autonomous.[40] On the other hand, they seem to view the criminalization of abortion in Brazil as an unchallengeable "fact of life," do not link the illegality of abortion to women's difficulties in achieving autonomy and respect, and fail to see that a humanization of illegal abortions might be a contradiction in terms. Their attitude contrasts with that of a Brazilian health professional in the 1990s who, during a debate on the use of misoprostol as an abortifacient, stressed that the main problem was not the off-label use of this drug but the criminalization of abortion.[41] The Atenas Project provides women who have started a self-induced abortion with support and care, but its organizers do not inform their patients that in countries where abortion is legal and free of charge women who wish to interrupt an unwanted pregnancy do not need to find themselves in a deeply distressing situation in the first place and that the termination of pregnancy itself is efficient, rapid, and safe.[42]

In several Latin American countries in which abortion is illegal or was illegal until recently, such as Argentina, Uruguay, and Chile, health professionals and feminist associations collaborated in providing practical help to women wishing to terminate a pregnancy. Support networks indicated reliable sources for purchase of misoprostol provided detailed information on how to use it, what to expect after taking it, and whom to call or where to go in case of complications.[43] As far as I know, there are no similar networks in Brazil and no groups that facilitate Brazilian women's access to services provided by organizations such as Women on the Web, which distribute by mail the more efficient abortive combination of misoprostol and mifepristone. Women on the Web receives approximately 1,800 requests for abortion pills from Brazil each year, a very small fraction of the estimated half million illegal abortions in Brazil annually.[44] Illegal termination of pregnancy continues to be a distressing and frightening event for many Brazilian women, especially the most vulnerable among them. Another strophe of Chico Buarque's poem, not quoted in the Atenas document, speaks about women who have no taste or desire, no defects, no qualities, no dreams, only omens, and who are scared.[45]

The Atenas Project was a response, however imperfect, to the difficulties of women in the situation of abortion arriving at a public hospital in northeastern Brazil, the region with the highest rate of induced abortions in the country.[46] A group of researchers led by Thália Velho Barreto de Araújo from the Federal University of Pernambuco in Recife published a text on the treatment of women in a situation of abortion (in 98% of cases before 12 weeks of gestation) in three state capitals, Recife (Pernambuco), Salvador (Bahia), and São Luiz (Maranhão) in northeastern Brazil. The study was published in 2018 but based on data collected between August and December 2010.[47] The researchers interviewed 3,064 women treated in public hospitals for consequences of pregnancy loss. One-third evoked shame and/or fear of being mistreated or humiliated by the health services. Less than half of the interrogated women were received in the first hospital where they sought help; a quarter went to two hospitals, and the remainder went to three or more, up to a maximum of eight hospitals. The delay between the start of worrying symptoms and admission for treatment increased with the number of hospitals visited, from a median of 15 hours if only one hospital was visited, to 48 hours if two were visited, to 72 hours if more than three were visited. The length of the delay correlated directly with the severity of postabortion complications. This study exposed the deep distress of women in northeastern Brazil who attempted to terminate a pregnancy five years before the Zika outbreak. Its coordinator, Thália Velho Barreto de Araújo, later played a key role in the study of Zika and congenital Zika syndrome in Pernambuco.

Abortion and Anencephaly

Following the May 2012 decision of the Brazilian parliament, a woman who learns that she is carrying an anencephalic fetus is allowed to terminate the pregnancy.[48] Not every woman is interested in doing this. For example, in a Porto Alegre maternity 12 out of 29 women who learned that their fetus was anencephalic elected to terminate the pregnancy, while 17 women elected to continue it.[49] One possible reason for the continuation of a pregnancy with a nonviable child might be that in Brazil diagnosis of anencephaly is frequently made late in pregnancy. Another might be that a woman told that her child would be born alive but would die soon after birth might decide to go ahead with the birth so that she could hold her child and say good-bye to him or her. Anencephaly is thus different from a fetal death in utero, when a woman who carries a dead fetus may feel that she is a "living tomb," and from situations such as, for example, a diagnosis of trisomy 18 (Edwards syndrome), when a woman learns that the child will be severely impaired but might live for an unspecific length of time, from days to years. In the latter case, the woman may justify a termination of pregnancy by a wish to prevent the suffering of her future child.[50]

After May 2012 a trajectory of a woman who elected to terminate her pregnancy following a diagnosis of anencephaly should have been very simple. Proof of a diagnosis of anencephaly is in principle sufficient to obtain an abortion in a public hospital. In practice, the trajectory of such a woman was often very taxing, physically and emotionally. An obstetrical nurse, Iulia Bicu Fernandes, interrogated 12 women who had been diagnosed with anencephaly in a public hospital; 7 women had decided to terminate the pregnancy and 5 to continue it.[51] The main impression Fernandes took from the interviews was, "damned if you do, and damned if you don't."

Women who decided to continue a pregnancy with an anencephalic fetus justified their choice by their religious faith; a wish to be a "real" mother and have a child who would be born alive, be given a name, and become a part of the family's history; a reluctance to be the person responsible for the death of her child; and fear of being criticized and ostracized. Their decision to continue the pregnancy was supported by their family and friends, but several women reported that they were negatively judged by health professionals who viewed their choice as "irrational." While some women received neutral information about their right to ask for an interruption of pregnancy, others felt pressured by their health providers to get rid of a "failed" pregnancy in order to rapidly start a "good" one. They also reported that some physicians told them that the continuation of pregnancy put their health at risk. Three among these women carried the pregnancy to term, and the child died shortly after birth. One woman had a stillbirth, and one fetus died in the womb.[52]

Women who elected to have an abortion got the impression that some health providers disapproved of their choice. In addition, some were harshly criticized by their families or other people. One woman reported that members of an evangelical church in her neighborhood called her a murderer for wanting to kill a child made by God. "They left antiabortion videos near my door. . . . When I was walking in the street they called after me, 'you want to kill your child! You have no shame!'" This made her very nervous; her blood sugar spiked, and she had to be hospitalized twice.[53]

The announcement of the fetal anomaly was often abrupt and sometimes brutal, with declarations like "the baby does not have a brain." None of the 12 interviewed women had heard about anencephaly before they learned that they were carrying a fetus with this condition. One woman said, "I have heard about babies with a too big head, but with a head like this—I did not know it existed." They were not offered more detailed information or counseling, and several women felt alone in deciding about the future of their pregnancy.[54] Some women also reported being told that the fetal anomaly was their fault because they had failed to take folic acid early in pregnancy.[55] Those who chose to end the pregnancy had to overcome additional obstacles. Theoretically, a woman who learned that the fetus was anencephalic should obtain permission to terminate the pregnancy without additional administrative steps. In practice, the women had to undergo additional interviews to confirm their wish to have an abortion, and then they had to find an institution willing to perform this intervention. One woman who opted to terminate her pregnancy was obliged to obtain the permission of a judge. This reinforced her guilt: "When I went to obtain the permission in the court, I felt very bad, because I found myself in a place where criminals go, like a thug, and a thug is a thug, so for me, it was really a very difficult situation; but now I've gotten over it."[56]

The abortion itself was described as a highly distressing event. It was distressing psychologically because women who aborted usually were not allowed to be accompanied during the procedure by a partner or a family member and because at the hospital the women there to terminate a pregnancy, as well as those giving birth to a nonviable child, were not separated from women giving birth to live babies. It was also a protracted and painful process.[57] The majority of the women interviewed by Fernandes praised the hospital staff who supervised their abortion. They were especially pleased that health professionals talked to them kindly and tried to help them. It is possible that these women expected ostracism or at best indifference and were surprised to be treated like "regular" patients. A few women were less satisfied with the staff's attitude and complained about the occasional rudeness of some professionals. However, none protested about the length of the induced abortion itself, usually taking several days and for some up to a week; about the fact that the process was very painful; or about the absence of anesthesia.[58]

Brazilian women who had a legal second- or third-trimester abortion in a public hospital did not know that in Western countries women having late abortions automatically are given epidural anesthesia unless they explicitly refuse it. The rationale is that while during a normal birth some women strongly wish to have a medication-free birth and others are encouraged by midwives to try to have such a birth, in an induced late abortion there is no reason for a woman to suffer physical pain (which may be more severe than the pain of normal childbirth) in addition to her emotional trauma. Brazilian women who underwent abortion for anencephaly also did not know that in Western Europe an induced late abortion performed in a hospital rarely takes more than 12 hours.[59]

The rapidity of induced abortion in countries like France relies on the systematic use of a combination of mifepristone with misoprostol (mifepristone is banned in Brazil, including for hospital use), detailed protocols for the abortion process, and probably above all the experienced medical staff—doctors and midwives—familiar with all the stages of induced termination of pregnancy.[60] Booklets distributed to women scheduled to undergo a late termination of pregnancy in France explain that the women will be hospitalized the evening before the intervention. In the early morning a physician will administer epidural anesthesia; then, if the fetus is more than 20 weeks old the physician will perform feticide (killing of the fetus), a routine step in induced abortion in the late second or third trimester.[61] The woman is invited to be accompanied during the whole procedure by her partner or another supporting person. She is closely attended by a midwife, who supervises the expulsion of the dead fetus. The midwife later helps the woman and the person who accompanies her to perform the mourning rites she desires, which may include taking photographs of the dead child (once expulsed it is regarded as a child, not a fetus) and collecting souvenirs such as the child's clothes and blanket.[62]

In Brazil, an induced abortion in a public hospital is frequently very different. Testimonies collected by Fernandes and analysis of files of numerous patients who underwent a legal late abortion in a public hospital exhibited complex and painful trajectories. The hospital had a protocol for an induced termination of pregnancy, but it was much less detailed than the French and Swiss ones. Interviewed gynecologists explained that the lack of detailed instructions was intentional: since each woman is different, it is better to leave the details of the induction of her abortion open. French gynecologists have a different opinion: they believe that it is important to have a detailed protocol based on their collective experience. They also believe that epidural anesthesia is an essential part of such a protocol. An additional problem is the absence of systematic transmission of abortion-related practical knowledge in Brazil. Legal abortions are relatively rare medical acts and are frequently performed by young temporary, part-time physicians (*platonistas*). Some physicians can learn on the spot how to induce abortions, but often their knowledge is not transmitted to others when they move on to their next job. This may reflect problems with staffing in public hospitals, but also the low status of this medical act, another aspect of the stigmatization of abortion. The criminalization of abortion in Brazil was usually framed as a question of women's rights and as a public health problem: the reduction of mortality and morbidity from unsafe abortions.[63] It was rarely framed as a medical problem, how to best employ technology and practical know-how to make the termination of pregnancy itself rapid and free of suffering.

Judges and Abortions for Fetal Indication in Brazil

According to Brazilian Health Ministry data, there were 11,318 legal abortions in Brazil between 2010 and 2016, 94% of which were justified by rape.[64] Anencephaly is the sole exception to the criminalization of abortion for fetal anomalies. In all other cases a woman who learns that the fetus she is carrying is severely impaired can request, with the support of her doctors, juridical permission to interrupt her pregnancy.[65] In the Brazilian context, *severely impaired* nearly always means incompatible with life. The accepted definition of a severe fetal impairment excludes anomalies induced by an infectious agent because such anomalies are highly variable and often are not lethal. This rule, established well before the Zika outbreak, was not modified by that outbreak.

Women who decide to apply for a juridical interruption of pregnancy face a protracted, potentially nerve-wracking juridical trajectory with an uncertain outcome. A nationwide meta-analysis published in 2020 found that between 2008 and 2018, 2,442 (40%) of the 5,075 Brazilian women who asked for juridical permission to interrupt a pregnancy for a fetal anomaly or a maternal indication failed to obtain such permission.[66] A woman's uncertainty about the fate of her future child is amplified by the very real possibility that she will make the difficult decision to interrupt her pregnancy, face a long period of waiting—with the fetus moving in her body, since the majority of diagnoses of severe fetal anomaly are made in the second trimester of pregnancy—and then learn that she has to carry her pregnancy to term or, not infrequently, until the fetus's death in the womb.

To strengthen the demand for an interruption of pregnancy for fetal anomaly, the geneticists or gynecologists who support the demand often add that continuing the pregnancy will put the pregnant woman's health at risk. This claim is not made merely to persuade the judge to agree to an abortion. In many cases, a gestation with an impaired fetus is linked with serious health risks for pregnant women. Many among the women who failed to obtain permission to terminate their pregnancies suffered from pregnancy-related complications. A study that compared the outcomes of 56 women diagnosed with a severe fetal anomaly with the outcomes of 38 women with similar anomalies who legally terminated the pregnancy found that women who elected to give birth to a nonviable child had much higher rates of complications during the pregnancy and the postpartum period. This was especially the case with women who carried fetuses affected by polyhydramnios (accumulation of amniotic fluid, often because of severe kidney malformation of the fetus), anomalies of the neural tube, and hydrocephalus.[67]

The case of conjoined twins is an especially dramatic illustration of the harms of continuing a pregnancy with a nonviable fetus. In the great majority of cases, conjoined twins cannot survive outside the womb. Only in a small number of cases are the twins born alive, and even more rarely do they survive after a surgical attempt to separate them.[68] An ultrasound diagnosis of conjoined twins can be made relatively early in pregnancy. It is also possible to assess at that stage the twins' chances of survival. Obstetricians at the São Paolo University Medical School suggested to all pregnant women diagnosed with conjoined twins who had very poor chances of survival outside the womb that they request juridical permission to terminate the pregnancy. Seventeen women, all less than 25 weeks pregnant, made such a demand; 12 obtained permission, while 5, with an identical indication, did not.[69] A follow-up article published by the same group presented the fact that 12 women were able to legally terminate a pregnancy as an important success for the medical team, not an illustration of the arbitrary nature of the juridical process, during which the outcome might depend on a given judge's whim.[70]

In 2020, obstacles to a juridical abortion in Brazil were highlighted by the especially dramatic case of a 10-year-old Black girl from São Mateus, a small town in the state of Espírito Santo, impregnated by her uncle, who had raped her repeatedly.[71] In early August 2020 the girl, found to be 22 weeks pregnant, was sent with her principal caregiver, her grandmother, to the main public hospital in Victoria, the capital of Espírito Santo, for an abortion. She had obtained a judge's permission to terminate the pregnancy, which was probably necessary because of her age.[72] The hospital's physicians refused to end her pregnancy, however, claiming (inaccurately) that it would be illegal since she was 22 weeks pregnant. In the meantime, the girl's name was revealed on social networks by an antiabortion activist closely linked with Brazil's conservative women and family rights minister, Damares Alves. Alves justified the decision of the physicians in Victoria, arguing (again inaccurately) that an abortion at such a young age would endanger the girl's life.[73] Conservative groups in São Mateus pressured the girl's family to prevent the abortion. Finally, the girl, her grandmother, and a social worker took a flight to Recife, the capital of the state of Pernambuco. They were met at the airport by the activist Paula Viana, a cofounder of the feminist group Curumim.[74] Fearing a violent intervention of antiabortion activists, who upon learning where the abortion was scheduled to take place organized a demonstration at the hospital's main entrance, the girl was hidden in the trunk of a taxi and smuggled into the hospital through a back door. The abortion itself was uneventful, and the girl was thankful for the care she received.[75]

Juridical Abortions in Rio de Janeiro: Trajectories and Justifications

An analysis of the files of 184 women who between 2011 and 2018 submitted petitions to a Rio de Janeiro regional court asking for permission to interrupt a pregnancy because of a severe fetal anomaly provides a glimpse of the process of pleading for such permission. All the files were from the archives of major maternity hospitals specializing in the follow-up of women with detected fetal anomalies or complications of pregnancy. The files have a standard makeup: a proof of the existence of an anomaly, nearly always ultrasound images displaying a structural impairment, a detailed description of the anomaly and its consequences, a statement that such an anomaly is incompatible with life, often an affirmation that the continuation of the pregnancy will put the pregnant woman's health at risk, and finally, a declaration that the institution's physicians support the woman's petition.

The average wait for the judge's verdict was around eight weeks. In exceptional cases permission was granted after a month; in other cases, the response arrived after three weeks, in one case after four months. Of the 184 women who submitted a petition to the court, 28 did not have an abortion. In two cases of women who continued their pregnancy, the files include an explicit mention of the rejection of the woman's petition by the judge. Both had children who died immediately after birth. The files of six women indicate that they changed their mind after submitting the petition, although it is unclear whether this happened before or after the judge's answer. Four among them gave birth to a child who died immediately after birth, one had a late miscarriage, and one gave birth to a live child with holoprosencephaly, a severe brain anomaly. Among the remaining 20 women, two gave birth to live children, one with holoprosencephaly and another with Patau syndrome (trisomy 13), a chromosomal anomaly that nearly always leads to the child's death during the first year of life. The remaining 18 women either miscarried late in pregnancy, gave birth to a stillborn child, or had a child who died immediately after birth. The hospital files were sometimes incomplete. It is probable that the petitions of some among these 20 women were rejected too, but the judge's opinion was not included in their files. In other cases, the woman might have miscarried or given birth while waiting for the judge's verdict. One such case is recorded: the judge's permission for an abortion was granted after the birth and immediate death of the woman's child. Since the waiting time for the judge's verdict was sometimes very long, it is possible that this happened in other cases as well.

In some cases, especially of severe structural malformations and conjoined twins, the diagnosis of the fetal anomaly was made in a private ultrasound facility. Prenatal care in Brazilian public health clinics and hospitals does not include routine ultrasound examinations. Official directives explain that ultrasound examinations are unnecessary because they do not improve pregnancy outcomes, defined as the reduction of perinatal or maternal mortality.[76] Despite the absence of an official endorsement, Brazil has exceptionally high rates of ultrasound examinations during pregnancy.[77] Private ultrasound facilities are not regulated, and the skills of their operators vary greatly. Some public hospitals also offer ultrasound examinations to pregnant women. Their quality is also variable. Some hospitals provide individualized attention, while in others the ultrasound examination takes place in crowded, impersonal facilities, and women who learn about serious problems of the fetus do not receive psychological support.[78]

Affluent women who are treated in expensive private maternity clinics have access to well-trained ultrasound experts and advanced equipment. These women want to learn whether the pregnancy is progressing well and above all whether the baby is "all right," and they are willing to pay a considerable amount of money for an expert's opinion.[79] Those who undergo an ultrasound examination in inexpensive street-corner facilities want to confirm the pregnancy and are especially interested to learn the fetus's sex and receiving the baby's "first photograph." When the sex is known, the future child receives a name and officially becomes a new member of the family.[80] Ultrasound examinations are thus often seen as a joyful family event.[81] When the ultrasound operator in a private facility detects a fetal anomaly, he or she may advise the woman to go to a public hospital.[82] Pregnant women are rarely prepared to receive bad news during a test they see above all as the first encounter with their future child. Some women minimize the gravity of fetal malformation by selectively assimilating only a part of the ultrasound operator's message. Other women, sent to a hospital for further tests, believe that they are going to see a specialist who will fix the detected problem. The latter belief may be related to religious feelings: the women hope that a combination of medical expertise and prayers will cure their future children.[83]

When the severity of the fetal malformation was confirmed by the hospital's specialists, usually by a detailed diagnostic ultrasound, the pregnant woman was directed to a genetic counseling session in which she, often together with her partner, received information on the nature of the fetal malformation as well as the possibility of applying for permission to interrupt the pregnancy. If the woman was interested in this possibility, physicians responsible for the genetic counseling produced a document for the court, which nearly always included ultrasound images of the fetus. These images were frequently selected to make the fetal anomaly easily visible and dramatic. Physicians know from experience that a judge is often more inclined to grant permission to terminate a pregnancy with a truly "monstrous" fetus.

The judge's verdict was often very brief, a mere statement that the court granted permission to interrupt the pregnancy. In some cases, the judge provided a much longer document that explained his or her decision, nearly always with the argument that the fetus had a lethal anomaly. The judge often added that since the fetus was not viable, this would not be a "eugenic" abortion. The decision about the fetus's programmed death was not made by the pregnant woman could not be understood as a refusal to give birth to an imperfect human being. The only motivating rejection of the woman's petition in this series employed a symmetrical argument: despite the presence of multiple malformations, the (male) judge was not persuaded that the fetus was not viable.

While some judges merely stated that they agreed to an interruption of pregnancy because the fetus was not viable and thus the case was similar to one of anencephaly, others judges further developed this argument. One (male) judge explained that obliging a woman to carry a pregnancy to term when she knows that the fetus will not survive is contrary to the dignity of human beings. Another (male) judge explained that continuing a pregnancy with a nonviable and severely deformed fetus produced intolerable maternal suffering. One (male) judge referred to the risk to the mental health of a woman who knew that the fetus she was carrying was "practically a stillborn." Another (male) judge maintained that asking a woman to wait until the end of pregnancy when it was certain that the fetus would die was contrary to natural law. One (female) judge extended the latter argument and explained that every pregnant woman hopes that after nine months she will become a mother. The only persons able to evaluate the frustration and the suffering of a pregnancy with a nonviable fetus (in that case, conjoined twins) are the parents of the future child. It must be insupportable to have a certainty of death instead of certainty of life. Another (female) judge explained that when the fetus cannot survive outside the womb, one cannot speak of a crime of abortion, and there is no reason to continue a pregnancy that puts a pregnant woman's health at a risk.

Only one verdict in this series was different. A (male) judge stated that the severity of the disruption to the central nervous system of the fetus might be incompatible with a fully dignified human life. This was the only verdict that pointed to the possibility of allowing a legal termination of pregnancy even if it was not certain that the child would die during the pregnancy or shortly after birth. This verdict was an exception. The view that every decision to terminate a pregnancy with a potentially viable child is "eugenic" and therefore totally inadmissible shaped all the debates on termination of pregnancy for fetal indication in Brazil, including those during the Zika epidemic. In public debates about abortion in Brazil, as in the judges' verdicts, the term *eugenic* was never problematized or historicized.[84] *Eugenic* was another way of saying "evil," and a woman could be granted the right to terminate her pregnancy for humanitarian reasons only if it was certain that the intent was not "eugenic."

Stories of Juridical Abortions: A Tangle of Rights, Faith, and Care

The study of files of women who submitted a petition to the court to obtain permission to terminate their pregnancy was followed by detailed interviews with 12 of those women. The great variability among the women's trajectories is striking, as are their diverse motivations, pregnancy outcomes, and reactions to these outcomes.[85] Their paths leading to a petition to the court were similar, but not the events that followed the petition or the ways the women experienced them. Unlike the women who carried anencephalic fetuses, who were certain to quickly obtain permission for an abortion, these women were confronted with a long waiting period during which the fetus continued to grow and move in their body. For some, this was a very difficult time. As one of the interviewed women, AC, explained, she waited for the judge's decision for a month, but it was like waiting two years: every single moment was torture. LS, who waited two months for the judge's decision and finally gave birth spontaneously to a stillborn child, said that the waiting period was the worst time in her life because she could feel the child growing in her belly, knowing that the child was condemned to die.

Other women felt differently. During the waiting period they continued to undergo routine testing for blood pressure and blood sugar, as well as ultrasound examinations, and some also participated in courses on breastfeeding. When I first found the comment "the patient successfully terminated a course on breastfeeding" in files of women who had asked for permission to end their pregnancy, I saw it as especially insensitive. Later I realized that for some women participation in a breastfeeding course might have helped them to perceive themselves as fulfilling their maternal obligations and becoming a "real" mother, although the mother of a child who died. Iulia Fernandes noted too that not infrequently women diagnosed with an anencephalic fetus who decided to continue the pregnancy decided to participate in all the activities offered to pregnant women, including activities that taught them how to care for their baby. Such participation allowed them to affirm their status as "real" mothers.[86]

For some women who received a diagnosis of a severe fetal anomaly, especially those who felt ambivalent about their decision to ask permission to terminate the pregnancy or hoped that the diagnosis of a fetal anomaly was not definitive, participation in pregnancy-related activities allowed them to remain in a state of suspension. Continuing routine checkups while not knowing what the outcome of their petition to the court would be might also have lessened their guilt about deciding to have an abortion. A liminal status might also be a blessing. This might have been the case for AL. After she learned in the sixth month of pregnancy that her fetus, diagnosed with extended gastroschisis (malformation of the gut), was not viable, she waited nearly two months before requesting permission from the court to end the pregnancy, because she hoped that the diagnosis would change. When she received court permission at the end of the eighth month of pregnancy, she perceived the death of her child as a stillbirth and not an abortion and thus felt less guilt about deciding to end the pregnancy.

Western feminists who discuss abortion speak about women's right to control their fertility and, if pregnant, to decide whether they wish to be mothers. But such a perception is very different from that deeply religious people who reject the individual-centered notion of human rights and elect instead to speak about their responsibility and their obligations to God, their family, and their community.[87] Listening to testimonies of deeply religious Brazilian women, whether evangelical, spiritist, or Catholic, I realized that thinking in terms of rights was alien to their way of thinking about abortion. Their discourse was centered on relationships—with their future children, their partners, their relatives, their friends, and, when relevant, their religious communities. Such relationships were built through dense networks of exchanges, mutual obligations, and positive and negative feelings, were changeable and situated, and were disconnected from the abstract notion of universal human rights.

Some women who initially saw the court's rejection of their petition for an abortion as harsh and callous later saw it in a positive light because it removed responsibility for the death of their child from them and put it firmly in the hands of God or Nature. CC, who defined herself as nonreligious, learned in the fifth month of her pregnancy that the fetus she was carrying was not viable because of a severe case of Cantrell pentalogy. Her doctors were persuaded that she would be allowed to end her pregnancy, as was the woman from the Public Defender's Office who presented her case to the judge. However, the judge rejected her petition. CC was initially very distressed, as was the presenter, who cried when she told CC about the judge's decision. In retrospect CC decided that it was for the best, because she would not have to face the decision whether to kill her child. The child was born at 34 weeks of pregnancy and died immediately after birth.

CW, a spiritist—thus belonging to a religious group that in Brazil is strongly opposed to abortion—learned in the fifth month of pregnancy that her fetus suffered from holoprosencephaly, a severe brain malformation. CW also had severe diabetes (diabetes may be a cause of fetal malformations). Believing that continuing her pregnancy would put her health in danger, her doctors encouraged her to ask for permission to end the pregnancy. However, despite the double legitimation—a nonviable fetus and a severe health problem—the judge, who was a very conservative Catholic, rejected her petition. In retrospect, CW was grateful for the judge's decision, which she believed saved her from committing the sin of abortion.[88] She believed that it had been God's will that she give birth naturally at seven months of pregnancy; the child was stillborn. MC learned when in the twelfth week of pregnancy that the child she was carrying had a brain anomaly. Her doctors suspected trisomy 13, a diagnosis confirmed a month later by amniocentesis. Even though this is nearly always a lethal condition, the judge rejected her demand for termination. The

Public Defender's Office appealed the decision, but the child was born at 36 weeks, before the court's decision, and died immediately after birth. MC and her husband were very affected by the court's refusal, but eventually MC, who was Catholic, thought that it was better that the child had been born and died naturally.

A recurrent theme in these narratives is the deep religiosity of some of the women and what they saw as God's intervention in their lives. AC, a Catholic, learned when she was five months pregnant with her third child that the fetus had a polycystic kidney, a malformation incompatible with life. Learning that the fetus was not viable was comforting in a way because she felt strongly that the decision about the fate of the pregnancy was no longer hers. The certainty of the future child's death made it easier to ask permission for an abortion. DZ, an evangelical, learned in the third month of her pregnancy that her fetus was anencephalic. When her doctors tried to persuade her to end the pregnancy, she hesitated but then finally requested permission for an abortion (this was before the law changed). The judge's permission arrived when she was in the fifth month of pregnancy, at which point she was reluctant to eliminate a fetus with a beating heart. She then prayed to God asking him to take the life of her child before the doctors did it. God answered her prayer: when she entered the hospital for the scheduled interruption she learned that the baby's heart had already stopped.

GV, also an evangelical, had a very different attitude. When she learned in the fourth month of pregnancy that her fetus was anencephalic, she felt relieved, because the decision what to do was taken from her hands. She saw the diagnosis itself, or rather her physicians' making the diagnosis, as a manifestation of God's will. God had made it possible for her to make the right decision without feeling guilty about it. She had no hesitation whatsoever about interrupting the pregnancy, and not only her family but also her pastor supported her decision. After the abortion, she wanted to see the child so that she could be certain that the diagnosis of anencephaly, was as well as her decision to have an abortion, had been correct. LS, who described herself as believing in God but not a regular churchgoer, had a similar attitude. When she learned in the fourth month of pregnancy that the fetus had an anomaly incompatible with life, she saw terminating the pregnancy as her only choice. Her religious family supported her decision. Alas, the juridical process was very long. She gave birth in the seventh month of pregnancy to a stillborn child, while still waiting for the judge's verdict. SF, a spiritist, learned in the second trimester of pregnancy that her fetus had a structural malformation incom-

patible with life (body stalk). She was very sad and cried a lot but soon decided to have an abortion, although her spiritist friends tried to dissuade her.
The juridical process was long, and she received permission for termination
when she was seven months pregnant. Despite her resolution to end the pregnancy, she felt guilty for a long time after the abortion.

AA, who described herself as evangelical and very religious, was the only
one among the interviewed women who gave birth to a live child. The fetus,
her second child, was diagnosed with hydrocephalus when she was four months
pregnant. She claimed that her doctors had told her that this anomaly was
incompatible with life. AA was initially reluctant to request permission to
end the pregnancy but finally agreed to do it. The child was born alive at the
end of the sixth month of pregnancy, while AA was still waiting for the judge's
verdict. AA saw it as a sign that God wanted a different fate for her baby boy.
Her son was hospitalized for three months. Initially, the doctors were not
very optimistic about his chances of survival, but the baby surprised them
when he started to breathe on his own. Nevertheless, he remained severely
handicapped: he feeds through a gastric tube, has very limited mobility, and
cannot be left alone. AA stopped working and now devotes all her time to the
care of her son.

All the interviewed women had male partners at the time they petitioned
the court, but only a few mentioned their partners in their interview. AL told
that she had not received any support from her husband, had already had
eight children with previous partners and was not very enthusiastic about her
pregnancy. CC's partner left her immediately after the stillbirth of their child.
MC and SK were supported by their husbands during the pregnancy and after
the loss of their child; MC added that her husband had been very affected by
the events. However, none of the interrogated women mentioned the participation of their husband or partner in the decision to request permission to
end the pregnancy. While several women spoke about positive or negative
reactions of relatives, friends, or their religious congregation and a few hoped
to receive God's direct guidance, none seemed to rely explicitly on the opinion of the father of their future child.

The abortion or childbirth itself was in many cases a long, difficult, and
solitary process. AC said that her abortion had been extremely painful: "I
probably scared the other women in the hospital, because I screamed so
much." AM testified that the staff at the hospital where she had an induced
abortion—of a fetus who died in the womb while she was waiting for the
judge's reply to her petition—were sympathetic and caring, but the expulsion

of the fetus was very harrowing. She refused to provide more details because it was something she wanted to forget. DZ's induced expulsion of a dead fetus was also slow and very painful, but she endured the pain patiently, knowing that her child had died by God's will, not because she had decided to end the pregnancy. LS, who gave birth naturally in the seventh month of pregnancy, testified that the premature birth that ended with stillbirth had been more painful than her previous two normal births, perhaps because of her knowledge that the child would not live. She also found it difficult to be alone: her husband was not allowed to stay with her. SF's abortion, induced when she was seven months pregnant, was very painful too. She remembered screaming for hours, because of the pain but also because of her sorrow, knowing that she was giving birth to a child destined to die.

AA, who gave birth to a child with hydrocephalus while waiting for the judge's verdict, had a C-section under general anesthesia because of the size of the child's head. Another woman, MC, also had a C-section for a medical reason (her first child had been born by C-section). She thus does not have painful memories from the birth of her stillborn child. Moreover, and this was especially important for her, her husband was permitted to assist at the birth and the death of their child. Only one among the 12 interviewed women, GV, who had an induced abortion in the fifth month of pregnancy, testified that the termination of her pregnancy had been relatively quick and smooth. In retrospective, the termination of pregnancy was seen as a tragedy by some women and as a difficult but finally positive experience by others. AC was depressed after her induced abortion and needed psychiatric help. AM was also depressed after the pregnancy loss and was hospitalized for severe depression. AC worked as a teacher before the pregnancy loss, but after her difficult experiences—a long period of waiting for permission to terminate the pregnancy, a harrowing abortion, and a postabortion clinical depression—she felt that she could no longer work with children and left teaching. CW's experience was just the opposite. She had previously worked as a salesperson in a shop, but the loss of her pregnancy, coupled with her decision not to have offspring of her own because another pregnancy could put her health in danger, led her to want to work with children. She went back to school, trained to be a teacher, and is very happy in her new profession.

SF, a teacher, decided to abort a nonviable fetus. She related that her pupils had known about her pregnancy and her lost child and had been wonderful about it, not asking questions but expressing sympathy and affection. When she later gave birth to a healthy child, her pupils openly showed their joy and bought many presents for her baby. For DZ, her loss of an anencephalic child, and especially the certainty that God had answered her prayer and by allowing her child to die naturally had sent her a direct sign of his grace, had fostered her spiritual growth. Thanks to this experience she was able to persuade other women not to have an abortion and to trust God. She was also able to comfort women who miscarried or lost a child. AA, the only woman in this group whose pregnancy ended with the birth of a living child, sees this birth and her son's survival as a miracle; she believes that thanks to her unwavering faith she received special help from God.

The decision to terminate a pregnancy for a fetal indication is always an extremely stressful one. Moreover, debates on this subject become entangled with the fraught issue of disability rights because some disability activists argue that a woman who elects such as abortion sends a strong message that impaired individuals do not have a right to live. When I became involved in a study of "juridical abortions" in Brazil, I assumed that in a conservative society characterized by strong religiosity, glorification of maternity, and a very negative perception of abortion the decision to terminate a pregnancy for a fetal anomaly would be especially difficult. I was not surprised to discover that Brazilian women who had chosen to have an abortion for a fetal indication faced numerous external obstacles, including pressure from family and friends, and had to cope with their doubts and remorse. Other elements were less predictable. I did not expect to find that because of the slowness of the juridical process, a high proportion of women who asked for juridical abortion ended by giving birth to a stillborn child or one who died immediately after birth. I was dismayed at the length and physical harshness of the abortion or stillbirth itself: women spent hours and often days in severe pain, usually alone. Finally, I was surprised by the importance for many women of their religious faith, perceived as a direct, nonmediated relationship with God.

Probably the main conclusion I drew from these interviews—to the extent that it is possible to draw a general conclusion from a study of a small, partly self-selected sample—was that the concept of a woman's "right to choose" is not very useful in a discussion of abortion for a fetal indication in Brazil.[89] Women who spoke about their decision to request permission to end a pregnancy frequently said that their options had been preordained by fate and/or God's will. Their stories, when negative, were about being overwhelmed by events they could not control, and when positive, they were about their ability to find meaning in dramatic events. Neither the "right to choose" nor repressive laws seem to have played a role.

Fetuses and Reproductive Injustice

This chapter focuses on trajectories of women who rely on the services of the Brazilian National Health Service (SUS), that is, approximately 75% of Brazilian women. Reproductive trajectories of middle-class women who use private health services are less visible, especially when they include illegal practices. The rule that "one counts only those who count" does not seem to apply to reproductive health in Brazil. Public hospitals provide data on women who were treated for complications of pregnancy loss, had an abortion for anencephaly, or terminated a pregnancy after receiving a judge's permission. For obvious reasons, there are no data on illegal interruption of pregnancy in private clinics, including second-trimester abortions for a fetal indication. In the latter case, a gynecologist might declare that the fetus died in the womb; or, occasionally, the gynecologist might propose that the pregnant woman undergo an invasive diagnostic procedure known to have a high risk of complications leading to the death of the fetus and then "allow" such complications to occur.[90]

Two distinct patterns of access to health care coexist in Brazil, the anthropologist Emilia Sanabria explains: health care as a right and health care as a choice. Users of public services have, in principle at least, the "right of health" granted by the Brazilian constitution.[91] SUS users are often seen by professionals as people who should "earn" this right by behaving responsibly, above all by submitting to medical authority. They evoke terms like *citizenship* and *rights* to get SUS patients to fulfill their obligations as good citizens. By contrast, users of private health insurance (*planos de saúde*) are seen as autonomous agents capable of self-discipline and entitled to individualized attention, tailored to their specific needs. They are not viewed as a homogenous mass of "citizens" but as unique human beings.[92]

Practically all the Brazilian political movements, including conservative ones, claim to support the SUS. At the same time, middle-class people, whatever their political orientation, take for granted the fact that they and their families have access to high-quality, individualized medical services. They may also be aware of the immense obstacles to providing access to such level of medical services to all Brazil's citizens. The debate on abortion in Brazil has to include the country's extremes of social stratification, including in health care. Such stratification is especially visible in the fraught area of reproductive health. Lower-class women who seek to control their fertility either conform to the state's law that proclaims that abortion is a crime or, as many poor women do, internalize as normal the harsh consequences of breaking this law. When a pregnant woman who relies exclusively on SUS services and is not opposed to abortion learns about a severe anomaly of the fetus, she knows, especially if the anomaly is not lethal, that she has either to accept the situation or, since the majority of fetal anomalies are discovered in the second or even the third trimester of pregnancy, to decide to have a risky late abortion. Few women choose the latter option.[93] The criminalization of abortion penalizes middle-class Brazilian women too. They have to travel abroad for a termination of pregnancy or use the services of upper-end but illegal clinics, a situation not entirely devoid of anxiety. Nevertheless, middle-class women are seldom confronted with the level of distress, fear, and pain faced by poor women who undergo illegal abortions. The possibility of escaping such distress and pain may be another expression of middle-class women's privilege to be recognized as unique individuals, not faceless, homogenous "citizens."

The young woman from a Rio favela who discovered feminism while working in a bookstore to pay for her abortion "adored" Caitlin Moran's book *How to Be a Woman*.[94] One reason for her enthusiasm might have been Moran's description of her termination of pregnancy: fully covered by the British National Health Service, uncomplicated, safe, and entirely guilt-free. Moran explains that the majority of the books about abortion, including those sympathetic to the feminist cause, claim that whilst a woman may try to persuade herself that she made an entirely rational decision, there will always be a part of her that rejects such rationalization, because women's bodies do not give up their babies so easily. Thus Moran waited for an unavoidable postabortion wave of misery and grief that never materialized. The only remarkable thing about her abortion was how unremarkable it was.[95]

Moran's matter-of-fact attitude toward abortion—she was very happy with her two children but certain that she did not want a third one—may be contrasted with the Brazilian view, shared by some prochoice activists, that the termination of a pregnancy is always a dramatic and traumatic event. The rallying cry of feminists who in August 2020 defended the right of a 10-year-old girl impregnated by a rapist to end her pregnancy as that women should have access to legal and safe abortions to stay alive (*para no morer*).[96] Moran's view of abortion might be especially attractive to a poor, non-white teenager who made the unusual decision to borrow money from drug dealers to have a safe abortion in an upper-end clinic. In making that choice, she boldly crossed the border between the favela and the *asfaltado* (neighborhoods with paved streets inhabited by middle-class people) and the gulf that separated women like her from middle-class women who, thanks to their money and social status, could escape the most distressing consequences of oppressive antiabortion laws. The omnipresent but rarely acknowledged chasm between reproductive choices and opportunities of middle-class and poor women was, this study proposes, one of the key elements that shaped the Zika epidemic in Brazil.

CHAPTER THREE

Surprises

"I've never seen anything like this"

"A Virus That Baffled the Experts"

All the narratives about the early days of the epidemic of microcephaly and the realization that it was probably linked to the outbreak of Zika several months earlier converge at one point: this was a total surprise. What made it surprising was not the arrival of a new virus, a frequent event, or that it was transmitted by *Aedes aegypti* mosquitoes, which carry numerous other disease-inducing viruses, but the entirely unexpected nature of the harm produced by this infectious agent in newborn babies—severe microcephaly, a condition in which the head is significantly smaller than usual and the astonishing "family resemblance" of these babies. Microcephaly is a well-known inborn anomaly, and it can have numerous causes, among them placental anomalies, chronic diseases of the pregnant woman, substances that are toxic to the fetus—probably the best-known cause of microcephaly is fetal alcohol syndrome—and infections during pregnancy. As a rule, however, it is rare for there to be multiple cases of microcephaly in a single maternity ward, and they tend to be diverse, some babies being born with pronounced and others with minimal microcephaly. Those newborns with microcephaly seen in maternity wards in northeastern Brazil beginning in August 2016 all looked alike: they had very small heads and severely deformed craniums; in some, it appeared that part of their brain was missing. Experienced gynecologists and pediatricians had the same reaction: "I've never seen anything like this." The striking similarity of the affected babies strongly indicated a common cause for these malformations. One possible explanation, an environmental toxin, was quickly ruled out: no candidate toxin was found in all the sites with microcephaly clusters. Epidemiologists quickly concluded that Zika, a new disease that had spread throughout the region several months earlier, was the origin of the observed anomalies. This was a truly scary prospect because there was no efficient way to control the spread of the Zika virus or to protect women from mosquito bites. Moreover, experts knew that the Zika virus could also be transmitted through sexual contact. Celina Turchi, a Fiocruz epidemiologist in Recife, who played a key role in investigating the links between Zika and inborn anomalies in northeastern Brazil, stated in an interview in the *Guardian*, "If I was a film-maker offering a scenario like this, people would say I was mad—a congenital disease transmitted by a vector that is everywhere and could also be sexually transmitted? From the first moment I had this feeling of being in a horror movie."[1]

The Early History of Zika: An Intriguing Virus

Emerging viruses, often viruses that for a long time circulated mainly among animals but suddenly broke out dramatically in humans, became visible beginning in the 1980s following the epidemics of the best-known virus, and up to the COVID-19 pandemic the most important among them, the human immunodeficiency virus (HIV), which causes AIDS. Scientists believe that HIV circulated for many years in African monkeys and occasionally infected humans until, in the early 1980s, a combination of air travel, increased sexual exchanges among selected social groups (such as some segments of the male homosexual community), the use of intravenously injected drugs, contamination of the blood supply, and poverty-driven unsafe practices in health care transformed AIDS into a pandemic that claimed tens of millions of lives worldwide.[2] Other emerging viruses, such as the Ebola virus, also circulated for a long time among animal hosts and probably produced localized human outbreaks until their diffusion among humans was accelerated by an increase in the volume of travel, and the disease was made more visible by more accurate and rapid diagnosis.

Before expanding into full-fledged human epidemic and reaching newspapers' headlines, the Zika virus was probably present for a long time in Africa and later in Asia. In Africa, scientists suppose, the Zika virus (ZIKV) circulated mainly among animals and only occasionally infected humans. ZIKV was believed to be a mild, essentially harmless pathogen. It was perceived as decidedly less dangerous than other viruses that belong to the same group of RNA viruses, flaviviruses (yellow viruses). Flaviviruses can be transmitted by numerous insects, but some of the best known among them—yellow fever virus, dengue virus, West Nile virus, Saint Luis encephalitis virus, and Japanese encephalitis virus—are mainly diffused by the mosquito *Aedes aegypti*. Until the Zika outbreak in Brazil, they were not known to be among the pathogens able to produce produced birth defects. The dengue fever virus was occasionally linked with malformations in newborns, but they were seen as a rare effect produced by an infection of a pregnant woman near her delivery date, quite different the from infection by viruses, such as rubella virus, known to be especially dangerous to the fetus early in pregnancy.

The history of Zika usually starts in 1947 with the first description of a new flavivirus by the Scottish entomologist and tropical disease expert Alexander Haddow (1912–1978). At that time, Haddow worked at the Uganda Virus Research Institute, then known as the Yellow Fever Research Institute, where he studied yellow fever and other viruses transmitted by mosquitoes (arboviruses). To capture infected mosquitoes, Haddow and his coworkers constructed in the jungle high towers with mosquito traps at their top. In 1947 Haddow first described in his notebook a new virus and named it Zika, after the Uganda forest where he found it. The first publication on the Zika virus dates from 1954, and the first fully documented description of human infection with this pathogen, from 1962.[3] In the second half of the twentieth century and the early twenty-first century scientists occasionally described cases of the Zika virus in Africa and Asia. The diagnosis of Zika was seen as important mainly to exclude the presence of other, more dangerous pathogens, especially the yellow fever virus. Since the Zika virus was found in the same geographic area and infected the same mammals (mainly jungle monkeys) and the same strains of mosquitoes as the yellow fever virus, it was important to avoid confusing the highly dangerous yellow fever virus with the presumably innocuous ZIKV.

A tower constructed in the middle of an African jungle and a small group of dedicated "virus hunters" who worked in difficult conditions to keep the population safe from dangerous germs and viruses constitute a good starting point for a dramatic story about a dangerous disease outbreak. One can, however, propose a different date—2008—as the starting point for the history of the Zika epidemic, and a different event—a surprising infection of an epidemiologist's wife. At that time, the Asian strain of the Zika virus, which until 2007 was seen as a pathogen that only occasionally infected humans, had already produced a massive outbreak on a tiny Pacific island, Yap (estimated population 11,000). The Yap epidemic was, however, viewed mainly as a curiosity and seemed to confirm that the Zika virus was a nuisance, not a public health risk.

The case of the infection of an epidemiologist's wife was different. After working in Senegal, two young epidemiologists returned to the United States and came down with fever, a rash, swelling of joints, and fatigue, not a rare event in the lives of people who conduct fieldwork in Africa. Then the wife of one of the epidemiologists, who had never left the United States, developed the same symptoms as her husband did; other members of his household and his colleagues remained healthy. At first the researchers infected in Senegal were unable to identify the mysterious pathogen that affected them. Because of their profession, they had access to a rich collection of antibodies to tropical diseases, but the results of all the tests they made were negative until both, and the infected spouse as well, tested positive for Zika. An article published in 2011, three years after the facts, employs a dry scientific language to tell about three patients with confirmed Zika. Male patients 1 and 2 in all probability acquired the virus during fieldwork in Senegal. The female patient, patient 3, spouse of patient 1, had stayed in the United States and in all probability was contaminated through sexual contact. Departing from the low-key tone of the article itself, its conclusion stresses that the observation that ZIKV could be transmitted through sexual contact was unexpected.[4] This observation, the article's authors explain, could potentially have far-reaching consequences. To the best of their knowledge, nobody had previously described a sexual transmission of an arbovirus in humans; if such a transmission was confirmed, it might change the understanding of ZIKV.

A more vivid version of the same story appears in the short film *Zika: The untold story*, produced by Tele Nova in 2016, at the height of the interest in the Zika epidemic.[5] The central personage of the film is Andrew Haddow, a tropical diseases expert and Alexander Haddow's grandson. Haddow explains that he chose to study viruses transmitted by mosquitoes, among them Zika, partly because of his grandfather's fascinating stories about the time he spent in the experimental station in Uganda. Haddow tells that while traveling in Asia, he talked by Skype with a US colleague who told him that he and his wife had been infected with a mysterious, apparently sexually transmissible virus. Haddow suspected that this mysterious virus might be Zika, and his friend confirmed his hunch. A single case of sexual transmission of a virus might be seen merely as one of the colorful stories that epidemiologists like to tell because it calls attention to their role as "virus hunters" and solvers of medical puzzles. However, as the authors of the 2011 article stressed, it was the first indication that the Zika virus was not, as researchers had assumed until then, merely a harmless relative of a more dangerous flavivirus and that it could have unique, sui generis properties.

2007–2014: Zika on Islands

Until 2007 all the known cases of Zika in humans were sporadic infections, usually detected by chance when looking for a different viral disease.[6] In the late twentieth century, Zika was viewed as a rare disease, although it is possible that this supposition was inaccurate. Symptoms of Zika can be easily confused with those of other diseases, and because of their relative mildness—a low fever and a rash that disappeared after a few days—not many people visited a doctor to complain about them. It is therefore possible that the frequency of infection with the Zika virus, especially in sub-Saharan Africa, was higher than suspected. The consequences of an occasional infection with the Zika virus in Africa are, however, difficult to detect because they occur among populations with limited access to advanced diagnostic technologies. In the second half of the twentieth century, ZIKV migrated from Africa to Southeast Asia. It changed during this migration. Molecular biology studies revealed that the structure of the Asian strain of Zika differs from that of the African strain.[7] It is also possible that the symptoms of the virus in infected individuals vary. Some virologists proposed that the African strain of the Zika virus might be more deadly to fetuses than the Asian strain that later infected Latin American countries, which did not induce fetal anomalies but miscarriages. Early miscarriages are frequent events. It is not easy to discover, especially in a resource-poor environment, that a woman miscarried because she was infected with a specific virus. If this hypothesis is correct, it may explain why it was not observed earlier that the Zika virus induces fetal anomalies.

The spread of ZIKV from Africa to Asia and then to Yap Island and beyond was probably driven by an increase in air traffic and intercontinental exchanges. It might have also been driven by climate change, which facilitates the proliferation of *Aedes* mosquitoes in more temperate zones. The 2007 Yap Island epidemic was the first demonstration that the Zika virus could produce a massive outbreak in an epidemiologically naïve population.[8] Yap Island physicians had observed a rapid increase in cases of rash accompanied by moderate fever. At first they thought the outbreak had been produced by a mild variant of dengue or chikungunya, but then they discovered that it had been caused by Zika. Although Zika was formally diagnosed in only 49 cases, epidemiologists estimated that more than 70% of Yap inhabitants had come into contact with the Zika virus. They also estimated that the majority of the infections were asymptomatic. Epidemiologists could provide this estimate because dengue fever, produced by a virus closely related to ZIKV, is relatively rare on Yap. Since antibodies against dengue cross-react with those against Zika, in places where dengue was widespread before a Zika outbreak it was much more difficult to know what proportion of the population had been infected with ZIKV.

The epidemic of Zika on Yap Island was an unexpected event, but it was discussed by only a narrow group of experts. The Zika outbreak in French Polynesia (estimated population 270,000) in 2013–14 had somewhat greater visibility.[9] It also might have indicated that the virus that reached the Pacific region was not identical with the one found in sporadic cases in Asia. It was later confirmed that the outbreaks on Yap Island and then in French Polynesia were probably linked with a mutation in the Zika virus that increased its neurotropism (affinity to cells of the nervous system) and therefore enhanced its capacity to induce neurological disorders.[10]

With the French Polynesia epidemic, Zika became a recognized public health problem. This epidemic reinforced the perception of Zika as a relatively mild disease in comparison with two other diseases propagated by the *Aedes aegypti* mosquito that produce similar symptoms: dengue fever and chikungunya. On the other hand, researchers in French Polynesia suspected that the Zika virus could result in a rare but severe neurological complication, Guillain-Barré syndrome, a paralysis of many muscles of the body that can last as long as several months and in some cases can lead to death. Guillain-Barré syndrome was linked with infections with numerous pathogens, among them cytomegalovirus, influenza virus, chikungunya virus, and HIV. The Zika virus was another likely candidate because scientists who studied it in laboratory animals in the 1950s and 1960s had already noted its tendency to infect nerve cells.

The likelihood that a person infected with the Zika virus would develop Guillain-Barré syndrome was not easy to estimate, because of the high prevalence of dengue in French Polynesia. Serological tests were unable to differentiate between infections with Zika and with dengue virus and thus to provide accurate data on the spread of Zika in populations. In the absence of a reliable serological test, the gold standard for diagnosis of Zika was a molecular biology test, the reverse transcriptase–polymerase chain reaction (RT-PCR). This test is, however, relatively expensive and has to be performed in a specialized laboratory. It is therefore not well adapted for large-scale epidemiological surveys. Moreover, the RT-PCR test for Zika is far from perfect because it detects the presence of the virus in body fluids and therefore is valid only as long as a person has an active infection. However, the period of active infection with ZIKV is usually short. By contrast, a serological test that detects antibodies against an infectious agent can also tell whether the tested individual had contact with a pathogen sometime in the past. The two tests are complementary: molecular biology tests indicate how many people are infected with a virus in a given moment, while serological tests indicate the prevalence of an infection in a population. The absence of reliable serological tests for Zika and the relatively elevated price of the molecular biology test greatly complicated epidemiological studies of this disease.

Virologists who studied the Zika epidemic in French Polynesia relied mainly on the RT-PCR test. They had discovered that often it is easier to isolate the Zika virus from secretions of infected people—urine, saliva, and semen—than from their blood. The presence of important quantities of the Zika virus in patients' semen was immediately interpreted as an indication that the virus could be transmitted through sexual contact.[11] Physicians also noticed that some men infected with Zika displayed symptoms such as swollen testes and blood in the sperm. These observations reinforced the supposition that the ZIKV multiplies in testes. Scientists who studied the Zika epidemic in French Polynesia proposed in early 2015 that sexual transmission might have contributed to the rapid spread of this infection on the island, a worrisome observation. The potential combination of two distinct patterns of diffusion of the Zika virus was perceived as a matter of serious concern. However, at that time (the first half of 2015) researchers were mainly preoccupied by the risk of Guillain-Barré syndrome.

January–June 2015: A Mysterious "Fever" in Northeastern Brazil

Scientists believe that the Zika virus arrived in Brazil, possibly from French Polynesia, in either 2013 or 2014. Virologists speculated about the possible role of sports competitions in the spread of Zika. They discussed three candidate events that might have brought this virus to Brazil: the Confederations Cup soccer tournament (June 15–30, 2013), the 2014 World Cup soccer tournament (June 12–July 13, 2014), and the Va'a canoe event (August 12–17, 2014).[12] Other researchers believe that an explanation that links the arrival of Zika to an international sports event makes a good story but is not necessarily correct. The Zika virus might have reached Brazil less spectacularly, such as by a visit of one or several infected people that led to the establishment of the virus in northeastern Brazil.[13] In all probability, the Zika virus later spread from the northeast to other parts of Brazil and other Latin American countries. Because it is highly probable that the Zika virus circulated in northeastern Brazil before it was identified by infectious disease experts, the label "2015–2016 Zika epidemic in Brazil" is imprecise. It is, however, a reasonably accurate description of an epidemic—a perceptible threat to the population's health and a multilevel reaction to this threat.

The early diffusion of the Zika virus in Brazil might have been invisible mainly because the clinical symptoms of Zika are similar to those of dengue fever and of chikungunya, another virus transmitted by *Aedes* that arrived in Brazil in 2014. In early 2015, physicians noted the rapid propagation of an "atypical dengue" in northeastern Brazil, first in the state Rio Grande do Norte and then in Parana and Bahia.[14] Molecular biology tests ruled out the dengue and chikungunya viruses as causes. Researchers from Salvador, Bahia, then formally identified Zika as the virus responsible for the outbreak.[15] In April 2015, the Brazilian Secretariat of Health Surveillance (SVS) included Zika in its monitoring of rash-producing diseases, while the Pan American Health Organization issued a warning about the presence of Zika in northeastern Brazil. A few months later, epidemiologists observed an increase in the number of cases of Guillain-Barré syndrome. They suspected, as their colleagues in French Polynesia had, that these cases were produced by an infection with the Zika virus. A supposition that ZIKV was responsible for an increase in the prevalence of Guillain-Barré syndrome was, however, not identical to formal proof that that was the case, especially since chikungunya virus was also linked with the induction of this syndrome. Moreover, epidemiologists suspected simultaneous or sequential infection with these two arboviruses. The latter hypothesis was confirmed by further studies.[16] Since the chikungunya virus and ZIKV belong to different families of viruses, serological tests can differentiate infections with these two pathogens. By contrast, it is much more difficult to detect a simultaneous or sequential infection with ZIKV and the dengue virus. Some specialists suspected that infection with these two flaviviruses could increase the harmful effects of each and thus explain some of the unusual aspects of the Zika outbreak in Brazil.

Microcephaly and Zika: August–October 2015

Guillain-Barré syndrome is a rare condition whose increased frequency was observed mainly by neurologists, who noted a statistical anomaly. The concentration of cases of very severe microcephaly in a small number of maternity hospitals in northeastern Brazil was novel, as was the almost immediate attribution of these cases to infection by ZIKV. The suspicion that Zika could produce anomalies in newborns did not arise in the void. In the first half of 2015 some Brazilian researchers were already concerned by the possibility that a pregnant woman who contracted Zika might transmit the infection to the fetus. They knew that infection with dengue fever and chikungunya, especially near pregnancy's end, led to complications such as miscarriage, preterm births, and the birth of low-weight babies. The pediatrician Patricia Brasil, of the Infectious Diseases Department at the Evandro Chagas Hospital, Fiocruz, Rio de Janeiro, followed for several years a cohort of women infected with dengue fever during pregnancy. When chikungunya arrived in Brazil, she included in this cohort also pregnant women infected with that virus. Patricia Brasil's cohort became an important reference group for research on the consequences of infection with ZIKV in pregnancy. Anomalies produced by the infection of pregnant women with dengue and chikungunya were, however, rare and diverse. The epidemic of microcephaly observed in northeastern Brazil in 2015 was very different: an impressive clustering of very similar inborn anomalies.

Perhaps the most striking thing about the testimonies of physicians and scientists who between August and October 2015 had noticed a multiplication of cases of severe microcephaly in northeastern Brazil was their immediate certainty that something truly unusual was going on. An immediate recognition of the existence of an anomaly was described by the philosopher Michel Foucault as a typical feature of the diagnostic mode of knowledge.[17] The Italian historian Carlo Ginzburg expanded this view. Hunters, physicians, detectives, and historians of art, Ginzburg proposed, share an acquired capacity to read traces as clues and signs. They can do it through a mainly unconscious process that is difficult to describe to outsiders. Thanks to an essentially nontransmissible, embodied knowledge, a hunter who observes traces in a forest will affirm that they were made by a small, wounded fox; a physician who strongly feels that something is wrong will recommend an immediate hospitalization of a healthy-looking child; a detective examining a car wreck will suspect that the reported traffic accident was staged; and an art historian studying a drawing will decide that it is an original work of a famous artist.[18] Thanks to a similar recognition mechanism, physicians and virologists in northeastern Brazil confronted with a cluster of cases of severe microcephaly quickly realized that they were observing an unfamiliar phenomenon in all probability produced by a new infectious agent. The Zika virus, a pathogen that only recently had reached Brazil and produced a massive epidemic in the northeast several months earlier, was the only infectious agent that fit this description and therefore the most likely culprit. Virologists and epidemiologists followed that intriguing lead. The Zika epidemic, Celina Turchi affirmed, "is a great tragedy but also a great opportunity."[19] Laura Rodrigues, an epidemiologist at the London School of Hygiene and Tropical Medicine, who, thanks to her close links with researchers in northeastern Brazil, also played a pivotal role in early studies of the Zika epidemic, similarly explained that the fast production of knowledge during the Zika epidemic provided a rare opportunity to observe science in the making.[20]

The first cases of microcephaly were observed in hospitals in Recife, Pernambuco, and Campina Grande, Paraíba, in August and September 2015. They rapidly attracted the attention of public health experts. Gynecologists like Adriana Melo, of the Pedro I Hospital in Campina Grande, who usually saw one or two cases of severe microcephaly in a year, began to see two or three cases every week and started to talk about them to colleagues.[21] Celina Turchi reported that she had first learned about severe microcephaly in newborns from a friend in the Health Ministry in Brasília, who had heard rumors about the multiplication of such cases and asked her to investigate. She was very surprised by what she saw. These cases did not look at all like the cases of microcephaly she had observed before. The heads of all the children had a very peculiar shape, squashed and deformed at the top.[22] Brain scans of the microcephalic babies as well as several aborted fetuses with similar features displayed severe brain anomalies such as microcalcifications (clusters of calcium deposits in the brain), a thin cerebral cortex (the part of the brain associated with thinking), lissencephaly (lack of typical "brain folds"), and ventriculomegaly (the enlargement of brain chambers). Taken together, such changes in the brain predicted severe neurological and cognitive disabilities in the affected children. The concentration of newborns with a highly distinctive pattern of deformities produced a growing feeling of alarm among researchers who observed them and stimulated an intensive search for possible causes.

A Discovery Made at the Periphery

In 2016, when Zika became a topic of intense concern in Western countries, some among the Brazilian researchers involved in the early stages of investigation of the northeastern microcephaly epidemic acquired overnight and international fame. Brazilian scientists studying diseases transmitted by mosquitoes have produced high-quality research, recognized in Brazil and abroad.

However, because the diseases they investigated were mainly present in developing countries, affected mainly vulnerable populations, and were not perceived as threatening to the inhabitants of the Global North, their research had relatively low visibility outside a small circle of specialists. With the advent of the Zika epidemic, some of the pioneers of studies of this disease suddenly received much wider attention. They were invited to give lectures at prestigious international institutions and published papers in top-level scientific and medical journals. Yet, such visibility was selective and did not benefit equally all the scientists who investigated Zika in 2015.

In her important pioneering study of the Zika epidemic in Brazil, the anthropologist Debora Diniz emphasized that the findings that the mysterious fever that erupted in Brazil in early 2015 was the Zika virus and that this virus was responsible for the epidemic of microcephaly were made in the impoverished regions of northeastern Brazil, and not in Brazil's major cities, São Paolo and Rio de Janeiro. She also contrasted the caring attitude of clinicians such as Vanesa Van der Linden and Maria Lucia Brito of Recife, Pernambuco, and Adriana Melo of Campina Grande, Paraíba, with the presumably more detached scientific approach of virologists and epidemiologists from the south.[23] The image of a conflict between underappreciated specialists from the "backward" north and those from advanced scientific institutions of southern Brazil, is, however, somewhat simplified. Salvador, Bahia, where the Rockefeller Foundation in the 1930s established a pioneering virology laboratory, has since become a major center of research in virology but also in epidemiology, while Fiocruz, Recife, and the Federal University of Pernambuco are also important centers of biomedical and epidemiological research. Zika, and then Zika-induced microcephaly, was first described by scientists from northeastern Brazil because cases of these pathologies were concentrated in the northeast, but also because the region was well endowed with high-quality scientific laboratories, no less competent to study arboviruses than those in São Paolo and Rio de Janeiro.

Once the importance of early studies of the Zika outbreak in Brazil was acclaimed internationally, several scientists and physicians from northeastern Brazil felt that their contribution was insufficiently recognized, while the studies made by researchers from the Brazilian south were given excessive importance. Debora Diniz's book reflects their view. Two articles that sum up the history of the Zika epidemic in Brazil display the tension between northern and southern research groups. One, written by an important group of scientists from Recife directly involved in Zika studies, attributes the description of the link between Zika and microcephaly mainly to this group.[24] Another, written by scientists from São Paolo University who did not take part in early studies of Zika, describes a much wider group of "pioneers of Zika studies" that includes experts from numerous Brazilian cities and the Health Ministry.[25] Tensions around credit for a scientific "discovery"—that is, a new development retrospectively recognized by the relevant scientific communities as an important first—are not new. The German poet Johann von Goethe explained in the early nineteenth century that "question of science are frequently career questions. A single discovery can make a man famous and lay the foundation of his career as a citizen. Every new phenomenon is a discovery, every discovery is property. Touch a man's property and his passions are immediately aroused."[26] This is probably no less true in the twenty-first century. One may add that one important difference is the scientist's gender: Goethe speaks about a man's property, but many among the Brazilian pioneers of Zika studies were women.

"Microcephaly" as a Scientific Puzzle

Tensions around priority and symbolic rewards arose only in later stages of the Zika epidemic. The early months of the investigation of the microcephaly epidemic in Northeastern Brazil were different; it was a period of an intensive collective effort to solve a troubling epidemiological puzzle.[27] In the first months, clinicians, virologists, and epidemiologists in northeastern Brazil worked together around the clock trying to validate their initial intuitions and prove that an outbreak of Zika had caused the concentration of cases of severe brain anomalies in their region. They felt that they had to work fast because the situation was very frightening. Epidemiologists did not know what percentage of women infected with ZIKV during pregnancy would give birth to severely impaired children. Some viruses, such as cytomegalovirus (CMV), induce fetal anomalies in only a small percentage of infected women, but other viruses, such as the rubella virus, induce such anomalies in the great majority of women infected early in pregnancy. They did know, however, that Zika was highly infectious, and the epidemic was spreading from the northeast to other parts of Brazil. Even if only 1% of the babies born to women infected with Zika during pregnancy developed severe brain anomalies, in a country with 3 million childbirths per year it would be a public health disaster.

Experts openly expressed their feeling of helplessness. The infectious diseases specialist Rivaldo Venâncio da Cunha, director of the Fiocruz Institute of Mato Grosso do Sul and one of the pioneers of Zika studies, explained in

November 2015 that there was no treatment that could be offered to a pregnant woman infected with the Zika virus, no vaccine against Zika, no efficient cure that can be proposed for children born with severe microcephaly, and no way to halt the spread of a disease transmitted by the omnipresent *Aedes* mosquito.[28] The persisting failure to prevent the spread of dengue fever and the recent unchecked spread of chikungunya attested to Brazil's incapacity to control viruses spread by *Aedes*. As another pioneer of studies of Zika, the virologist Pedro Vasconcelos, of the Instituto Evandro Chagas in Ananindeua, Pará, affirmed in an interview published in the journal O Globo in December 2015: "It is a terrible situation for a physician. I feel desperate when I see so many pregnant women unprotected and scared, while we are bound hand and foot because we know so little. . . .We need first of all rapid, inexpensive, and efficient diagnostic kits; we also need to better understand this virus."[29]

In September 2015, researchers in northeastern Brazil unofficially transmitted their concerns about the multiplication of cases of severe microcephaly in their region to experts in the Brazilian Health Ministry. They reinforced this message in October 2015. They also increasingly pointed to the Zika virus as the most probable cause of the increase in cases of microcephaly and other brain anomalies.[30] Carlos Brito, of the Federal University of Pernambuco, who rapidly became one of the most visible propagators of the Zika hypothesis, in December 2015 published an article with an ambitious title: "Zika Virus: A New Chapter in the History of Medicine." Brito affirmed that all indications—the high concentration of cases in a short period, their simultaneous occurrence in numerous states, the similarity of the observed cerebral malformations, the exclusion of other maternal infections as producing the malformations, and the fact that many among the mothers of affected children reported that they had typical symptoms of Zika (rash, conjunctivitis, and moderate muscle pain, but no high fever)—led to the inescapable conclusion that microcephaly in newborns was caused by an infectious agent. Moreover, the first cases of microcephaly appeared five to seven months after the peak of the Zika epidemic in northeastern Brazil, another indication that they were produced by infection with the Zika virus early in pregnancy.[31]

The Microcephaly Epidemic and the Brazilian Health Ministry

On October 22, 2015, the health department for the state of Pernambuco officially notified the Secretariat of Health Surveillance of the Brazilian Health Ministry to investigate 26 cases of children with microcephaly. On November 11, the ministry issued a special alert about the risk of Zika infection for pregnant women. Zika was declared a Public Health Emergency of National Importance (Emergência em Saúde Pública de Importância Nacional, or ESPIN), and a special task force, the Centro de Operação de Emergência em Saúde Pública (COES), was established to deal with the new epidemic. On November 17, the Health Ministry also began publication of a weekly bulletin, the *Boletim Epidemiológico*, with cumulative data on suspected cases of microcephaly. The rapid increase in the number of suspected cases—more than 1,000 cases in November and December 2015—and their visibility, since these numbers were widely circulated in the media, amplified women's fears and their feeling of impending doom. In late 2015, physicians noted that babies born with small heads displayed numerous other neurological anomalies, and they started to talk about congenital Zika syndrome (CZS). They feared that the number of babies born with CZS would increase rapidly. Rivaldo Venâncio da Cunha stated in early January 2016 that 16,000 cases of Zika-induced microcephaly were projected for 2016 and that specialists estimated that the Zika outbreak in Brazil, which at that time was expected to last several years, would lead to the birth of 40,000 to 50,000 children with CZS.[32]

The Zika epidemic was seen as especially alarming because of a widely shared opinion that not much could be done to prevent or control it. The Health Ministry's interventions followed a long tradition of reaction to arboviruses, focusing exclusively on the danger of mosquito bites. The efforts to control yellow fever played a key role in the shaping of public health responses to epidemics in Brazil.[33] Unsurprisingly, they also shaped the reaction to an outbreak of a new pathology transmitted by mosquitoes. The ministry employed martial language, derived from previous episodes of dealing with mosquitoes. It proclaimed a "war on mosquitoes," declared the *Aedes* mosquito Brazil's number one enemy, and distributed educational materials—posters and leaflets—to instruct the population on how to fight this enemy.[34] The ministry also organized campaigns of fumigation of mosquito-infested areas in northeastern Brazil by units of the Brazilian army. The media displayed images of soldiers dressed in impressive protective gear pulverizing insecticides. The pulverization of insecticides provides at best partial, short-term relief.[35] On the other hand, it sends a strong signal to the population: the government is concerned about your health. During the Zika epidemic, it sent an additional signal: since the government was willing to engage the army in a massive anti-mosquito intervention, it was persuaded that the frightening increase in the birth of babies with small heads had been caused by Zika. This message was probably well received, or at least not opposed, by concerned populations. In Puerto Rico, by contrast, the government's proposal in early 2016 to aerially spray the insecticide Naled was met with strong protests, and representatives from the scientific, academic, professional, agricultural, cultural, religious, and other sectors organized a Frente Unido contra la Fumigación Aérea (United Front against Aerial Fumigations). The Puerto Rico state government was obliged to cancel the plan.[36]

Another key focus of the governmental intervention was the surveillance of inborn anomalies. On December 5, 2015, the Health Ministry promoted a national plan to deal with the Zika outbreak, and on December 14 the ministry published a protocol for surveiling the occurrence of microcephaly in relation to infection with the Zika virus.[37] In the following two years, the Health Ministry issued 17 ordinances, 6 technical notes, 4 protocols on microcephaly, and 60 weekly reports on cases of this inborn anomaly. The two protocols promulgated in December 2015 provided guidelines for monitoring pregnant women who displayed symptoms of Zika during pregnancy. They also provided detailed instructions to guide the supervision of all Brazilian newborns through an elaborate system of sentinel laboratories, expected to trace CZS cases and send biological samples to reference laboratories. The protocols allocated special funds for the supervision of pregnant women and newborns and defined criteria for the collection of data on the prevalence of Zika in pregnancy. They also outlined the medical and social support the Brazilian state would provide to children born with microcephaly related to an infection with the Zika virus and their families. The proposed surveillance and support measures were detailed and exhaustive. In practice, however, their implementation was uneven and partial.[38]

At the very heart of the surveillance proposed by the ministry was the systematic measurement of newborns' heads. Measuring heads is a very simple activity for which no specialized knowledge is needed. This first sign that something might be wrong with a baby, the ministry's experts assumed, would lead to a more systematic investigation of suspected cases. A small head is a very imprecise sign of the presence of Zika-related birth defects in a newborn. The presence of brain anomalies is seen as a much more accurate sign of the presence of CZS. Moreover, the detection of such anomalies has a prognostic as well as a diagnostic value: it helps to predict the extent of the child's impairment. A diagnosis of brain malformation was, however, possible only in leading hospitals that had the expertise and the appropriate medical imaging equipment, while even the smallest maternity clinics have a measuring tape and can provide data on head size.

The Health Ministry's decision to use a small head size as the sole sign of potential Zika-induced birth defects was based on the supposition that diagnosis of microcephaly has low specificity (it produces many false positives) but high sensibility (it produces only a few false negatives). While further investigation of babies born with smaller than average heads would show that many among these babies were not affected by Zika, an investigation of all the babies born with abnormally small heads would lead to an identification of nearly all the babies with CZS. The ministry's initial decision to provide a very broad definition of microcephaly that included borderline cases may have reflected the belief that children with a less severe Zika-induced microcephaly might benefit most from medical and educational interventions in infancy.

The protocols of the Brazilian Health Ministry prudently spoke about "microcephaly related to an infection with Zika virus" rather than about microcephaly induced by an infection with this virus, but the experts who promulgated this protocol did not seem to question the assumption that the sharp increase in the number of babies born with small heads in northeastern Brazil was a direct consequence of a Zika epidemic. It was not easy, however, to provide formal proof of this assumption, because the Zika virus is more difficult to isolate from blood, body fluids, and tissues of the affected fetuses and newborns than other infectious agents that cause birth defects. Nevertheless, on November 17, 2015, Adriana Melo, Ana Bispo de Filippis, and their collaborators isolated the Zika virus in the amniotic fluid of a woman in her fifth month of pregnancy whose fetus was diagnosed with severe microcephaly (this severely affected fetus later died in the womb) and in the amniotic fluid of another patient who later gave birth to a live child with Zika syndrome.[39] Then on November 28 Pedro Vasconcelos and his colleagues isolated the Zika virus in the blood and tissues of two stillborn children who displayed a typical clinical image of microcephaly with severe brain malformations.[40] These findings were interpreted by Brazilian researchers as a confirmation of what they already knew: the Zika virus was the cause of the Brazilian epidemic of microcephaly.

The results of the studies of Melo, Bispo, and their collaborators and of Vasconcelos and his coworkers, first circulated within Brazil, were later published in major international scientific journals. Another study, published in February 2016 by a group of Slovenian and North American scientists, reported the isolation of the Zika virus in an aborted fetus with severe microcephaly. In that case, the fetus was aborted by an Italian woman who had been infected with Zika during a stay in northeastern Brazil and then returned to

Europe.[41] The latter study independently confirmed the results of the investigations made by Brazilian researchers. An additional confirmation that the
Zika virus induced fetal anomalies came from a new analysis of the data collected in French Polynesia during the 2013–14 Zika outbreak. When Brazilian
scientists linked microcephaly with Zika, researchers from French Polynesia
on November26, 2015, notified the European Centre for Disease Prevention
and Control (ECDC) about the existence of a cluster of 17 rare neurological
anomalies potentially linked with the Zika outbreak.[42] This cluster was not
spotted earlier because several of the women who learned of a severe fetal impairment elected to terminate their pregnancy.[43]

The introduction to a text published in 2017 by the Brazilian Health Ministry that summarizes the role of the Brazilian National Health Service in the
Zika epidemic explains that the isolation of the Zika virus from the amniotic
fluid of two of Adriana Melo's patients in November 2015 put an end to uncertainty about the origins of the mysterious epidemic of small heads. From
that moment on, the ministry's text states, the link between Zika and microcephaly was proven.[44] The key point in this statement was that ZIKV "was
responsible for serious sequelae in babies." Evidence that in selected cases the
Zika virus was directly linked with brain anomalies of an investigated fetus (a
weak claim about causal links between Zika and inborn impairments) is not,
however, definitive proof that the Zika virus was the sole cause of the epidemic of microcephaly reported by the Brazilian authorities. The latter claim
was questioned in early 2016.

Zika and Microcephaly: The Rise of Doubts

In late 2015 Brazilian scientists' and physicians' strong conviction that the
microcephaly epidemic in northeastern Brazil was the result of infection with
the Zika virus seemed to be widely accepted by foreign specialists. On November 17, 2015, PAHO published a short report about the possible links between Zika and microcephaly. A more detailed report published by PAHO on
December 1 extended the warning about potential risks of Zika. It affirmed
that infection with the Zika virus during pregnancy might be dangerous for
the fetus. PAHO's document stressed the importance of an accurate epidemiological reporting of all the abnormal findings in newborn babies, careful
monitoring of babies with microcephaly and other inborn impairments, and
help for affected families. It also stated that if fetal anomalies were detected
during pregnancy, the pregnant woman and her partner should receive accurate information about the risk of unfavorable outcomes, although it stopped

short of mentioning the possibility of termination of pregnancy.[45] On November 24, the ECDC published a document that stated that since there was a strong suspicion of a causal link between Zika and fetal anomalies, women traveling to zones where Zika was endemic needed to protect themselves from mosquitoes. The ECDC document also raised the question of the safety of the blood supply and the possibility that the Zika virus could be transmitted through sexual contact.

Neither PAHO's nor the ECDC's document questioned the causal link between ZIKV infection and fetal and newborn anomalies. Some experts were more prudent. One of the first scientific texts on the multiplication of cases of microcephaly in Brazil, a short article published in December 2015 in the medical journal *The Lancet*, explained that Brazilian scientists had isolated the Zika virus from affected fetuses, then hinted that the story might be more complicated than it seemed because of the lack of clear-cut correlation between the prevalence of microcephaly in a given geographic area and the prevalence of confirmed cases of infection with the Zika virus in the same area.[46] A more detailed report written by Brazilian scientists and published in January 2016 in the *Morbidity and Mortality Weekly Reports* of the US Centers for Disease Control and Prevention (CDC) explained that while the Brazilian studies provided strong circumstantial evidence that Zika was behind an increase in the frequency of inborn anomalies, many questions about the epidemic of microcephaly remain open. One problem is the equation of microcephaly with CZS. Another is the lack of reliable data on the prevalence of microcephaly before the Zika outbreak. The Health Ministry stated that the prevalence of this condition in Brazil increased twenty times in the fall of 2015, but many experts questioned this statement. They estimated that microcephaly was systematically underreported in the Brazilian registry of birth anomalies, the Sistema de Informações sobre Nascidos Vivos (SINASC). The Zika-induced increase in the number of cases of microcephaly in Brazil, the article concluded, was undoubtedly a real phenomenon, but in the absence of a reliable baseline, the magnitude of the phenomenon was unknown.[47]

Microcephaly, like fever or paralysis, is not a disease but a symptom. The abnormally small size of a baby's head can be produced by an infection, health problems of the pregnant woman, malnutrition, or toxic substances. Images of babies with severe fetal alcohol syndrome closely recall those of newborns with microcephaly attributed to Zika. The well-studied link between toxins absorbed voluntarily or involuntarily by a pregnant woman and microcephaly of the newborn favored a hypothesis that the Brazilian microcephaly epidemic had been produced by intoxication. Moreover, a frightening epidemic of anomalies in newborn babies was a perfect breeding ground for rumors that attributed the microcephaly epidemic to corrupted batches of vaccine, chemical fertilizers, or an antimosquito product. The last hypothesis gained short-living fame in early 2016.

In February 2016 a report from a group of Latin American (mainly Argentinian) physicians, Team Reduas, coordinated by Dr. Medardo Avila, published a document that argued that the Zika story was but a coverup for an environmental scandal: the toxic effect of insecticides, especially pyriproxyfen, a substance produced by the Japanese firm Sumitomo Chemical and widely employed to eliminate the mosquito *Aedes aegypti*.[48] The Team Reduas report, widely circulated through social media, claimed that there was a close correlation between the diffusion of this insecticide and the prevalence of microcephaly in Brazil, and that the reason why no cases of microcephaly had been found in other countries with important Zika outbreaks, such as Colombia, was that they did not use pyriproxyfen. The Team Reduas report argued that insecticides, presented as crucial to the elimination of human diseases, are dangerous environmental toxins aggressively pushed by multinational corporations interested only in profit. It also strongly criticized biological approaches to the mosquito problem such as the use of genetically modified insects to fight Zika and other mosquito-borne infections or the infection of *Aedes* mosquitoes with the bacterium *Wolbachia*. The reliance on bioengineering in the "war" against *Aedes* mosquitoes is but another profit-driven strategy of disease control. It detracts attention from the real causes for the presence of diseases disseminated by mosquitoes in Latin America, namely, poverty, inadequate sanitation, lack of access to clean water, and systematic neglect of the environment.

To support its claim about environmental causes of the microcephaly epidemic, the Team Reduas report quoted a statement on Zika by the Brazilian Association for Collective Health (ABRASCO). ABRASCO's statement of February 2016 indeed criticized Brazilian health authorities' exclusive focus on the "war against mosquitoes," the excessive use of insecticides, and systematically neglected broader societal and environmental issues that led to an increase in the prevalence of mosquito-borne diseases.[49] ABRASCO did not contest the existence of a causal link between the Zika virus and microcephaly. Its main goal was to attract attention to social determinants of health and disease and to argue that making improvements to sanitation was a much more efficient long-term solution to the control of diseases spread by mosquitoes than the use of insecticides and insect repellents. Following the buzz around the Team Reduas report, ABRASCO's leaders declared that their original statement had discussed the broad social background to the spread of mosquito-borne diseases and did not back the claim that a specific larvicide had produced the microcephaly epidemic.[50]

A hypothesis that pyriproxyfen might have been responsible, at least partly, for the increase in severe brain anomalies in babies born in northeastern Brazil in the fall of 2015 was not unreasonable. Environmental toxins had been reported to produce such anomalies. In addition, the ZIKV hypothesis and the pyriproxyfen hypothesis were not mutually exclusive. One possible interpretation might have been that the increase in microcephaly cases in northeastern Brazil had two unrelated causes, Zika and pyriproxyfen. An alternative hypothesis might have been that pyriproxyfen increased the capability of the Zika virus to induce fetal anomalies. Both hypotheses were, however, disproved through epidemiological investigations. Pyriproxyfen was employed only in selected municipalities in northeastern Brazil. It was therefore possible to compare municipalities that employed this insecticide with those that did not. Brazilian epidemiologists made such a comparison and found no correlation between the geographic distribution of pyriproxyfen and the prevalence of microcephaly.[51]

A small number of scientists continued to support the pyriproxyfen hypothesis even after the publication of epidemiological data contradicting it.[52] Nevertheless, Team Reduas's claim that the Brazilian microcephaly epidemic had been produced by an insecticide circulated mainly among activists and left-leaning political groups concerned about environmental issues and opposed to powerful multinational corporations. In all probability it had only a limited impact, if any, among scientists and public health experts who studied the Zika outbreak. Another critique of the claim that the Zika virus had produced an epidemic of microcephaly in northeastern Brazil in the second half of 2015 had a much greater impact among experts. This critique, issued by scientists from the Latin American Collaborative Study of Congenital Malformations (ECLAMC), contested not only the reliability of epidemiological data published by the Brazilian Health Ministry in late 2015 but the very existence of a Brazilian epidemic of microcephaly.[53] ECLAMC is a non-governmental organization that, from the mid-1970s, systematically records inborn anomalies in Latin America.[54] Despite its nongovernmental status, ECLAMC participates in all international coordination of inborn impairments and is perceived as an important and reliable source of information. In a report published on December 30, 2015, ECLAMC experts affirmed that before 2015 SINASC had seriously underreported the frequency of microcephaly in Brazil. The new focus on newborns' head size, the ECLAMC's report argued, had led to an opposite mistake. The Health Ministry's *Boletim Epidemiológico* had reported in December 2015 a total of 1,153 cases of microcephaly. This number, ECLAMC experts argued, was very likely grossly inflated, produced by an active search for children born with small heads and the classification of children at the lower end of normal values for head size as confirmed cases of microcephaly. Since neither the past nor the present data on the frequency of microcephaly published by Brazilian authorities were reliable, the ECLAMC document concluded, it was not possible to determine the magnitude and the cause(s) of the epidemic of microcephaly in Brazil or even to ascertain its existence.

The ECLAMC report was widely distributed among mainstream researchers inside and outside Brazil. Articles published in major scientific journals in January and February 2016 echoed some of the doubts expressed in this report.[55] At the time, these articles explained, it was impossible to know how many babies with microcephaly had been born in northeastern Brazil between August 2015 and January 2016 and what the magnitude of the increase in their number had been. The authors of these articles did not doubt that Brazilian scientists had observed a cluster of babies with very severe microcephaly in northeastern Brazil and that in selected cases they had demonstrated the presence of the Zika virus in affected fetuses. They also believed the affirmations of Brazilian experts about the highly unusual character of fetal brain anomalies observed in newborns with severe CZS.[56] It was less clear, however, whether there had also been a significant increase in cases of moderate brain anomalies, and if there had been, whether it had been related to the Zika outbreak. Moreover, while the isolation of the Zika virus from impaired fetuses and the amniotic fluid of women who carried such fetuses was a strong indication of links between this virus and microcephaly, it was not formal proof that Zika was the cause, or the only cause, of all the observed changes in the fetal brain.

An Undecided Diagnosis: Scientists and Parents

Brazilian scientists knew that the data on the frequency of microcephaly in Brazil before 2015 published by SINASC were not always reliable and that some cities and regions had better systems of recording such defects than others.[57] The imperfection of the SINSAC system was indirectly recognized by the Health Ministry too. Following the first reports on the microcephaly epidemic, the ministry established a parallel system of registering inborn anomalies, the Registro de Eventos em Saúde Pública (RESP), and advised clinicians to register microcephaly cases with RESP rather than with SINSAC. Brazilian researchers were also aware of the difficulty of formally linking a symptom, microcephaly, with a well-defined cause, an infection with the Zika virus.[58] Finally, they knew that the adoption on November 17, 2015, of a very broad definition of microcephaly, as a head circumference of less than 33 centimeters in a baby born at term, was problematic and might have led to the overdiagnosis of this inborn anomaly. The ministry's definition of microcephaly was later modified twice, first on December 12, 2015, when microcephaly was redefined as a head size of less than 32 centimeters, and again on March 13, 2016, when Brazil adopted the WHO's definition of microcephaly.[59] Yet, despite their awareness of problems with the microcephaly registry and with a diagnosis of CZS based on the size of newborns' heads, Brazilian scientists strongly disagreed with the conclusions of the ECLAMC report, which put into doubt the very existence of the microcephaly epidemic and the causal link between Zika and birth defects. These conclusions, Brazilian scientists believed, were not only false but harmful. The need to respond to the ECLAMC report and disprove its conclusions led to important delays in the research on Zika in Brazil.[60]

One of the main reasons for doubts about the existence, or in a more moderate version of this argument the size, of the Brazilian Zika-related microcephaly epidemic was practical obstacles to a reliable diagnosis of Zika in newborns. A major issue was the absence of reliable laboratory tests to demonstrate infection with ZIKV. Moreover, babies with very small, dramatically deformed heads at the origin of the alert about an epidemic of microcephaly had highly distinctive traits, difficult to miss. By contrast, many babies included on ministry registers and investigated by health authorities were borderline cases. The investigations of babies classified as "undecides cases" frequently were long and stressful. According to the *Boletim Epidemiológico* for September 2018, 5.1% of the children first investigated for microcephaly in 2015 and 11.6% of those investigated in 2016 were still under investigation.[61] Some parents received a confirmation of Zika syndrome in their children and learned that they were entitled to specialized medical and social services. Coordination between these two categories of services wase facilitated by a series of orders issued in late 2015 and early 2016 that promoted the coordination of the responses to Zika of the Brazilian Health Ministry and the Social Development Ministry. Other parents learned that the investigations had not confirmed the presence of Zika syndrome in their child. This was excellent news when the child was healthy at birth and continued to do well later. But if the investigations showed that the child was not affected by CZS and then the child did display health problems and developmental delays, because of her or his exclusion from the group of children with a confirmed Zika syndrome, the child could not benefit from special medical and socioeducational help provided by the state or by local health authorities.

The diagnostic odyssey of many parents of children with suspected Zika syndrome increased their confusion and anguish. In March 2016 the *New York Times* published a long interview with Germana Soares, of Pernambuco, a mother of a child with CZS. The article was accompanied in the web edition by a video that depicted the daily life of Soares and her family.[62] Unlike the majority of articles on mothers of babies with Zika syndrome published in 2016 in the Brazilian and the international media, which depicted poor women living in very difficult conditions, this interview presented an upwardly mobile couple. Germana Soares—who later became one of Brazil's best-known Zika activists—was a real-estate agent, and her husband was a welder on an oil rig. They lived in a house provided by the oil company and had a car, a large-screen TV, and private health insurance, which was important to Soares because it gave her access to quality hospitals and clinics and allowed her to avoid the overcrowded and understaffed SUS facilities. However, their comfortable middle-class lifestyle unraveled rapidly, which was not unusual in Brazil, where people born to established upper-class families generally hold on to their birth privileges, while the status of lower-class people tends to be more fragile. Soares's husband lost his job, and with it the family's private health insurance, and when her son developed serious health problems Soares was obliged to leave her work to dedicate herself to his care.

Another feature that distinguished the interview with Soares and her husband was visual: their son, Guillermo, did not look like a typical infant with severe microcephaly. The *New York Times* showed a cute baby with no external signs of impairment. Germana Soares's son was born with a near-normal head size, but because she knew that she had contracted Zika during her pregnancy, her child underwent additional tests, which revealed brain anomalies. It was not immediately clear, however, whether these anomalies and the child's health problems, such as convulsions and feeding difficulties, had been induced by Zika. Only after several months of tests, frequent visits to the hospital, and parents' vacillating between hope and despair, Guillermo was "officially" classified as having CZS. For Germana Soares and her husband, the long period of uncertainty about their son's diagnosis was one of the most distressing aspects of their experience.

In early 2016, Brazilian researchers' initial certainty that infection with the Zika virus had caused a microcephaly epidemic in northeastern Brazil was weakened. The difficulty of proving that a baby diagnosed with microcephaly indeed had CZS, or that a child who was born with a normal-size head but then developed health problems had this syndrome, left many families facing an undecided diagnosis and an uncertain future.

CHAPTER FOUR

Zika in Brazil

Producing Partial Knowledge

Did the International Response to Zika Let Women Down?

Scientists who wrote about the Zika epidemic in late 2016 and 2017 frequently stressed the important achievements of researchers and doctors who investigated this disease: the rapid display of the links between Zika and microcephaly; elucidation of the effects of ZIKV on fetal tissues; the construction of "genealogical trees" of the virus that made possible detailed studies of its migration from Africa to Asia, the Pacific Islands, and South America. Some experts have called impressive how much we know now about a virus practically unknown before 2013.[1] However, the *New York Times* journalist Donald McNeil, who followed the Zika epidemic from the very beginning and wrote a well-researched popular book about it, had a different opinion.[2] In early 2017 McNeil asked several renowned experts to evaluate progress on Zika. The majority of the interrogated scientists believed that the international response to the Zika epidemic, far from being an unqualified triumph, represented a series of missed opportunities for efficient sanitary intervention.

Some leading Western specialists at first showed little faith in data provided by their Brazilian colleagues, even though the latter were often internationally recognized experts on arboviruses. Dr. Peter J. Hotez, the dean of the National School of Tropical Medicine at Baylor College of Medicine, explained that the initial reluctance of the Centers for Disease Control and Prevention (CDC) to accept Brazilian scientists' results slowed the international response to the Zika outbreak. Even when the Brazilians found the Zika virus in two women's amniotic fluid and in the brain of a microcephalic fetus, "the

C.D.C. would not accept it until they had done it themselves," Hotez said. "I saw that as hubris." Dr. Albert I. Ko, a Yale epidemiologist who had worked for many years in Salvador, Bahia, and Dr. Ernesto T. A. Marques Jr., an infectious disease specialist at the University of Pittsburgh and the Oswaldo Cruz Foundation in Brazil, believed that Brazilian scientists and public health experts who had made a key contribution to the understanding of Zika epidemic felt let down when they looked for outside help. "The local researchers' role was mainly to collect samples," Dr. Marques said bitterly. The overall international response to Zika was, the experts interviewed by McNeil felt, at best a mixed bag. "The greatest failure, all agreed, was that while tourists were warned away from epidemic areas, tens of millions of women living in them—many of them poor slum dwellers—were left unprotected. . . . Trucks sprayed pesticides that often did not work. Admonitions from on high to wear repellent and long sleeves were given with no studies proving that they could protect indefinitely. And health authorities, fearful of offending religious conservatives, never seriously discussed abortion as an alternative to having permanently deformed babies—even in countries where abortion is legal." The response to the Zika epidemic in Latin America, McNeil concluded, had really let women down.[3]

Uncertainty as a Risk: Zika and the WHO

In early 2016, the Brazilian microcephaly epidemic had an uncertain status. Brazilian researchers, clinicians, and public health experts were persuaded that the significant increase in the number of children with birth defects was the consequence of an infection with the Zika virus during pregnancy. Many international experts agreed with this interpretation, even though some questioned the reliability of Brazilian data.[4] In January 2016 the *Lancet* published a collective text, signed by numerous leading epidemiologists and public health specialists, "Anticipating the international spread of Zika virus from Brazil," which strongly recommended the intensification of international research on the Zika epidemic.[5] This call might have influenced World Health Organization experts. On February 1, 2016, the WHO declared Zika a Public Health Emergency of International Concern (PHEIC).[6] In all probability the WHO, strongly criticized for the slowness of its response to the Ebola epidemic in 2014, aspired to avoid the repetition of its failure to rapidly recognize an important threat to public health. The international reaction to Zika, WHO experts argued, needed to be faster and smarter. Zika and Ebola were perceived as global health threats with potentially dramatic consequences. Yet, the two

PHEICs were different, not only because of important biological dissimilarities between these two pathologies but also because the reasons given for declaring Zika and Ebola as public health emergencies were not the same. There were no doubts about the presence of the virus Ebola in Guinea, Liberia, and Sierra Leone or the disastrous consequences of infection with this virus. The main reason given by WHO experts for defining Zika as a PHEIC was the uncertainty whether Zika indeed induced microcephaly. It was crucial, they explained, to rapidly assess whether an infection with Zika virus was a global threat and, if it was, what precisely the magnitude of the threat was. Zika was declared a PHEIC not to halt an immediate danger but to rapidly dispel health-related uncertainty.[7]

The declaration of Zika as a PHEIC transformed this disease from a Brazilian problem into an international one. While the declaration also mentioned an association between Guillain-Barré syndrome and the Zika virus, the main reason for the WHO's response was the risk of infection with ZIKV during pregnancy. The focus on this risk linked Zika with the knotty issue of women's reproductive rights, especially their right to decide whether to continue a hazardous pregnancy. The WHO elected to sidestep this issue. The PHEIC declaration was accompanied by the statement that "pregnant women who have been exposed to Zika virus should be counseled and followed for birth outcomes based on the best available information and national practice and policies." The expression "based on . . . national practice and policies" could have been interpreted as accommodating the repressive antiabortion policies of many Latin American countries. The WHO document mentioned in addition the importance of protecting people traveling to zones where Zika was endemic, the need to prepare health care systems in countries affected by Zika for a predicted increase in the number of children with severe neurological syndromes, and the key role of international collaborations and the sharing of data about Zika among all the researchers investigating this disease.

The declaration of Zika as a PHEIC was probably motivated by the fear that the Brazilian epidemic of microcephaly might spread to other parts of the world. Some experts believed that such fears were greatly exaggerated. Steven Hatch, a physician who in 2014 was involved in the control of the Ebola epidemic in central Africa, argued in March 2016 that the declaration of Zika as a PHEIC was a typical case of institutional overreaction, in this case to the accusations that the WHO had failed to efficiently respond to the Ebola epidemic. The current estimate, Hatch claimed, was that Zika might produce microcephaly in one live birth per thousand (0.1%), a number he probably had extrapolated from the early data on the prevalence of Zika in northeastern Brazil. These data, he argued, indicated that the threat of Zika-induced microcephaly was not greater than the threat of microcephaly induced by the most frequent cause of this inborn impairment in the United States, excessive alcohol consumption during pregnancy. Although thousands of babies with fetal alcohol syndrome–related microcephaly were born in the United States during the peak of the epidemic, public health authorities did very little besides issuing propaganda against alcohol intake by pregnant women. Such propaganda successfully persuades women with no alcohol-related issues that even a single drink when pregnant can have terrible consequences for their future child, but it does very little to help women with a real alcohol problem control their drinking during pregnancy. The implicit tolerance of children born with microcephaly induced by fetal alcohol syndrome contrasted with a strong reaction to a small risk of children born with microcephaly induced by Zika. The danger of Zika during pregnancy, Hatch concluded, was far from negligible, but it did not justify its declaration as a PHEIC.[8]

Hatch's estimate of one birth with Zika syndrome per 1,000 live births was decidedly low given the frequency of Zika syndrome in strongly affected areas of Brazil. Of children born in Salvador, Bahia, in December 2015, the highest point of the CZS epidemic there, 2.24% had significant brain anomalies; between April 2015 and June 2016, 0.34% of children born in Salvador were diagnosed with such anomalies. According to the data published in the Health Ministry's *Boletim Epidemiológico*, the frequency of Zika syndrome during the peak of the microcephaly epidemic in northeastern Brazil was 49.9 per 10,000 live births (0.5% live births).[9] The number quoted by Hatch, one in 1,000 live births (0.1%), was higher than the proportion of children born with confirmed Zika syndrome in Brazil as a whole (approximately 0.04% live births in 2015 and 0.03% in 2016), but in March 2016 Hatch had no way of knowing that other regions of Brazil would have a much lower incidence of CZS than the northeast.

Hatch's view was atypical. In the early stages of the epidemic the majority of international experts held a pessimistic view of the risks of Zika. In February and March 2016, many among them feared that Zika would produce in Latin America a generation of children with severe neurological anomalies. The first prospective study (a study following events as they unfolded) of the effects of Zika in pregnancy, conducted at the Instituto Fernandes Figueira, Fiocruz, Rio de Janeiro, reinforced the notion that Zika was indeed strongly linked with fetal malformations, as well as experts' apprehension. This study followed 42 women who had contracted a laboratory-confirmed Zika infection during pregnancy; they were then monitored through frequent ultrasound examinations. Researchers who conducted this study found that the fetuses of 12 of the women failed to develop normally: they displayed either anomalies of the brain or a "failure to thrive" (slower than normal growth in the womb). Two women in this group miscarried. In a matched control group—women who became pregnant at the same time but did not have symptoms of Zika—researchers did not observe anomalies of development of the fetus or miscarriages.[10]

The Rio de Janeiro study was an important step in the refutation of the argument that Zika was not responsible for the microcephaly epidemic, or more precisely, for the increase in the number of babies born with inborn impairments in Brazil in late 2015 and early 2016. The publication of its results in March 2016 amplified the fears that Latin America would face the challenge of caring for a generation of severely disabled children. The virologist Rivaldo Venâncio da Cunha argued in late February 2016 that the Zika problem had barely begun: Brazil was facing a "sanitary tsunami." Thirty years of failure to limit the spread of dengue fever in Brazil had shown that the existing methods of mosquito control did not work, while sanitary interventions had failed to halt the spread of diseases transmitted by *Aedes aegypti*. It was therefore likely that Zika too would become "naturalized" in Brazil and integrated into the national landscape, already rich in preventable disasters. It was not surprising that Brazilians, living in a country where 50,000 people were murdered every year, were not scandalized by 1 million cases of dengue fever each year with 1,000 deaths. They would probably learn to live with Zika too and adapt to a significant increase in the number of children born with neurological anomalies. Alas, da Cunha concluded, much more human suffering could be expected in the near future.[11]

Two well-known US experts from the National Institute of Allergy and Infectious Diseases, Antonio Fauci and David Morens, agreed with da Cunha's pessimistic evaluation, predicting that it would be very difficult to halt Zika's spread, especially in crowded urban areas.[12] A review article by Brazilian experts published in the *American Journal of Public Health* in April 2016 similarly stated that while it was not possible at the time to predict the number of microcephaly cases in Brazil or in other Central American and South American countries, things looked bleak.[13] Pessimistic evaluations of the potentially negative effects of the massive spread of Zika were reinforced by an observation published in June 2016 that some babies classified as normal based on their head size displayed severe neurological impairments several months later.[14] Since babies born with a normal-sized head escaped further epidemiological investigation, the number of children diagnosed with Zika syndrome, this article indicated, may have been underestimated rather than overestimated. Microcephaly, some Brazilian scientists feared in early 2016, might be but the tip of the iceberg in terms of the harm produced by infection with Zika virus during pregnancy.[15]

In the spring of 2016, pessimistic predictions about a rapid spread of the epidemic of inborn anomalies reached mainstream Western media. In November and December 2015, when the Brazilian media first reported the concentration of cases of severe microcephaly in northeastern Brazil, this subject, although widely covered in Brazil itself, received relatively little attention outside this country. In March and April 2016, Zika was omnipresent in newspapers and on television, mainly in emotionally wrenching images of babies with severe microcephaly and their mothers, often poor, non-white women from northeastern Brazil. A long article on Zika published in the British journal the *Guardian* in April 2016, entitled "On the frontline in Brazil's war on Zika," was accompanied by striking photographs. One photograph showed a baby with severe microcephaly held by a doctor; a second, a man in white protective gear that made him look like one of the sanitary workers who treated people with Ebola, approaching a poor neighborhood, probably in Pernambuco, with fumigation equipment; a third, a soldier inspecting a courtyard in another or perhaps the same poor neighborhood; and a fourth, a pool of stagnant water and heaps of trash in Linha de Tiro favela in Recife. The article described the two approaches to the Brazilian war against Zika: efforts to control *Aedes aegypti* mosquitoes and to rapidly develop research on Zika. Laboratory studies, the article stated, had already provided important information about this virus. Controlling mosquitoes was, however, very difficult, and in 2016 experts agreed that developing an effective vaccine against ZIKV, probably the best hope to limit the harm produced by this pathogen, might take many years. In the meantime, a rapid spread of Zika in Latin America could lead to the birth of tens of thousands of severely disabled children. In a few months, the *Guardian* article concluded, it would be clear whether Colombia and other Latin American countries affected by the Zika epidemic were also going to witness the birth of an unprecedented number of brain-damaged babies and whether the disease might also affect the southern United States and Europe.[16]

In 2015 and 2016, Zika-induced birth defects were concentrated mainly in northeastern Brazil. The geographic concentration of babies with Zika syndrome in the northeast became more evident when the introduction of a more stringent definition of microcephaly in March 2016 reduced the number of reported cases of microcephaly in central and southern Brazil. Initially the concentration of cases of inborn Zika syndrome in a single region was seen as an indication that the Zika epidemic in the Americas had started in that region. When Zika later moved to other parts of Brazil and other Latin American countries, experts expected the number of babies with CZS to rise there too. They also believed that unlike the relatively short Ebola epidemic, the Zika epidemic would last several years. Ebola's progress was stopped thanks to an efficient interruption of circulation to and from affected areas. It is more difficult to halt the circulation of mosquitoes. The persistence of obstacles to the control of other mosquito-borne diseases such as dengue and chikungunya foretold the difficulty of containing Zika. Epidemiologists estimated that the Zika epidemic would burn ou" in the end, but only when a sufficient number of people had developed immunity against ZIKV, a process that might take three or four years. In the meantime, the world needed to be prepared for the possibility of living with this epidemic and its potentially disastrous consequences for newborn children. Time would probably define the emergence of Zika, Enny Paixao and Laura Rodrigues affirmed in an editorial in the *British Journal of Hospital Medicine* in March 2016, as one of the decade's biggest personal tragedies and scientific challenges for international public health.[17]

The Puzzle of the Microcephaly Epidemic in Northeastern Brazil

In the spring of 2016, many publications about Zika in Brazil focused on a looming public health disaster. On the other hand, since mosquitoes are much less active in cooler weather, experts expected an important drop in new cases of Zika between June and October. Brazil hosted the Olympic Games in August 2016. The Brazilian government attempted to reassure potential visitors to the games, explaining that during the tropical winter the risk of being infected with the Zika virus was very low. The main exception was pregnant women or those who wanted to become pregnant: they were advised not to visit Rio. Participants in the games and tourists traveling to Rio for the games received detailed instructions on how to protect themselves from mosquitoes and the sexual transmission of Zika. Men who visited Rio for the Olympic games were also instructed to protect their female partners upon their return.

Exhaustive information about sexual transmission of Zika diffused to visitors to the Olympic Games contrasted with the paucity of information on sexual transmission of Zika available to Brazilians.

The Zika epidemic did not impede the Olympic Games. In hindsight, the games marked a turning point in the story of Zika in Brazil. After the games, Zika became much less visible in the Brazilian media. One important reason for its lower visibility may have been the severe political crisis that culminated with the impeachment of President Dilma Rousseff on August 31, 2016. Another reason may have been the decrease in the number of children born with CZS. Beginning in May 2016, epidemiologists noted a sharp fall in the number of children born with severe brain anomalies in northeastern Brazil. Physicians from Recife who in November and December 2015 had observed up to ten cases of severe microcephaly per week reported that during the tropical winter of 2016 they saw only one case per month. The decline in the frequency of CZS in northeastern Brazil was attributed to an earlier decline in the frequency of infection with the Zika virus. The Zika epidemic peaked in this region in the first half of 2015; CZS in newborns peaked nine months after ZIKV infections peaked.

On the other hand, the precise links between the prevalence of Zika and the birth of children with CZS were not always obvious. Zika outbreak in Brazil started in the northeast, then spread to many other regions of the country.[18] The reported frequency of Zika in some of these regions, such as the southeast and the central west, was similar to its reported frequency in the northeast.[19] Officially registered cases of Zika probably represented only a small portion of real-life encounters between humans and ZIKV. It is reasonable to assume that the majority of people with typical symptoms of Zika, such as a rash, conjunctivitis, and a low-grade fever, did not bother to see a doctor, while many others had a silent (asymptomatic) infection. But it is also reasonable to suppose that the reliability of epidemiological data collected in northeastern Brazil was not different from the reliability of the data collected in other regions. Yet, the reported frequency of confirmed cases of CZS in other parts of Brazil was much lower than in the northeast. Moreover, only a few among the babies diagnosed with Zika syndrome outside the northeast were affected by a very severe form of microcephaly that included a partial collapse of the cranium. The gradual increase in the number of highly unusual, visually striking cases of microcephaly played a key role in the initiation in October 2015 of an intensive search for possible links between Zika and the microcephaly epidemic.[20]

Some Brazilian researchers argued that the presumably puzzling concentration of cases of birth defects linked with infection with the Zika virus during pregnancy in northeastern Brazil was not mysterious at all. It could be explained by the particularly high number of people infected with Zika in that region in the first half of 2015, coupled with the fact that women from northeastern Brazil were, in the words of the anthropologist Debora Diniz, the "first generation of Zika."[21] Pregnant women of this "first generation" were unaware that a disease perceived as a minor nuisance was very dangerous for their future child. The Brazilian Health Ministry made its announcement about the dangers of Zika to the fetus in November 2015, while the majority of children with CZS in northeastern Brazil were born between September 2015 and February 2016. Thus, either they were born before the ministry's announcement or their mothers were already several months pregnant when they learned about the danger. By contrast, women who belonged to the second generation of Zika, those who became pregnant after November 2015, knew that the Zika virus was dangerous for the fetus. Since Zika reached other regions of Brazil several months after it hit the northeast, the majority of women in these areas, this argument goes, aware of the danger of infection with ZIKV, took protective steps, such as delaying pregnancy and avoiding mosquitoes. These protective steps, probably coupled with a somewhat lower frequency of Zika, are sufficient to explain why the prevalence of CZS in other parts of Brazil was much lower.

Other specialists rejected this explanation. They argued that while it contained accurate elements, it could not fully account for the exceptionally high concentration of cases of severe microcephaly in a small number of Brazilian states. In 2015 and 2016 the great majority (more than 80%) of the confirmed microcephaly cases were in the northeast. The difference between the first and second generations of Zika women cannot by itself explain the concentration of CZS in a single region, especially because women from lower socioeconomic strata in other parts of Brazil had limited opportunities to protect themselves from the consequences of infection with Zika virus.[22] Moreover, the Zika epidemic started in some parts of Brazil well before November 2015. In some states where the prevalence of CZS was relatively low, such as Mato Grosso, the Zika outbreak occurred almost simultaneously with outbreaks of this disease in states with the highest prevalence of affected babies, that is, Paraíba, Pernambuco, Sergipe, Bahia, and Rio Grande do Norte.

Researchers advanced numerous possible explanations for the concentration of cases of CZS in northeastern Brazil.[23] The first explanation suggested, and probably the most popular, was the intensity of the Zika epidemic in the northeast in the first half of 2015. The second was that the concentration of cases of CZS in that region reflected its great poverty. Poor women were more exposed to mosquitoes and might also have been more susceptible to infection with the Zika virus. A third possible explanation suggested was that vaccination with the yellow fever virus, a pathogen that belongs to the same family as ZIKV, protected against CZS, but the uptake of yellow fever vaccine in northeastern Brazil was especially low. A fourth possible explanation was that a simultaneous infection of a pregnant woman with Zika virus and dengue virus or with Zika virus and chikungunya virus might magnify ZIKV's capacity to harm the fetus. Such double infection was certainly possible in areas of high levels of circulation of all three viruses. A fifth explanation, a variant of the fourth, was that when a woman was first infected with dengue virus and later with the Zika virus, antibodies against dengue facilitated infection of the fetus with ZIKV. A sixth explanation linked a high probability of Zika-induced fetal anomalies with a co-infection of the pregnant woman by bovine diarrhea virus. Researchers also looked for possible environmental factors that might have potentiated the effects of ZIKV on the fetus. All these possibilities were thoroughly investigated by epidemiologists, but none were proven.[24]

The exceptionally high frequency of birth of babies with Zika syndrome in northeastern Brazil between October 2015 and March 2016 seems to have been an anomaly. Epidemiologists warned that Brazil should be prepared for a long war against this virus, but such a war did not occur either in Brazil or in other Latin American countries.[25] In early 2016, there was indeed an apparent increase in the prevalence of Zika, especially in northeastern Brazil. It was accompanied by a rise in the number of cases of Guillain-Barré syndrome but not by an increase in the frequency of CZS. Some experts proposed that the disease observed in this region in the tropical summer of 2016–17 was not Zika but chikungunya.[26] The clinical symptoms of the two diseases are similar, and both can cause Guillain-Barré syndrome, but chikungunya does not induce fetal anomalies. Other researchers argued that the presumed second wave of Zika in the northeast was not followed by a surge in the frequency of CZS because women successfully implemented preventive measures. Still other researchers proposed that in 2015 unknown amplifying factors increased the risk for the fetus in northeastern Brazil, whereas these putative factors no longer existed in 2016.[27]

The three hypotheses—that women delayed pregnancies and took precautions to avoid mosquito bites, that many cases of Zika were confounded with chikungunya, and that unknown amplifying factors aggravated the risk for fetuses during the first wave of Zika in the northeast—are not mutually exclusive. All could have contributed to the absence of a second wave of "microcephaly" in that region. Alternatively, the absence of a "second wave" of CZS in 2017 might have had a different yet unknown cause. In 2023 scientists still do not know why only a few babies with congenital Zika syndrome were born in Colombia despite the severity of the Zika epidemic in that country; one should add, however, that termination of pregnancy for a severe fetal anomaly was legal in Columbia. As the Brazilian Health Ministry publication *Zika Virus in Brazil: The SUS Response* stated in 2017, it was not clear why the Zika virus has been so cruel to Brazil, while sparing other Latin American countries.[28]

The high rate of birth of babies with brain anomalies in northeastern Brazil is but one among several Zika puzzles. Another, incompletely understood aspect of this epidemic is whether ZIKV was propagated exclusively by the *Aedes* mosquito or by other mosquitoes as well. Brazilian health authorities presented *Aedes aegypti* as solely responsible for the spread of ZIKV. A group of entomologists from Fiocruz, Recife, affirmed that other mosquito species, especially members of the widely diffused genus *Culex*, might have contributed to the rapid spread of the Zika virus in Brazil.[29] They claimed that they had been able to infect mosquitoes from this genus with the Zika virus in the laboratory but also to isolate this virus from *Culex* mosquitoes captured in the wild. Researchers from another group of entomologists, based at Fiocruz, Rio de Janeiro, strongly disagreed.[30] The infection of *Culex* mosquitoes with the Zika virus, they argued, was a laboratory artifact. The majority of specialists did not believe that *Culex* mosquitoes played an important role in the dissemination of Zika, but in 2023 this question is still partly open, as is the question whether the observation that the *Aedes* mosquito can be simultaneously infected with two different arboviruses is a mere curiosity, or whether such double infection can play a role in the propagation and severity of Zika.[31] Finally, the precise role of the sexual transmission of ZIKV in the spread of Zika and the rise of cases of CZS is still unknown.

Sexual Transmission of Zika: Brazil's Selective Blindness

The possibility of transmission of Zika through sexual contact, first postulated in the United States in 2008, was corroborated during the Zika outbreak in French Polynesia.[32] However, during the 2015–16 epidemic there was little evidence of sexual transmission of Zika in Brazil. Control of Zika was equated with control of *Aedes* mosquitoes, an attitude perhaps linked to the importance of efforts to curb yellow fever in shaping public health responses in Brazil.[33] Analysis of public health messages issued by the Brazilian government during the Zika epidemic confirmed the absence of references to sexual transmission of ZIKV, while interviews with women in northeastern Brazil and with their male partners confirmed the absence of information about sexual transmission of this virus.[34] Many Brazilian women attested that they had been unaware of the risks of transmission of Zika from an infected sexual partner, while some among those aware of this risk explained that they had been unable to persuade their partner to use a condom.[35] The paucity of information about the sexual transmission of Zika in Brazil may be contrasted with the widespread awareness of the importance of sexual transmission of this virus in Puerto Rico, where 83% of interrogated people mentioned the use of condoms as a way to protect themselves from this virus.[36]

The low visibility of sexual transmission of ZIKV in Brazil may be surprising in a country that circa 2000 was known for its effective control of AIDS and other sexually transmitted infections owing to the progressiveness of public health experts and their close collaboration with civil organizations such as homosexual groups and organized sex workers.[37] On the other hand, the efficient control of sexually transmitted pathologies in Brazil started to unravel in the second decade of this century, accelerated by the turn to the right in Brazilian politics.[38] The Zika epidemic unfolded against the background of the return of religious and political conservatism. In the new political climate, it might have been simpler to speak about controlling mosquitoes or women's individual responsibility to avoid mosquito bites than about the sexual transmission of Zika.

Another reason for the low visibility of sexual transmission of Zika might have been that many researchers assumed that this mode of propagation of ZIKV was important in northern countries, where in the absence of *Aedes* mosquitoes sexual contact was the only path of dissemination of this disease, but played a modest role, if any, in countries with a high density of *Aedes*. The centrality of the war against *Aedes* mosquitoes in public health interventions in Brazil in the twentieth century might have been an obstacle to viewing Zika as a sexually transmitted infection. The reluctance to examine the role of sex in propagation of ZIKV might have been further reinforced by health authorities' tendency to present Zika as a women's or mothers' problem, their potential reluctance to speak about male responsibility in infecting women through sexual contact, and women's disempowerment in heterosexual relations.[39] The supposition that sexual transmission did not play an important role in the transmission of the Zika virus in Brazil was, however, contested by some Brazilian researchers.[40] An indirect approach, a comparison between the reported prevalence of Zika and that of dengue in Rio de Janeiro in 2015 and 2016, these researchers claimed, revealed that while more women than men were diagnosed with dengue during that period, the difference between the sexes was not very big (approximately 30%). It was much greater (approximately 80%) in the case of the Zika diagnosis. Since the two diseases produce similar clinical symptoms, the comparison between reported rates of infection with Zika and dengue neutralized the obvious hypothesis that women, worried about the possibility of contracting Zika when pregnant, were more inclined than men to consult a doctor about a suspicious rash or fever. The most logical explanation for the higher incidence of Zika among women was the transmission of this pathology through sex. The authors of this study estimated that as many as 40% of Zika cases in Rio de Janeiro might have resulted from the sexual transmission of ZIKV. The same group studied the frequency of Zika in Rio de Janeiro in 2017, when this disease was less prevalent, and again found higher rates of infection with Zika among women than among men.[41]

Retrospective studies conducted in Brazil indicated that men who had many casual sexual relationships had a higher level of anti-ZIKV antibodies than did men who had few such relationships, confirming the potential role of sexual transmission in the propagation of Zika.[42] Retrospective epidemiological studies conducted in Puerto Rico and Brazil suggested that the role of sexual transmission of Zika might have been greater than previously assumed. These studies employed a direct approach, comparing the transmission of Zika (as attested by the presence of specific anti-ZIKV antibodies) among people who shared the same household but did not have sexual relations and those who did have sexual relations. Sexually involved couples, the researchers found, had a much greater chance of being infected with Zika than other persons living in the same household. No such effect was shown for chikungunya. The authors of the Puerto Rico study concluded that for a given couple, the risk of Zika transmission via sexual contact might be twice as great as the risk of being contaminated by a mosquito bite.[43] The authors of the Brazilian study—among them Brain Foy, the first researcher to describe a sexual transmission of ZIKV—explained that the *Aedes* mosquito was very efficient in transmitting chikungunya. The presence of one case in a given household was a good indication of the presence of other cases. By contrast, *Aedes* was less efficient in transmitting Zika. Only rarely did other people in the household of a person infected with Zika become infected too. The only exception was the sexual partner of the infected individual. Even if the *Aedes* mosquito had only a moderate capacity to disseminate ZIKV, this did not mean that once a given locality reached a high threshold of infections with this virus, its further propagation was accelerated through sexual relationships.[44]

Some researchers proposed, based on clinical observations and studies conducted in laboratory animals, that a disease produced through the sexual transmission of ZIKV was not identical to the one produced by the transmission of this virus by a mosquito bite, and it might have different consequences for the fetus.[45] ZIKV has a tropism for male and female sexual organs and can remain fixed in the female reproductive tract. Such fixation may be facilitated by its sexual transmission.[46] Studies in laboratory animals indicated that pregnant females infected with Zika through sex or the deposition of infected semen in their vagina gave birth to abnormal fetuses more often than those infected through a mosquito bite or a direct injection of Zika virus into their blood.[47] In areas with a high level of transmission of ZIKV, there might be not only a considerable risk of catching Zika virus from a sexual partner but an additional risk that this pattern of propagation of ZIKV might increase the probability of contamination of the fetus.

If sexual transmission increases the risk of ZIKV for the fetus, it may be especially important to protect pregnant women. Even if it does not increase the risk for the fetus, it may still be important to limit the danger of infection of pregnant women with Zika through sex. This is not an impossible task. Thanks to the widespread diffusion of pregnancy tests, many women know rapidly that they are pregnant. Other women "feel" that they are pregnant shortly after fertilization. Epidemiological studies indicate that the majority of mothers of children with CZS who recalled having Zika when pregnant contracted the disease at the end of the first trimester, and about a quarter of them recalled contracting it during the second or even the third trimester.[48] Moreover, some women reported that their partner had had Zika too. Pregnant women in epidemic zones were strongly urged to guard themselves against mosquito bites through the use of protective clothing and insect repellents. They and their male partners might also have been strongly urged to refrain from unprotected sex, especially during the early stage of pregnancy.

Another Sex-Linked Risk to the Fetus: Syphilis in Zika Times

Visitors to the Olympic Games in the summer of 2016 were warned about the risk of sexual transmission of Zika. The Brazilian sanitary authorities did not mention, however, the exceptionally high prevalence of another sexually transmitted infection harmful for the fetus, syphilis. While the Brazilian media amply covered the danger of ZIKV infection in pregnancy, the parallel danger of infection with *Treponema pallidum*, the etiological agent of syphilis, was seldom mentioned. One notable exception was an article published in August 2016 in an English-language web-based journal, *Quartz*, that explained that syphilis presented a much greater danger to pregnant Brazilian women than Zika. It pointed to the rapid increase in the prevalence of syphilis among pregnant women in Brazil and explained that the disease led to pregnancy loss, newborn deaths, and severe inborn impairments. The rise in the prevalence of syphilis was attributed to shortages in the supply of benzathine penicillin, the most effective drug for treating the disease; a decrease in the use of condoms, especially among young men; and the decline in the quality of prenatal care. Dr. Rosana Camargo, of the Brazilian Society of Infectious Diseases (Sociedade Brasileira de Infectologia), interviewed by *Quartz*, concluded that since syphilis was treatable, it was very sad that the occurrence of syphilis in pregnancy was so high.[49]

The prevalence of congenital syphilis (syphilis in newborns or stillbirths) in Brazil indeed increased greatly in the second decade of the twenty-first century. The *Boletim Epidemiológico Sífilis* of 2019 reported rates of 6.5 cases of congenital syphilis per 1,000 live births in 2015, 7.4 in 2016, 8.5 in 2017, and 9.0 in 2018.[50] In October 2017 the Brazilian Health Ministry started a national "Green October" campaign to increase awareness of risks of infection with syphilis and congenital syphilis. This campaign did not seem to have notable results, at least in the short term. The *Boletim Epidemiológico Sífilis* of October 2020 indicated that the frequency of syphilis and congenital syphilis decreased in selected Brazilian states but that the overall prevalence of the disease in Brazil continued to be very high, with an average of 8.2 cases per 1,000.[51] In 2019 the popular magazine *Veja* asked why cases of syphilis continue to increase in Brazil. Another article in the same magazine in 2020 stated that Brazil had 18 new cases of syphilis per hour, while information collected in the northeast indicated that data on the incidence of syphilis might be undercounted.[52]

The sharp rise in the incidence of syphilis in the second decade of the twenty-first century was paralleled by the decline in Brazil's efforts to contain AIDS. Circa 2000, Brazil's successful program for the prevention, detection, and cure of AIDS was perceived as a model for other middle-income countries.[53] But during the following decade Brazilian achievements in controlling AIDS were weakened by the decrease in funding from targeted international programs and the rise of religious conservatism.[54] Thanks to the solid support structures for HIV-infected people established in the late 1990s, in the second decade of the century Brazilian sanitary authorities continued to provide diagnosis and care to the majority of AIDS patients. The dramatic rise in the incidence of syphilis was probably a more sensitive indicator of the collapse of public health measures in the area of sexual and reproductive health.

The high prevalence of congenital syphilis in Brazil was explained mainly by the inadequate prenatal care in the public sector. According to Health Ministry data, in 2019 17% of pregnant women whose children were classified as suffering from congenital syphilis at birth did not receive any prenatal care, and only 27% of those who did receive such care had access to rapid syphilis testing.[55] Studies conducted in numerous Brazilian states confirmed that the high incidence of congenital syphilis reflected inadequacies of prenatal care in SUS hospitals and clinics. Many infected women were diagnosed only in the third trimester of pregnancy, and some were not diagnosed until birth. The increased frequency of syphilis in pregnant women led to high numbers of miscarriages and neonatal deaths, premature births, and neurological complications in children. Moreover, the sexual partners of the infected women were rarely identified and treated, a corollary of women's disempowerment. Consequently, even if a pregnant woman was successfully treated for syphilis, she had an elevated probability of being infected again by her partner.[56] Until 2014, northeastern Brazil had lower rates of congenital syphilis than other regions, but in the years 2015–17 the prevalence of syphilis in that region increased rapidly, an indirect indication of the declining quality of prenatal care at the time of the microcephaly epidemic.[57] With the advent of Zika, some families were affected by both diseases. Maria, who helps her daughter take care of a granddaughter born with CZS, reported that another of her daughters had just lost a fetus in the eighth month of pregnancy owing to congenital syphilis.[58]

The Failure to Develop Diagnostic Tests for Zika

The rapid rise and fall of the Zika virus left unanswered many questions about the epidemiology and pathophysiology of the ZIKV outbreak and its social consequences.[59] One of the main reasons for the persistent gaps in the understanding of the Zika epidemic was a failure to develop inexpensive and dependable diagnostic tests. The diagnosis of discrete and durable entities called "specific diseases," the historian of medicine Charles Rosenberg explained, became the foundation of modern scientific medicine. It played a central role in the rise of medical specialties, a new division of medical labor, the concentration of patients and resources, and the entry of powerful new actors in medicine, in particular public and private insurance providers. It also contributed to the rise of public health policies and knowledge: "The very possibility of modern epidemiology," wrote Rosenberg, "is in some measure dependent on standardized disease categories as employed in aggregate morbidity and mortality statistics and hospital and government statistics."[60]

Brazilian experts recognized as early as December 2015 the importance of reliable, inexpensive, and efficient diagnostic tests for Zika.[61] When the WHO declared ZIKA a PHEIC on February 1, 2016, one of the main goal was to develop a reliable and inexpensive test for ZIKV. This goal was not achieved during the peak of the epidemic in Latin America or in the following years. The Zika virus was first detected in Brazil in April 2015 via the reverse transcription PCR test (RT-PCR) to identify the virus. This method, accessible only in specialized laboratories, remained the primary method for detecting the virus during the Zika outbreak. Reliance on PCR technology effectively restricted the capacity to detect viral genetic material to a network of around 12 well-equipped laboratories across the country. Reagents to perform PCR had to be bought from foreign suppliers, at considerable cost: even major research institutions had to scramble to afford their purchase. After the declaration of Zika as an ESPIN on November 11, 2015, the Brazilian Health Ministry ordered that all suspected cases of ZIKV infection reported to the National Notifiable Disease Information System (Sistema de Informação de Agravos de Notificação, or SINAN) had to be confirmed through a PCR test. However, the national testing infrastructure struggled to cope with the rapid increase in demand for this test. Upper-end private hospitals developed their own in-house PCR tests, as did some blood banks concerned with the possibility of contamination of blood transfused through ZIKV, but these efforts remained sporadic and uncoordinated, and the data they produced were not included in the national system of epidemiological surveillance.[62]

Recognizing the urgent need for better, more accessible diagnostic tools, the Brazilian regulatory agency in charge of registering new commercial medical products, the Agência Nacional de Vigilância Sanitária (ANVISA), announced in January 2016 its willingness to fast-track applications for new Zika in vitro diagnostics, both molecular and serological. That same month, Fiocruz researchers announced the development of a new rapid molecular test capable of simultaneously detecting Zika, dengue, and chikungunya viruses. Fiocruz considered its new diagnostic an in-house test and therefore exempt from the standard regulatory review for market products. ANVISA disagreed, arguing that since the diagnostic was to be used in more than one laboratory, it could not be classified as an in-house test. Furthermore, because the Health Ministry would need to buy the test from Fiocruz before distributing it to other public laboratories, the test had to be registered with ANVISA before it could be legally procured. The latter view prevailed, and the test was subjected to a full review. It was finally accredited in December 2016, when the Zika epidemic had already receded. The Fiocruz test was also judged by some Brazilian virologists as less efficient than the foreign-produced tests.[63]

The status of serological tests—which were essential for epidemiological studies because they revealed past contact with ZIKV, while an RT-PCR test was positive only during the short time an individual had an active infection—was even more convoluted. The main obstacle to the development of an efficient serological test for Zika was the cross-reactivity of antibodies against ZIKV with those against other viruses, above all the closely related dengue virus.[64] In November 2015, when Brazil declared a national public health emergency, there was no test capable of detecting Zika antibodies. In January 2016, ANVISA authorized the use of the first serological test for anti-ZIKV antibodies, developed by the German firm Euroimmun. However, the cost of this test, around US$33 per unit, made it unsuitable for widespread adoption by SUS or for use in epidemiological surveys. In May, ANVISA approved the first Brazilian serological test for ZIKV, a rapid antibody test developed by the Bahia Foundation for Scientific Research and Technological Development (Bahiafarma). This test was described as a game changer in the Zika diagnostic landscape because it was four times cheaper than foreign commercial tests. In October 2016 the Health Ministry ordered around 3.5 million kits of the Bahiafarma test.[65] However, these kits did not arrive in health care facilities until January 2017, by which time the number of reported cases of Zika had declined dramatically. Moreover, the use of this test was soon hampered by claims of low sensitivity and insufficient accuracy. A similar test developed by Fiocruz's Immunology Technology Institute, Bio-Manguinhos, did not receive approval from ANVISA until April 2019, two years after the official end of the Zika epidemic.[66]

The patchwork of imperfect diagnostic capabilities meant that during the Zika epidemic in Brazil testing was expensive, sporadic, and often equivocal. This had immediate consequences for the production of reliable epidemiological knowledge. Pregnant women at risk of developing ZIKV-induced congenital abnormalities frequently had reduced access to accurate diagnosis in

SUS facilities. It was not unusual for women in some of the hardest-hit areas of the northeast to wait weeks or months for their RT-PCR results—if they arrived at all. In addition, the meaning of a negative result was often uncertain, given the short time the virus was present in the blood and the practical difficulty of detecting low quantities of RNA in blood or urine. The situation in the private health sector was different: pregnant women followed in private facilities had access to imported serological tests and had the possibility of employing a combination of several diagnostic methods to arrive at a more definitive conclusion about their status.[67]

In the absence of widespread testing, epidemiologists struggled to develop an accurate picture of the prevalence of Zika in different regions of Brazil.[68] Thus while Brazilian epidemiologists proposed that in 2016 Zika had been widespread in the majority of Brazilian states, an international group of epidemiologists and infectious disease modelers led by specialists from the London School of Hygiene and Tropical Medicine argued that the circulation of ZIKV had been largely restricted to the northeast, with 94% of an estimated 8.5 million total cases occurring in that region.[69] The publication of radically different estimates of the prevalence of Zika during the 2015–16 outbreak is evidence of the dearth of dependable epidemiological data. The question that led to the definition of Zika as a PHEIC by the WHO in February 2016, whether the Zika virus was responsible for anomalies in newborn babies, was quickly answered rapidly answered yes. By contrast, since it was difficult to know how many pregnant women were infected with ZIKV, there was no way to estimate the probability was that such an infection would lead to the birth of an impaired child.[70]

The Microcephaly Epidemic: Still Many Unknowns

The main consequence of the 2015–16 Zika epidemic was the birth of a significant number of children with CZS, but there are still no accurate data on their number. One of the main difficulties of studying the scope of the microcephaly epidemic was the initial exclusion of children with heads of "normal" size from further investigation. The choice of head size as the main criterion of possible Zika syndrome in a newborn was dictated by practical considerations: a measuring tape was available everywhere, while advanced diagnostic tests were not. This choice may, however, have hampered the detection of numerous cases of infection of babies with Zika. Prospective studies in which women in whom infection with Zika virus was confirmed early in pregnancy underwent numerous ultrasound examinations during pregnancy and then researchers investigated the fate of their children indicated that some among the children born with normal-sized heads nevertheless had health and developmental problems. Some of these problems appeared immediately after birth; others were revealed only later.[71]

Another difficulty was the variability of criteria employed to ascertain that a child who entered a Health Ministry–sponsored investigation because of his or her smaller than average head size had a "confirmed" case of Zika syndrome. Such criteria combined, in different proportions, data from laboratory tests; clinical findings; data produced by medical imaging, such as brain scans; and self-reported information about the mother's infection with Zika during pregnancy.[72] Brazilian states varied in their definitions of confirmed Zika syndrome. In some states, such confirmation had to include evidence of structural changes in the brain, while in others evidence of brain anomalies was not obligatory for confirmation of a diagnosis of CZS. An additional problem was the varying quality of laboratory tests and diagnoses based on medical imaging, as well as, for some of those tests, the absence of nationwide standards of good clinical practice or imperfect implementation of such standards. All these elements might have affected the official diagnosis of CZS. The percentage of investigated babies who received such a diagnosis was not very high. According to the Health Ministry data, 24.4% of the babies investigated in 2015 and 16.5% of those investigated in 2016 were finally classified as "confirmed" cases of CZS.[73] The ministry did not provide data on the "discarded" babies; it is difficult to know how many among them continue to have health and developmental issues.

The variability of definitions of confirmed microcephaly in a child might have led to the inclusion in this group of children with microcephaly or brain anomalies produced by other causes and the exclusion of children with birth defects produced by the Zika virus. Some experts who evaluated suspected cases might have tended to provide a less stringent definition of Zika syndrome so that more families of children with developmental problems could gain access to resources allotted for the use of children with confirmed Zika syndrome. By contrast, researchers who collected data on Zika syndrome in the framework of clinical trials might have favored a stringent definition of CZS. The use of more restrictive criteria made sure that they studied only children with birth defects induced by Zika and therefore produced an accurate knowledge about Zika syndrome. The use of a stringent definition of Zika syndrome by these researchers might have been facilitated by the fact that they usually had access to resources of leading teaching hospitals. They were thus able to perform advanced diagnostic tests, such as magnetic resonance imaging (MRI).

The observation that different professional groups define a given disease or condition differently was made as early as 1929 by the pioneer of social studies of science, Ludwik Fleck. Fleck gave an example of epidemiologists and bacteriologists who studied an outbreak of scarlet fever. Bacteriologists, interested in fundamental research on this disease, provided very stringent bacteriological criteria for the classification of suspected cases as scarlet fever and excluded all borderline cases (high specificity) because they wanted to be absolutely sure that they included only "true" cases of scarlet fever in their study and thus produced dependable scientific knowledge on the disease. Epidemiologists, interested above all in halting the spread of an infection in a given locality, provided a much broader definition of scarlet fever that included all the borderline cases (high sensitivity). It was better, they believed, to impose an unnecessary quarantine on some children than to risk an infected child's contaminating many of her or his peers.[74] How to define a "true" disease or condition was, Fleck argued, far from a purely academic problem. It had important consequences for research, clinical practice, public health interventions, and people living with the consequences of these interventions. It was important to remember, however, that such a definition was produced by a specific group of professionals and reflected their training, opinions, goals, and the means at their disposal.

In Brazil, the difficulty of deciding whether a given child had Zika syndrome mirrored shortages of public funds for diagnosis, monitoring of patients, medical and paramedical care of the affected children, and financial help for their families. In a resource-rich and socially progressive environment, all the children born during an epidemic would have been thoroughly evaluated for signs of inborn anomalies, and all, including those declared "normal" at birth, would have been carefully monitored for additional problems in infancy. And in such an environment all the families with children with developmental difficulties, whatever their cause, would have received appropriate medical, educational, and financial support. Brazil is proud of many accomplishments of its National Health Service, especially in areas such as primary care, but it is far from being a resource-rich environment. The coincidence of the Zika epidemic with a severe economic and political crisis amplified the difficulty of proving adequate care to all the children with developmental delays and favored a focus on a single, highly visible subgroup of such children.[75]

The decision to provide the state's help only to children with confirmed CZS was problematic because whether Zika was the only cause of the epidemic of microcephaly in Brazil remained an open question. After an initial period of doubt, practically all the experts agreed that infection with the Zika virus was a key cause of the sharp rise in the number of microcephaly cases in 2015–16. Nevertheless, some researchers argued that some of the microcephaly cases observed during that period might have had a different cause. Zika syndrome was confirmed in only 23% of the children investigated for microcephaly in 2015 and in 22% in 2016. The cause of small head size in "discarded" children was frequently unclear.[76] A Latin American Collaborative Study of Congenital Malformations (ECLAMC) text published in the fall of 2017 affirmed that between 2005 and 2014 the prevalence of microcephaly in Brazil more than doubled and that this phenomenon was especially visible in the northeast.[77] In 2015–16, the advent of Zika led to an additional, sharp increase in the prevalence of microcephaly in this region, from 0.106% to 0.5%. But if this information on the increase in the number of children born with small heads in northeastern Brazil before the Zika outbreak is accurate, it is possible that additional elements aggravated the microcephaly epidemic in that region.

Epidemiologists who conducted a longitudinal survey of changes in birth defects in two Brazilian municipalities, one in the center-south region (in the state of São Paolo) and another in the northeast (in Maranhão) had independently confirmed the existence of a "silent epidemic of small heads" among Brazilian babies. The authors of this study extracted from the data they collected in 2010 information about the prevalence of microcephaly in the surveyed sites. They found a higher prevalence of severe microcephaly among children of women from lower socioeconomic strata, especially evident in the northeastern municipality. The most likely explanation of the observed higher prevalence of severe microcephaly in women from the lower classes, they proposed, were undetected infections during pregnancy (numerous infections can lead to smaller head size in newborns). Undetected infections might have mirrored the shortcomings of prenatal care in resource-poor settings.[78] They might also have accounted for the elevated proportion of children with inborn neurological impairments who failed to be officially diagnosed with CZS.[79]

Microcephaly epidemic is an emotionally loaded term. The declaration of an ESPIN by the Brazilian government on November 11, 2015, and the definition of Zika as a PHEIC on February 1, 2016, were probably reactions to fears of a rapid extension of a scary phenomenon. Epidemics are almost by definition frightening events.[80] An outbreak of birth defects is even more likely to produce anxiety. The study of fetal impairments was originally called *teratology*, that is, the science of monsters. During the outbreak of Zika in Brazil and its aftermath, researchers accumulated an impressive amount of knowledge on the Zika virus itself—its history, its properties, its circulation worldwide, and the physiological effects of an infection with this pathogen—but there is still no satisfactory explanation of the phenomenon that led to the investigation of links between Zika and fetal anomaly, namely, the very high concentration of cases of severe CZS in northeastern Brazil.[81]

CHAPTER FIVE

Stratified Reproduction

Class, Ethnicity, and Risk

Men, Sex, and Zika

Zika was presented in Brazil as a women's problem. Women were instructed to protect themselves from mosquito bites and to delay pregnancies. They were also seen as responsible for cleaning their houses and keeping them mosquito-free.[1] Sexual transmission of Zika was presented as a problem that concerned mainly male visitors to Brazil, who, if infected with ZIKV, could contaminate their female partners.[2] Few initiatives aimed to increase women's awareness of the risk of transmission of Zika through sex. One of the rare sites of diffusion of information on this topic was a small-scale initiative, the campaign "More Rights, Less Zika," conducted by the United Nations Population Fund (UNFPA) in Pernambuco.[3] Messages elaborated by this campaign were diffused on community web radio, TV stations, and social media. One of its more imaginative aspects was the mobilization of young, often Afro-Brazilian artists to propagate the campaign's message. A song by the popular funk group Dream Team do Passinho, "The Mosquito Is Not the Only One to Blame," pointed to men's responsibilities during the Zika epidemic:

> You gotta be aware
> You gotta take care
> Zika in the quiet water
> Zika at the time of love
> She felt like getting pregnant
> More rights, please
> The mosquito is not the only one to blame

So take care of whom you love
Use the condom
Don't take Zika to bed
Black girl who got pregnant in the favela with no sanitation
And the baby with microcephaly
His father got away quickly . . .
The world must be ready to support whoever needs it
So, let's go get together for more rights, less Zika.[4]

It was not clear how effective the song was. According to a representative of one of the main groups involved in the UNFPA program, the Recife-based Grupo Curumim, the Passinho song took the country by storm and encouraged people to talk about the sexual transmission of Zika with the campaign's agents. Other reports about the efficacy of this song were less upbeat. The representative of Gestos, another nongovernmental organization based in Recife, claimed that the song was popular mainly in the southeast of Brazil and few people in the northeast were aware of it. More to the point, studies of the Zika epidemic in Brazil indicate that the efforts of small groups of activists notwithstanding, the overwhelming perception was that Zika was a women's problem, first for those who might get pregnant and then for the mothers of children with CZS, whose fathers "got away quickly."[5]

"Democratic" Mosquitoes and Selective Pathology

Children with CZS were born mainly to lower-class, non-white women. This fact was emphasized by the media, especially foreign, social sciences publications on this topic, but also by associations of mothers of children with Zika syndrome, who employed it to justify their demand for special state support for their children. The concentration of children with CZS among poor women was often explained by their greater exposure to the disease-carrying mosquitoes. Mosquitoes do not respect boundaries, whether between countries, states, or neighborhoods, and when they have an opportunity , they will bite any human being they come across. The key point is that they will do so *when they have an opportunity*. Mosquitoes have fewer opportunities to multiply in affluent areas, and people who live in these areas have more possibilities to protect themselves from insect bites.[6] This may be even more true in the case of the "domesticated" *Aedes aegypti*, found mainly within and near humans' habitation. Moreover, *Aedes* is a day mosquito. Mosquito nets, effective in shielding people from the *Anopheles* mosquito, the vector of malaria, cannot protect people from *Aedes*.[7] Diseases disseminated by the *Aedes* mosquito, such as dengue fever and chikungunya, affect all the social classes but are more frequent among inhabitants of poor neighborhoods. Zika was no exception to this rule.[8]

One of the first articles about the Brazilian Zika epidemic to appear in a major medical journal, a short text, "A new mosquito-borne threat to pregnant women in Brazil," published in the *Lancet* on December 23, 2015, affirmed that all 40 women from Pernambuco who gave birth to children with microcephaly between August and October 2015 belonged to low-income families.[9] Later data confirmed that there was a strong link between CZS and social class. Thus approximately 97% of children with "microcephaly" in Pernambuco were born in public hospitals, while middle-class women very rarely gave birth in SUS hospitals.[10] When the Zika epidemic in northeastern Brazil became a hot topic in the Brazilian and foreign media in early 2016, articles, videos, and reports presented the plight of mothers of children with severe microcephaly: nearly all were poor, Black or Brown. But not all. The Zika activist Germana Soares, although not white, could have been described as middle class (according to the US definition of this term), at least before she and her then husband lost their jobs. The same was true for several women depicted in the documentary *Zika, the film*, made by ANIS in late 2015, and some of the mothers active in organizations that defend the rights of children with CZS. Still, activists and health professionals agree that the great majority of children with CZS were born to women of color from low socioeconomic strata.[11]

Epidemiologists who studied children born with CZS in northeastern Brazil confirmed that the majority of these children had been born in deprived neighborhoods.[12] One study indicated that in the early stages of the microcephaly epidemic a few children with Zika syndrome were born in middle-class neighborhoods of Recife. Later, with the elucidation of the link between Zika and birth defects, it was determined that all the children with CZS had been born in the less affluent parts of the city.[13] Class and ethnicity differences in the distribution of Zika syndrome in newborns were often attributed to differences in the probability of a pregnant woman being bitten by an *Aedes* mosquito. Middle-class and poor Brazilians often occupy distinct "ecological niches," especially in cities. Middle-class people frequently live in high-rise buildings (*Aedes* usually cannot fly higher than four floors) and, especially during the tropical summer, spend their time in climatized spaces—apartments, workplaces, cars, upper-end shopping centers. (Climatization make it possible to keep the windows closed, so that mosquitoes cannot enter.) The lower classes live in areas with blurred boundaries between inside and outside, as well as poor sanitation. Consequently, they often share their living quarters with the "domesticated" *Aedes* mosquito.[14]

The poor also are less likely to use repellents to protect themselves from mosquito bites.[15] Manufacturers of repellents saw the Zika epidemic as an excellent commercial opportunity. They increased the publicity for their products and hiked up their prices. The repellent Exposis, developed by the Brazilian army and considered to be especially effective, was sold in São Paolo for 46 to 100 reais a bottle (US$10 to $24); despite its step price, it was heavily purchased by middle-class women.[16] Affluent pregnant women, especially those in the most affected areas of Brazil, were also reported to move abroad temporarily or to southern Brazil. The Brazilian government decided to purchase a protective antimosquito repellent and distribute it to women who received monthly financial support through the Bolsa Familia program, but the distribution of this repellent did not begin until November, a year after the declaration of Zika as an ESPIN, when the prevalence of Zika and CZS had already greatly decreased. Moreover, two months later the Brazilian Federal Court of Accounts ordered the Health Ministry to conduct additional laboratory tests of the repellent because some experts believed that the high concentration of its active component made it unsafe for pregnant women.[17]

The argument that poor women in northeastern Brazil were at higher risk of giving birth to children with CZS because their living conditions exposed them to *Aedes* bites is probably correct. That it is a sufficient explanation for the exceptionally high concentration of CZS among lower-class women is less certain. Poor women were at much greater risk of giving birth to children with this condition than of contracting other mosquito-borne diseases—dengue fever, Zika, chikungunya.[18] Experts therefore proposed additional, nonexclusive explanations. One explanation was that poverty increased susceptibility to infections. Poor nutrition, poor general health, and chronic stress can impair immune mechanisms and weaken the body's response to viruses. In a pregnant woman, it may increase the probability of transmission of a pathogen to the fetus.[19] A second explanation was that poor women were more likely to be infected with more than one pathogen, which might have increased the risk of ZIKV infection of the fetus. It is thus probable that not only was a pregnant woman from a lower socioeconomic level more likely to be infected with ZIKV but such an infection might have more dramatic consequences for her than it would for a middle-class woman.[20] The third explanation was that women from lower social strata were not sufficiently informed about the Zika risk in pregnancy, and for those who *were* sufficiently informed the possibilities for avoiding the risk were limited.[21]

The last explanation linked the risk of giving birth to a child with CZS to a woman's capacity to control her sexuality and reproduction. In 2015 and 2016, lower-class women had few options for reducing their risk of giving birth to a child with CZS. To understand why that was the case, it might be easier to examine the skewed distribution of CZS cases by asking how middle-class women were able to reduce the probability of having a severely impaired child. The truly interesting question may not be how poverty harmed women but how privilege protected a specific segment of middle-class women, those of reproductive age. Such protection relied on a combination of several approaches. Each approach was imperfect, but together they were effective. One important means of protecting middle-class women from Zika was an especially strict avoidance of mosquitoes. Women who were pregnant or who thought that they might be pregnant avoided mosquito-infested places and used high-quality insect repellents. In a hot climate, it is very uncomfortable to wear long pants and long-sleeved blouses outside climatized areas. During the tropical summer, the period of maximal activity of *Aedes* mosquitoes, middle-class women could limit their time in nonclimatized zones and therefore were able to wear protective clothing. A rigorous avoidance of mosquitoes was combined with other protective means: control of fertility to prevent unwanted pregnancies or to delay wanted ones; prevention of contamination with Zika through sex, especially of women who were pregnant or suspected they might be; testing for ZIKV infection during pregnancy, especially in the first trimester; checking for brain anomalies of the fetus in the second trimester of pregnancy; and access to a safe abortion. Poor women had very limited access to these multiple layers of defense against the consequences of infection with the Zika virus. They were less well protected against the risk of giving birth to a child with CZS, but also against the stress and fear generated by the awareness of such a risk.

Women Who Control Mosquitoes: Community Health Workers

On the local level, the elimination of *Aedes* mosquitoes is delegated to community health workers (*agentes comunitários de saúde*). Control of mosquitoes is but one of many activities of the community health workers, a body of nearly 300,000 lower-level SUS workers. Their task is to serve as a bridge between the health system and its users, particularly the most marginalized and vulnerable among them. Their responsibilities include the elimination of *Aedes* breeding places, but also other health promotion activities—keeping records of individuals and families in their area; making regular household visits to monitor the vaccination of children; scheduling appointments with specialists; and teaching the correct use of medication. Community health workers are predominantly (more than 75%) female and are often recruited from the communities in which they work. They have at least nine years of education (the majority graduated from a public high school), do not need to have formal training, and are hired with a great variety of contracts, temporary or permanent. Their salary is lower than that of the mostly male endemic disease control agents (*agentes de combate a endemias*), who specialized in targeted campaigns to eliminate disease vectors.[22] The mainly male disease control agents were direct heirs of the long tradition of yellow fever control, considered an exemplary Brazilian public health success. The mainly female community health workers did not benefit from such a prestigious heritage.

Community health workers are expected to identify all the sites where mosquitoes can breed. They check vacant lots and trash deposits, verify that empty bottles are turned upside down, garbage bins and bags are securely shut, and plant pot saucers contain sand to prevent water from accumulating there. They are also expected to fill out detailed checklists during the household visits, a tradition probably inherited from the RF-controlled Yellow Fever Service of the 1920s and 1930s. Their situation is highly ambivalent. They may be close to the poor women they supervise and are occasionally seen by them as "friendly police." On the other hand, because of their multiple surveillance tasks, community health workers may also be seen as partly hostile street-level bureaucrats. Moreover, their ability to make a difference within their areas of intervention is very limited, while the heavy paperwork can increase their frustration and accelerate their burnout. In many sites, community health workers may be aware of the limited effectiveness of their antimosquito interventions, which may increase their ambivalence about their work.[23]

While the official task of community health workers is to mediate between SUS institutions and the users of SUS services, they are not expected to express their own opinions. Thus they are not involved in decisions on how to organize mosquito control in the areas where they work. This was true during the Zika epidemic too. Community health workers remained practically invisible during the discussions about efficient ways to contain Zika.[24] In early 2016, the Brazilian government decided to increase the scale of antimosquito intervention through heavy spraying of insecticides, an approach perceived by many experts as having a strong symbolic value (showing the government or the municipality taking a spectacular action) but a weak practical effect (if larvae were not eliminated, the mosquitoes would come back after a short time). This more visible antimosquito intervention was conducted by civilian men, vector control agents, and soldiers. Photographs of men dressed in futuristic combinations and masks and carrying spraying equipment became symbols of the fight against Zika. There were no photographs of female community health workers patiently searching for mosquito breeding sites.

André Novais Oliveira's 2018 film *Temporada* (A Season; the English title is *Long Way Home*) is a poignant, fine-grained portrait of a community health worker, Juliana.[25] Juliana leaves a small town, Itaúna, in the interior of Minas Gerais state, to become a community health worker in a bigger town in the same state, Contagem, a satellite city of the state's capital, Belo Horizonte. The film shows her arrival at a new place and her integration into a group of sanitary workers, mostly, like her, lower-middle-class, non-white women. Upon her arrival, Juliana receives rudimentary instructions from female low-level bureaucrats, a vest, and a bag bearing the service's logo, and she is assigned a fixed inspection area. At the end of each day she is expected to fill out numerous forms, but in the work she performs she does not seem to be supervised. The film shows Juliana walking through modest neighborhoods of Contagem, visiting houses and gardens, sometimes alone and other times with a coworker. The image of Juliana leisurely chatting with people (mostly women) who live in the houses she inspects is very different from that of the uniformed male agents of the Yellow Fever Service in the 1930s, whose job was to police the inhabitants and punish transgression. On the other hand, while Juliana and her colleagues dutifully strive to fulfill their inspection tasks, the film strongly hints that their work can have at best a modest effect on the density of *Aedes* mosquitoes and that neither slogans nor the modest work of community health workers will solve the *Aedes* problem.

Zika and Stratified Reproduction: Contraception

The term *stratified reproduction* points to the key role of differences in class, race, ethnicity, religion, or citizenship status in defining women's capacity to control their reproduction and the conditions under which they perform their maternal and care tasks. This term was initially proposed to describe the contrast between the situations of affluent North American women and the immigrant nannies who take care of their children. These immigrant women frequently have children of their own, left in the care of their families while they seek work abroad. Economic circumstances force them to abandon their children to take care of those of other women. The nanny's inability to be a good mother contrasts sharply with her employer's ability to "have it all"— motherhood, a fulfilling job, and free time. The term *stratified reproduction* was later extended to include other kinds of reproductive injustice: the difficulties of women from lower socioeconomic strata to control their fertility because of obstacles to the use of efficient contraceptive means and, in many settings, limited access to abortion; violence against women; and fragile sexual health.[26] This term also includes differences in women's access to medically assisted reproduction, and to quality pre- and postnatal care. Reproduction is stratified because it is not merely a biological event but also, to an important degree, a socioeconomic one.[27]

One possible reaction to a frightening epidemic that threatened pregnant women was to delay pregnancy until after the threat disappeared. In the winter of 2015–16 the US Centers for Disease Control and Prevention and the Pan American Health Organization, or PAHO, advised women to postpone planned pregnancies. Facing the prospect of an epidemic of severe birth defects, the Brazilian government as well as countless health professionals repeated this advice. Cláudio Maierovitch Henriques, the director of infectious disease surveillance at the Health Ministry, told women in November 2015: "Don't get pregnant now. This is the soberest advice that can be given." Although the ministry denied that this recommendation represented official policy, the same advice was conveyed publicly by many policymakers, including the minister of health, Marcelo Castro, who on November 18 declared to the newspaper *Folha de São Paulo* that "sex is for amateurs, pregnancy is for professionals." Women, Castro explained, should be responsible for their pregnancies, and those who were pregnant should be especially careful—hinting that individual women should be charged with preventing births of impaired children.[28] The Frente Parlamentar da Saúde, an influential group of deputies in the National Congress, issued similar advice: "Whoever is planning to have a baby now should postpone that plan."[29]

Health care professionals and feminist activists strongly criticized an approach that put the onus of reducing the burden of the Zika epidemic on individual women.[30] They also pointed out the incongruity of calls for a "responsible maternity" in a country where more than 50% of pregnancies were unplanned.[31] The Zika epidemic, the activists argued, was an especially telling example of the neglect of pathologies that disproportionally afflicted poor populations, exposing the persistent geographies of inequality. Instead of making poor women responsible for eliminating mosquitoes from their environment and accountable for the birth of children with Zika syndrome, the state should provide clean water for all, eliminate trash heaps, and improve sanitation in impoverished neighborhoods.[32] Activists' protests again holding women accountable for the birth of children with CZS were undoubtedly justified. On the other hand, an exclusive focus on the state's failure to implement structural reforms that could have limited the density of *Aedes* mosquitoes in poor neighborhoods was problematic. In late 2015 and early 2016, Brazilian sanitary authorities faced an emergency and multiple unknowns. In such a situation it was not entirely unreasonable to propose that women delay pregnancies, at least until the nature and the magnitude of the Zika risk was better understood. But when such advice was not accompanied by concrete steps to help lower-class women control their fertility, it merely made visible the gap between the haves and the have-nots.[33]

Statistical data from Brazil indicated a 20% decrease in the number of pregnancies in 2016. This sharp drop in fertility may have reflected women's decision to postpone pregnancies, induced abortions, spontaneous miscarriages induced by ZIKV infection, reactions to a severe economic crisis, or a combination, in unknown proportions, of all of these. It is nevertheless reasonable to assume that the main reason for this drop in childbirth in Brazil in 2016 was a voluntary restriction of fertility through contraception and induced abortion, because in 2017 the fertility rate in Brazil returned to its previous level despite the continuing economic crisis.[34] There are no accurate epidemiological data on the distribution among social classes of the decrease in fertility in 2016. Social scientists discovered that in 2016 Brazilian women of all social classes attempted to avoid pregnancy, but only upper-class women successfully controlled their fertility. While lower-class women were also aware of the risks of Zika for the fetus, only a small fraction among them used contraception to delay pregnancy.[35] Data provided by Women on the Web, an organization that provides a safe combination of abortion pills, indicate that in 2016 this organization saw an important increase in the Brazilian demand for its services, which it attributed to the Zika epidemic.[36]

The Brazilian National Health Service, the SUS, provides contraceptive means to women who wish to use them. Poor women have more limited access to reliable birth control, however, and are seldom free to seek the contraceptive method that best fits their body and their needs. Moreover, they face obstacles, such as the costs of transportation to health care clinics; limited access to reliable information about the full range of contraceptive methods;

reduced possibility of obtaining the contraceptive means of their choice; and difficulties in obtaining guidance from professionals in primary care clinics. A Health Ministry protocol in March 2016 that outlined guidelines for the health care system's response to "a Zika-related microcephaly epidemic" discussed women's right to be informed about risks of Zika in pregnancy and the use of contraception, but the ministry did not acknowledge the specific difficulties faced by poor women who wish to postpone pregnancy and did not suggest concrete steps to reduce such difficulties.

Visiting a SUS clinic to obtain contraceptives, sociologists and anthropologists reported, could be a distressing and occasionally humiliating experience.[37] Women who visited public clinics for contraception advice complained about a lack of privacy. They described staff joking and gossiping about the clinic users or revealing out loud the results of pregnancy tests. The fear of stigma and violation of privacy was exacerbated by the fact that the clinic workers commonly lived in the same community as their patients. Women explained, "We go to the public clinic and everybody will know about your life. Why didn't I go there when I lost the baby? If I went there, then the whole place would know, 'oh, that little girl is already a woman [no longer a virgin]. . . . Clinics are full of gossipy women. As for your pregnancy test. You are sitting there: instead of calling you inside the room, they call you out loud and say: here it is, go there and pee here [showing the container to be used]. Then, they give you a huge paper and say out loud: go to the reception and schedule your prenatal care."[38]

Women from lower social strata were occasionally blamed for their "irresponsible" behavior: "So, when I went to the clinic, the nurse turned to me there and said, 'For God's sake, why did you get pregnant now?' I said: 'Okay, but is it any problem for me to get pregnant now?' She said: 'Because we have a mosquito problem there and we are in the focus area.' Then I said: 'How so?' She said: 'You're going to have to wear a lot of long sleeves, long pants and whatever, and repellent, because Zika virus is this and that, it can happen this way, so with the baby, etc.' I said, 'My goodness!'" This in principle sound advice was very difficult to follow for women who did not have access to air conditioning. As another woman explained: "I did not wear long sleeves . . . how could I walk covered in this heat?"[39]

Sexual Transmission of Zika

During the Zika epidemic, Brazilian health authorities rarely, if ever, discussed risks related to the unequal power dynamics in intimate relationships, especially for women from lower socioeconomic strata. Such unequal power relationships hampered the women's capacity to protect themselves from unwanted pregnancies and the sexual transmission of the Zika virus. When it became generally known that the Zika epidemic presented a threat to newborns, men often saw this as a women's problem. They were reluctant to help their female partners to control their fertility or to reduce the risk of contracting Zika through sexual contact. Some women suggested that their partner's indifference stemmed from the fact that ZIKV had largely been portrayed by the Brazilian Ministry of Health as an illness that was transmitted by mosquitoes and affected pregnancy, not as a sexually transmitted pathology.[40]

Low-income women who participated in focus groups in Recife explained, "Men don't worry! Men only want sex. And the silly [girls] are giving in." They added that Zika had not changed the behavior of men they knew. One low-income woman reported, " I talked to my partner [about Zika being sexually transmitted], . . . but he categorically refused [to use a] condom, calling it 'that plastic.'" Another woman added that there was no information on the sexual transmission of Zika; all the posters showed only mosquitoes or women. "I didn't see anything about that; that fathers and husbands who intend to have children should be careful with Zika not to transmit it to their partners through sex. At no point was there talk about that. . . . When men hear at length that Zika causes microcephaly, then they create a barrier in their minds that they don't need to protect themselves, because it's all about the baby." Recife women in a high-income group agreed that their male partners were not concerned about Zika and dislike sex with condoms, but they added that when a woman insisted that she did not want unprotected sex, she got her way.[41]

Feminist organizations, such as the nongovernmental organization Grupo Curumim, based in Recife, attempted to fill the void left by the absence of official support for women's sexual and reproductive rights.[42] Activists from this group pointed to the double social injustice of putting the onus of responsibility for the birth of children with Zika syndrome on women and the absence of state interventions that might have helped women from less privileged social strata to better control their fertility. The Curumim group distributed educational materials about contraception, such as leaflets, and posted information on its website. Such information often specifically targeted young women. Curumim also collaborated with the UNFPA's campaign "More Rights, Less Zika."[43] Curumim was one of the few organizations that disseminated information about the sexual transmission of Zika. During the Zika epidemic Curumim opened a hotline that provided information on reproductive and sexual rights, especially in the context of Zika. On the other hand, Curumim is small, and its intervention had a limited scope. To amplify its reach, the group organized a seminar—"Contraceptive Methods and the Prevention of Sexually Transmitted Diseases during the Zika Epidemic"—in Goiânia in October 2017. One of the main topics discussed in the seminar was the total absence of public health interventions directed toward men. Health Ministry protocols for testing pregnant women for Zika did not mention their male partners, and there were no attempts to inform men that they could transmit Zika through sex or even to persuade them to be tested for the presence of the Zika virus.[44] Curumim continued its effort to protect women against Zika after the epidemic disappeared from the news, and in January 2019 it issued a "Summer Alert" poster that explained that Zika was a sexually transmitted disease.[45]

Zika and Stratified Reproduction: Abortion

Friday, Dr. Adriana Melo, an obstetrician and pioneer of studies of congenital Zika syndrome in newborn babies, told a BBC journalist, had become the day of the week she dreaded most because that was the day she performed ultrasound scans on women infected with the Zika virus during their pregnancy. Women in her waiting room were terrified. The majority were reassured to learn that the ultrasound image of their future child was normal. But in some cases the fetal head was small and the brain looked abnormal. Afraid to receive a diagnosis of a severe anomaly, some women elected to avoid altogether ultrasound examinations during pregnancy.[46]

In late 2015 and early 2016 many Brazilian women found themselves pregnant—and terrified. The Zika epidemic raised the issue of abortion for the risk of fetal impairment. This was a general problem in Latin America, where abortion is criminalized in the majority of countries. During the Zika epidemic, the thorny issue of abortion rights was carefully avoided by most international organizations, with one notable exception: in April 2016 the Pan American Health Organization, in the document *Zika Ethics Consultation: Ethics Guidance on Key Issues Raised by the Outbreak,* clearly stated that a woman's capacity to make reproductive decisions based on her beliefs, values, situation, and concrete reality should include the option to terminate a pregnancy.[47] On the other hand, while pregnant middle-class women who were afraid they had contracted Zika had access to diagnostic tests to detect the presence of this virus, poor women who relied exclusively on SUS services had very limited access to such diagnostic tests.[48]

With the sole exception of those who participated in prospective clinical trials of ZIKV risk, Brazilian women who relied on SUS services seldom had an opportunity to undergo a diagnostic ultrasound (*ultrassom morphológico*), which could reveal severe anomalies of the fetal brain as early as 18–20 weeks of pregnancy. The WHO's guidelines of May 16, 2016, on pregnancy management in the context of the Zika epidemic state that "regardless of a history of illness consistent with Zika virus infection, all women in areas of ongoing Zika virus transmission should be requested to have a fetal anomaly scan between 18 and 20 weeks or at the earliest possible time if the first visit occurs after 20 weeks."[49] However, when the Brazilian Ministry of Health allocated resources to state and municipal secretaries to increase the access of women at risk of Zika infection to diagnostic ultrasounds, such funds were earmarked for tests performed in the seventh month of pregnancy.[50] Municipal and state authorities confirmed that they had hired or trained sonographers or gynecologists to perform diagnostic ultrasounds at 30 to 35 weeks of pregnancy, that is, well beyond the threshold of fetal viability.[51]

The debate on abortion in Brazil was strongly influenced by the contradictory effect of, on the one hand, the very negative image of women who "eliminate their babies" (*tirar o bebê*) and, on the other hand, the high number of induced terminations of pregnancy. Women who had abortions might be against abortions in general and feel guilty about having had one. Eva, a single mother of a daughter with CZS (and four other children), who had an abortion before having her disabled child, recalled that "after I had the abortion, I suffered a lot. What had I done to a child that hadn't done anything? I was going to go mad, even after I had the abortion. Then I held on to God, I held on to God, my life improved. I got pregnant again, then I thought: 'My God! It was a punishment.' What I did . . . I took out my . . . so, you know, I killed my son. God gave me another one."[52]

The debate over whether abortion after infection with the Zika virus during pregnancy should be decriminalized in Brazil revolves around two distinct configurations, each raising a different set of questions. In the first configuration, a pregnant woman contracts Zika early in pregnancy and wants to have an abortion because she feels unable to continue the pregnancy knowing that the fetus may die in the womb or be born with an unknown degree of impairment. In this configuration, abortion is justified mainly by the pregnant woman's stress and mental suffering (a maternal indication for termination of a pregnancy). An argument against abortion in such a case is that it may lead, especially if the risk for the fetus is not very high, to the elimination—for the opponents of abortion, the killing—of a great number of unaffected fetuses.

In the second configuration, a pregnant woman, typically in the second trimester of pregnancy, learns during a diagnostic ultrasound that the fetus has a severe brain anomaly and is persuaded that the birth would lead to insurmountable difficulties for the child, herself, and her family. In this configuration, abortion is justified mainly by the predicted consequences of the birth of a severely disabled child (a fetal indication for the termination of pregnancy). An argument against abortion in this case is that it might be understood as an indirect statement that people with disabilities have no right to live or as a selfish decision of a woman who rejects her moral obligation to take care of her child.

In the early stages of the microcephaly epidemic in Brazil, in late 2015 and early 2016, Brazilian media, as well as professional publications, debated whether women who contracted Zika during pregnancy should be allowed to have an abortion. At that time, the understanding of Zika was strongly shaped by fear. The combination of alarmist data on the rapid rise in the number of children diagnosed with microcephaly published in the Health Ministry weekly *Boletim Epidemiológico* and the frightening images of children with severe microcephaly that regularly appeared in the media was highly unsettling. Women were afraid to get pregnant, and those who found themselves pregnant were afraid to continue the pregnancy. Women or the experts who advised them could not know that the number of children born with Zika syndrome in Brazil was already declining; it had diminished since April 2016. They also could not know that the risk of giving birth to a child with Zika syndrome was much higher in northeastern Brazil than in other parts of the country. Many women who found out that they were pregnant, especially, but not exclusively, if they suspected that they might have been infected with Zika, wanted to end their pregnancy. In the face of women's acute distress, some physicians, social scientists, and activists openly called in early 2016 for the liberalization of Brazil's restrictive abortion laws. It is highly probable that many women indeed elected to terminate their pregnancy at that time, although there is no way to quantify a possible increase in the frequency of illegal abortions.[53]

Medical experts and social scientists who contributed to a special issue of *Cadernos de Saúde Pública* in May 2016 on women's reproductive rights during the Zika epidemic noted that the guidelines issued in the Health Ministry protocol of March 2016 did not mention dangers associated with an illegally terminated pregnancy. Affluent women, afraid to have a child with CZS, could have a safe abortion, while poor women risked their health, indeed their lives, by having unsafe ones. The Health Ministry's protocol failed to acknowledge the realities faced by these women and their right to make their own reproductive choices. It was time, several texts published in the special issue of *Cadernos* stated, to put end to such blatant social injustice and the hypocrisy around this topic and start an honest debate on abortion laws in Brazil.[54] In February and March 2016, several Brazilian personalities, such as the ex-minister of health José Temporao and the physician and TV personality Drauzio Varella, strongly criticized the fact that a safe abortion was freely accessible only to affluent women and stated that the Zika epidemic had exposed the fundamental injustice of the situation. The criminalization of abortion, Varella stated, punished women who had no money.[55] However, in mid-2016, when the worst fears about a rapid propagation of the epidemic of microcephaly in Brazil had receded, debates on the legalization of abortion disappeared from the media. Fear of Zika opened between January and April 2016 a window of opportunity for wider support for the decriminalization of abortion, but it was closed again in the (tropical) winter of 2016. This development was privately bemoaned by more liberal Brazilian doctors as a missed opportunity.

The early 2016 debate about the legitimacy of abortion for a woman who contracted Zika when pregnant may recall the 1950s and 1960s debates on the possibility for a woman who contracted rubella early in pregnancy and had, therefore, a high risk of giving birth to a disabled child to terminate her pregnancy. In 1941 an Australian ophthalmologist, Norman Gregg, observed a link between congenital blindness and infection with the rubella virus during pregnancy.[56] Gregg's observations were rapidly confirmed and extended by other physicians. In 1947, the US pediatrician Douglas Murphy, author of an influential textbook on congenital malformations, argued that women infected with the rubella virus early in pregnancy should be allowed to legally terminate the pregnancy.[57] This point of view was adopted by many doctors, especially in Europe. UK physicians estimated that infection with the rubella virus produced major fetal malformations in 10 to 20% of the affected pregnant women, and probably an early pregnancy loss in many others. Some physicians believed that such risk was not sufficient to justify abortion; many others held the opposite opinion.[58]

In her widely debated 1959 paper on rubella and abortion, the British pioneer in medical genetics Julia Bell, of the Galton Laboratory, University College, London, stated that "now the facts of the situation have accumulated so that one can state without doubt that rubella in the early weeks of pregnancy is such a menace to the normal development of the fetus that it constitutes a risk one cannot allow to be taken for the unborn child."[59] Answering her critics, Bell added that the problem of birth defects induced by infection with the rubella virus is at the same time individual and collective: "There are three main aspects of this problem, concerned with (a) the risks of a severe handicap to the unborn child, (b) the risks of acute distress and difficulty for the potential parent, perhaps for the rest of her life, (c) the burden likely to rest upon the Welfare State. I appreciate the difficulty in deciding certain cases, but these must be very rare and do not touch the main problem."[60] Bell explained in 1959, that is, ten years before the decriminalization of abortion in the United Kingdom, that women at risk of fetal malformation induced by infection with the rubella virus very often had an abortion. "To such an extent has this become a routine treatment," she wrote, "that maybe we can no longer hope to get a measure of the risk involved, or discover what proportion of such occurrences can be expected to result in a normally developed child."[61]

In the 1960s, obstetrical ultrasound was in its infancy. There was no way of knowing whether infection with the rubella virus affected the fetus. The main reason why doctors in the United Kingdom and France agreed to women's demands to have an abortion if they contracted rubella was their conviction that a woman should not be forced to continue a pregnancy when they were terrified about its issue. "There is widespread agreement," the British obstetrician Bevis Brock, of St. Bartholomew's Hospital, London, wrote in 1959, that "when a pregnant mother, having had rubella, is aware of the risks and is prepared to face them, then no one would try to persuade her to accept termination. But if she feels unable to face the appalling anxiety of a pregnancy overshadowed by fear of a blind or deaf child, then it requires strong convictions to refuse this request." Brock's statement was grounded in his own experience. "As a father of a boy trebly handicapped following maternal rubella I would ask only that we do not adopt a too rigid attitude to this problem, that we treat each mother who finds herself in this situation as an individual problem, and that we do not allow statistics to blind us to what we are asking of these patients."[62] In the 1950s and 60s, despite the criminalization of abortion, British and French women infected with rubella who wanted to end their pregnancy were nearly always able to find a physician who would perform an abortion, in the majority of cases in a public institution.[63] Brazilian doctors, unlike their British counterparts, did not openly admit that they helped women who wanted to end a pregnancy because they feared giving birth to a severely impaired child. It is nevertheless reasonable to assume that physicians provided such a service, and that they provided it mainly to women who could afford to pay for it.

Other women who feared the birth of a child with CZS might have elected to undergo a risky abortion method.[64] Leticia Marteleto and her colleagues conducted focus groups among low- and high-income Brazilian women to study their reproductive intentions and their behavior during the Zika epidemic. They discovered that many women had been ready to have an abortion following infection with the Zika virus. As one low-income woman explained, "My friend got pregnant right at the top of the Zika epidemic. She said she was going to do the ultrasound and if it was positive, she would take the baby out. I said: oh, don't do that! And she said: Do you know what it feels like to have a child like that for the rest of your life?" The woman who told her friend's story added that her friend's words had given her the courage to admit that she too was in favor of abortion in such circumstances. Another low-income woman testified, "Many of my relatives took the tea. Pinga [a local alcoholic drink] with that stink flower, Aarruda [common rue]. Or they stick in mamona [*Ricinus*]." Another woman explained, "I got the Pau Brasil [Brazilian native tree] around here, cut down the bark, made the tea and smoke"; she had an abortion but later developed severe health problems. Unsurprisingly, while women from the low-income group told harrowing stories about abortion, those from the high-income group were convinced that if necessary, they would be able to find a doctor who would perform a safe abortion. Middle-class women believed that they would be able to reduce their risk of giving birth to a child with CZS through contraception, the use of a condom by a sexual partner, or an abortion. Those from lower-income groups were less confident of their ability to be in charge and more afraid of Zika.[65]

Juridical Struggle over Abortion in Zika Times: ADI 5581, Habeas Corpus 124.306, and ADPF 442

In early 2016 experts feared that the microcephaly epidemic, already intense in northeastern Brazil, would rapidly spread to other parts of the country. They also suspected, on the basis of early data, that a woman infected with Zika during pregnancy might have an elevated risk of giving birth to a severely disabled child.[66] On August 24, 2016, the National Association of Public Defenders, ANADEP (Associação Nacional dos Defensores Públicos), together with the ANIS Institute of Bioethics, a human rights organization linked with the University of Brasília, submitted a petition to the Brazilian Supreme Court (Supremo Tribunal Federal, STF) asking for a change in the law that would allow women infected with Zika virus during pregnancy to end the pregnancy in order to protect their mental health. Infection with this virus, the petition explained, exposed pregnant women to intense mental suffering produced by the uncertainty about the fate of their future child. Such suffering could be described as psychological torture; therefore, forcing women to continue their pregnancy under these conditions violated their fundamental rights.[67] The right to abortion following a ZIKV infection was only one of the demands of the petition ADI (Ação Direta de Inconstitucionalidade) 5581. The petition included other demands too, such as prevention and educational campaigns about the Zika risk; rehabilitation for children with CZS in centers in close proximity to the homes of the affected children; training of health professionals to care for CZS children; increasing the availability of prenatal examinations; and offering women long-term, reversible contraceptives. Another demand of ADI 5581 was a permanent state pension, the Benefício de Prestação Continuada (BPC), the equivalent of one monthly minimum wage (in 2016, 880 reais, approximately US$260), to all children with congenital Zika syndrome.

From the very beginning of the Zika crisis, conservative Brazilian politicians strongly resisted calls to decriminalize abortion laws as a possible answer to this crisis. Thus on February 16, 2016, a National Congress member from Pernambuco, Anderson Ferreira, introduced a bill that would increase sentences for women who had abortions because of fears of microcephaly or other fetal anomalies.[68] Unsurprisingly, in a long document published on September 16, 2016, Rodrigo Janot Monteiro de Barros, attorney general of Brazil, rejected the claims developed in ADI 5581 as unproven, and as going beyond the legal limits of an ADI.[69] After the initial hearing, the Supreme Court adjourned debates on ADI 5581 numerous times; the final hearing took place in 2020.[70] In April 2019 the Brazilian Senate discussed the possibility of the Supreme Court legalizing abortion for risk of microcephaly. Several senators strongly opposed this. They evoked the evil of "eugenic abortions" and the (presumed) severe psychological harm of termination of pregnancy. Senator Eduardo Girão quoted a "US research" of 2004 that had shown that 77.9% of women who "destroy their baby" deeply regret this act and feel guilty for the rest of their lives, while 55.9% among them stated that part of them died following the abortion. Many among these women, he claimed, became depressed and alcoholic and abused drugs; they were also at a high risk of suicide.[71]

During the four-year interval between the initial and final hearings on ADI 5581, two other important events shaped the debate on abortion in Brazil: Habeas Corpus 124.306, which discussed the legality of early terminating a pregnancy, and debates on ADPF (Arguição de Descumprimento de Preceito Fundamental, or Argument of Noncompliance with a Fundamental Principle) 442, a petition submitted to the STF in March 2017 asking for formal decriminalization of early abortion by the court. ADI 5581 was submitted in August 2016, shortly after the Supreme Court unexpectedly declared in favor of decriminalization of first-trimester abortion. At the time, the court was considering a seemingly unrelated case. The owners of an illegal abortion clinic in the town of Duque de Caxias, in the state of Rio de Janeiro, had complained of unfair treatment by a lower court. They had been arrested in a police raid of their clinic on March 14, 2013, before the October 2014 Operation Herod in Rio de Janeiro. The Duque de Caxias raid led to the arrest of five employees of the clinic, a policeman who acted illegally as the clinic's security guard, and a young woman who recruited new clients. Four women who were at the time undergoing a termination of pregnancy at the clinic were detained too. One, bleeding heavily, was taken off the operating table; she needed urgent medical help.[72] The arrested employees submitted a habeas corpus petition to the Supreme Court protesting that their long detention had been illegal. The habeas corpus was not related to the Zika epidemic, nor was it directly linked to the accusation that the clinic had performed abortions: the accused did not contest the fact that their activity was illegal. Nevertheless, the STF's verdict stated that an abortion up to 12 weeks of pregnancy should not be criminalized.

The main author of Habeas Corpus 124.306 was the progressive justice Luis Roberto Barroso, who before being named to the Supreme Court had been a well-known human rights lawyer. The document, published on August 9, 2016, and officially ratified on November 29, 2016, is an impressive defense of abortion rights. It declares:

> It is necessary to construe Criminal Code articles 124 to 126—which define the crime of abortion—following the Constitution, resulting in the exclusion from its scope of the voluntary termination of pregnancy carried out in the first trimester. The criminalization, in this case, violates several fundamental rights of women, as well as the principle of proportionality. The criminalization is incompatible with the following fundamental rights: the sexual and reproductive rights of women, who cannot be forced by the State to maintain an unwanted pregnancy; the autonomy of women, who retain the right to make their own existential choices; the physical and psychological integrity of the pregnant woman, who is the one that suffers the consequences of pregnancy in her own body and mind; and gender equality, given that men do not get pregnant and,

therefore, it is necessary to respect the woman's will on this matter to achieve full gender equality. Beyond these considerations, we must add the impact of criminalization on poor women. The treatment of abortion as a crime, provided for by Brazilian criminal law, prevents these women, who do not have access to doctors or private clinics, from turning to the public health system to obtain the appropriate procedures. As a consequence, cases of self-mutilation, serious injuries, and death multiply. . . . Finally, virtually no developed and democratic country in the world considers the termination of pregnancy during the first trimester a crime, including the United States, Germany, the United Kingdom, Canada, France, Italy, Spain, Portugal, the Netherlands, and Australia.[73]

Habeas Corpus 124.306 accepted practically all the arguments of advocates of the liberalization of abortion in Brazil. It is not surprising that external observers drew a parallel between this document and the *Roe v. Wade* verdict of the US Supreme Court in January 1973, which legalized abortion in the United States.[74] However, unlike the verdicts of the US Supreme Court, STF decisions are not binding (*súmula vinculante*) unless the judgment explicitly states otherwise. Legislators and judges are free to consider them—or not. Habeas Corpus 124.306 was virulently attacked by conservative members of parliament as a license to murder children in their mothers' wombs.[75] As a consequence, Brazilian legislators and judges elected to reject its recommendations. This led in turn to the initiation of a specific juridical action in favor of a binding decision of the Supreme Court to legalize abortion.

On March 6, 2017, ANIS, together with the left-wing party PSOL (Partido Socialismo e Libertade), submitted to the Supreme Court ADPF 442, which explicitly requested the decriminalization of abortion before 12 weeks of pregnancy.[76] This initiative was supported by Brazilian feminist organizations. The PSOL parliament member and law professor, Luciana Boiteux, one of the lawyers who submitted this petition, explained that while she is aware of the fact that the conservative political climate is not unfavorable to abortion rights, it is precisely in such moments a window of opportunity for progress may arise.[77] The public Supreme Court hearing on ADPF 442 was conducted in August 2018. The plea for the legalization of early abortion was presented by STF judge Rosa Weber, known for her liberal views; she had also been one of the main supporters of Habeas Corpus 124.306.[78] The hearing was conducted in a very charged atmosphere. Supporters and opponents of abortion clashed in the traditional and social media, and militants for abortion rights, such as Debora Diniz, received death threats.[79] The hearing became a public display of the tensions around the abortion question in Brazil. There were powerful testimonies of specialists and laypeople in support of both sides.[80] The tribunal then adjourned its verdict.

The long trajectory of ADI 5581 ended in failure. At the April 24, 2020, plenary session the Supreme Court unanimously rejected the petition and declared that a woman infected with the Zika virus during pregnancy could not terminate the pregnancy because of mental anguish. The STF accepted the argument of the Advocacia Geral da Union (Public Defender's Office) that decriminalizing abortions of women infected with the Zika virus during pregnancy would be a retrograde move that would make possible a eugenic selection of human beings of the kind performed by the Nazi regime in Germany. Allowing abortion in such cases would open the doors to decriminalization of abortion for other fetal anomalies. The court's opinion took effect on May 1, 2020.[81] The Union of Catholic Jurists of Rio de Janeiro presented the verdict as an important victory. Raphael Câmara, a conservative obstetrician at the Federal University of Rio de Janeiro, explained that when an attempt had been made in 2016 to allow abortion in Zika cases, little was known about the virus, but "since then, we have answers to many of the issues raised in ADI 5581 in support of allowing abortion. . . . Recent studies show that fetuses of infected mothers are affected only 5 to 14% of the time, and the majority have mild problems only. . . . In addition, a study recently released by the Center of Disease Control (Atlanta) showed that 73% of Brazilian laboratories are unable to provide a reliable diagnosis of an infection with the Zika virus." The request to allow abortions for women infected with the Zika virus, Câmara concluded, was therefore meaningless: "We cannot talk about a woman 'infected by Zika,' but rather 'may be infected by Zika.' It is unacceptable to kill fetuses on the basis on such inaccurate diagnosis."[82]

In the summer of 2023 the STF had not yet decided the fate of ADPF 442. Brazilian activists were encouraged by the legalization of early abortion in Argentina, an important victory of Argentinian feminists. Nevertheless, there was an important difference between the struggles to decriminalize abortion in Brazil and in Argentina. In Argentina, feminists and health professionals constructed powerful networks that provided practical help to women who wished to terminate a pregnancy.[83] The struggle of Brazilian feminists was conducted in the courts, the parliament, and public spaces, but with a handful of exceptions, it did not include offering practical help to women who wished to terminate their pregnancy.

A Difficult Subject: Zika and Late Abortion for a Fetal Anomaly

The debate on ADI 5581 ended in 2018 with a rejection of the proposed motion. The one on ADPF 442 continues (in early 2023). The decriminalization of abortion up to 12 weeks of pregnancy, demanded by ADPF 442, would not, however, solve the problem of Zika-related anomalies detected during the pregnancy. Abortion for a fetal indication, especially beyond the first trimester of pregnancy, is a very difficult choice. Yet, in countries in which an abortion is legal, many women have made this choice. Experts who studied the Zika epidemic in French Polynesia explained that they had failed to notice a rise in microcephaly or brain anomalies following the epidemic because many women who had received a diagnosis of a severe brain anomaly of the fetus had elected to end the pregnancy. When Brazilian physicians linked the epidemic of microcephaly in northeastern Brazil with infection with the Zika virus, their colleagues in French Polynesia reviewed their epidemiological data, which included abortions for a malformation of the fetal brain, and realized that French Polynesia also had had an epidemic of microcephaly.[84]

Brazilian media in early 2016 debated the legalization of abortion for the risk of Zika syndrome. There was no parallel debate on the legalization of abortion of a fetus already diagnosed with a brain anomaly. Social scientists presented testimonies of women who said that their doctors had suggested to them, and occasionally pressured them, to have an abortion following a diagnosis of ZIKV-induced fetal anomaly. A Recife woman told the anthropologists Rosamaria Carneiro and Soraya Fleischer that "the doctors wanted me to do an abortion. They offered the abortion option, saying that the child would not be born, that if it was born, it would vegetate, etc. I did not want this at all. They said, 'You don't want this? So you are crazy.' They told me that I was crazy, and they called a psychologist to convince me. It was my child! I wanted my child. During the ultrasound exam, I was looking at that baby; I saw he/she had a finger in the mouth. I said, 'Look, he/she has a finger in the mouth, that is so beautiful!' The woman doctor looked at me, and thought that I was crazy. She said that I was crazy, that I needed the professional help of a psychiatrist. Just because I was observing the ultrasound exam, seeing my child, admiring him/her in my belly." Another woman also reported that her doctor had insisted that she should terminate a pregnancy with a brain-impaired fetus and saw her refusal to do so as irrational. She was dismayed and hurt by their cruel and unfeeling attitude. Still, another woman reported that she "saw two abortions, one was a baby with micro, where she saw the professionals wrapping the dead child up in a cloth. And taking advantage of the anesthetized state of the mother, made her sign a term of consent making the stillborn available for study."[85]

Accounts of women who learned that they were carrying an anencephalic fetus, as the study of Iulia Fernandes attests, revealed that some doctors treated with disrespect "irrational" women who refused an abortion for anencephaly.[86] Testimonies collected by anthropologists who relied on women's willingness to tell their stories might, however, be biased. Since abortion is viewed in a very negative light by many Brazilians, a woman who resisted a proposal to terminate a pregnancy might have been eager to share their negative feeling about this proposal, while a woman who decided to end a pregnancy with an impaired fetus might have been unwilling to talk about it.[87]

A major difficulty when dealing with CZS-induced fetal anomalies is the timing of the abortion. Unlike the highly teratogenic rubella virus, which induced fetal anomalies in the majority of the women infected early in pregnancy, the Zika virus induced such anomalies in only a small fraction of the infected pregnant women (estimates vary between 1% and 15%; their variability reflects the lack of reliable diagnostic tests for Zika). It may make sense for a woman infected with ZIKV early in pregnancy to delay the decision about an abortion until she knows whether the fetus is affected. But because the Zika virus attacks the central nerve system, anomalies it induces become evident only relatively late in pregnancy.

The late diagnosis of Zika syndrome in the fetus, several physicians argued, was a major obstacle to an abortion following a diagnosis of brain anomaly. This statement needs to be qualified, however. Microcephaly—which often became shorthand for Zika syndrome in the newborn—is indeed often visible only in the third trimester of pregnancy, and except in extreme cases its severity is not easy to determine before birth. It is also not a very reliable prognostic sign. By contrast, microcalcifications and major changes in the structure of the brain can be diagnosed by a competent ultrasound expert earlier, usually in the middle of the second trimester (at 20–24 weeks). Prenatal diagnosis of brain anomalies is not 100% reliable. Scientists estimate that about 10% of children born with ZIKV-related microcephaly and microcalcifications (although usually not the most severe ones) develop normally later and that a similar percentage of ZIKV-exposed children who do not display brain anomalies at birth develop neurological impairments in the first year of life. Still, an 80–90% risk of severe neurological impairment is very high. In France, interdisciplinary ethics committees in hospitals usually agree to late termination of pregnancy when the estimated risk of a serious intellectual impairment is more than 10%. If the second-trimester diagnostic ultrasound of a Brazilian woman treated in the private sector reveals suspicious changes in the brain, she often undergoes additional tests, such as magnetic resonance imaging.[88] A woman who knows that she had contracted Zika when pregnant and then learns that the fetus's brain looks perfectly normal cannot be sure that her child will not have CZS, but a woman who learns that the fetus displays important brain anomalies can be almost certain that her child will have serious neurological problems. However, the majority of pregnant women treated in SUS clinics had no access to reliable diagnostic tests that could confirm infection with ZIKV or to ultrasound and MRI diagnosis of anomalies of the fetal brain.[89]

International organizations such as the WHO carefully avoided mentioning abortion when discussing Zika, whether for risk of anomaly or for an already diagnosed anomaly.[90] The topic of abortion is especially fraught because of the objection of disability rights associations to "eugenic abortion." The PAHO document of April 2016, the only statement of an international organization that explicitly affirmed women's right to terminate a pregnancy because of the risk of Zika, justified this right on the basis of the "significant mental anguish about reproductive issues that women experience during the Zika virus outbreak." It therefore seems to refer, as did ANIS's petition to the Brazilian Supreme Court, to the mental suffering induced by the unknown risk of anomaly rather than to abortion following a diagnosis of an anomaly.[91] If abortion in general was the elephant in the room in many debates on Zika, an abortion for an already confirmed fetal impairment was a creature the size of a blue whale.[92] In August 2018 a symposium on Zika, part of the ABRASCO meeting, gathered together scientists, epidemiologists, public health experts, social scientists, and representatives of associations of mothers or parents of children with CZS. The two days of discussions between professionals and activists led several months later to publication of a detailed "chart of recommendations" for dealing with Zika and CZS. One of the recommendations was to improve prenatal diagnosis, especially to test all pregnant women for infection with Zika at the beginning and the end of pregnancy (recommendation 4-B) and to perform a quality ultrasound examination of every pregnant woman, especially in areas of a high prevalence of arboviruses (recommendation 4-D).[93] In the absence of a possibility to terminate a pregnancy for a fetal indication, it is not clear what the goal of the diagnostic ultrasound will be. As one WHO official stated, "If the use case is to diagnose and treat, then for Zika it was really—how can I say—a borderline issue. Because if you want to diagnose a woman with Zika in pregnancy, what are you offering? Are you offering abortion? Are you offering a solution? This is where everybody freezes again. They don't want to discuss this matter. We have to avoid the discussion."[94]

Abortion, Expressivist Objections, and Emotionally Charged Narratives

Debora Diniz is a dedicated and courageous advocate of women's reproductive rights in Brazil. Nevertheless, probably because of her equally strong commitment to disability rights, she seems to reject the argument that a child's disability, be it so difficult as a severe case of Zika syndrome, can lead to the suffering of children with this disability and/or their families. In response to an article on the Zika epidemic in Brazil published in the *American Journal of Public Health* that mentioned the possibility of interrupting a pregnancy after a diagnosis of CZS in a fetus, Diniz stated: "I am leading a group who will demand that the Brazilian Supreme Court protect women's fundamental rights violated by the epidemic. The right to terminate a pregnancy will be included in our demands, but the ethical reasons for our petition are largely different from the authors' arguments: women have the right to decide to be freed of psychological torture imposed by the epidemic. It is not the fetus's future impairments or the 'extremely negative consequences for the families affected' that moves our demand."[95] Another Brazilian scholar, Pablo Valente, similarly argued that decriminalizing abortion for malformations produced by the Zika virus was highly problematic because "legal instruments that allow abortion only in cases of fetal malformations may promote stigmatization of people with disabilities."[96]

Diniz's and Valente's arguments against terminating a pregnancy for ZIKV-induced anomalies are grounded in the *expressivist objection* to selective abortion. Such an objection is a relatively new development. In the 1960s and 1970s, an abortion for "social reasons" (the refusal of a child) was often perceived as less legitimate than abortion for "medical reasons" (the refusal of this child). The latter was often justified by the pregnant woman's wish to spare her child the difficulty of a life with a severe impairment. Activists of the religious antiabortion movement, especially in the United States, advanced the opposite argument, however. In their view, a refusal to be a mother is less blameworthy than a refusal to give birth to a disabled child because in the latter case pregnant women classify human beings along a scale of perfection and decide who is not entitled to live.

In the 1980s and 1990s, this argument was adopted by disability rights activists, who argued that termination of pregnancy for a fetal malformation was an implicit statement that life with a disability was worthless and equivalent to the practice of eugenics. The claim that abortion for a fetal anomaly hurt all people living with disabilities was coupled by disability activists with a critique of a utilitarian, neoliberal society in which only "productive" individuals were seen as entitled to full human rights, while those unable to contribute to the collective well-being were viewed as a burden. Disability, these activists proposed, was a social and not a medical condition, and a just society should provide an environment that allows all its members, able-bodied or not, to live happy, fulfilling lives. Terms such as *suffering* and *negative consequences* are accordingly banned from the vocabulary of activists for disability rights. It is not difficult to understand why activists strongly reject a vocabulary that perpetuates a pessimistic view of life with disability and indirectly legitimates the discrimination of disabled people. The expressivist objection is an emotionally powerful argument. It is also a problematic one. It lumps together different conditions and degrees of impairment and presents "exemplary disabilities" frequently compatible with an autonomous life, such as limited mobility, deafness, or impaired sight, as representative of all disabilities. It also carefully avoids, except for a vague claim that "society" should provide for all its disabled members, the question of care for severely disabled children and adults. In practice such care is frequently provided by the child's mother; this is probably even more true in resource-poor societies.[97]

The story of Amanda Loizy illustrates the complexity of debates on abortion for Zika-induced impairments. Loizy's prenatal examination opens the documentary *Zika, the film*, made by Debora Diniz and her colleagues at the ANIS Institute. The film shows Loizy entering the consultation room of Dr. Adriana Melo at the Pedro I Hospital in Campina Grande, Paraíba. During an ultrasound when Loizy was 22 weeks pregnant, the operator who examined her noticed the fetus's small head and sent her to the hospital for further evaluation. The ultrasound performed by Melo confirms the diagnosis of microcephaly. Melo then explains to Loizy that indeed the fetus has a small head, but it is not possible to draw definite conclusions from this finding, because the head's size is not a decisive variable. The most important element is changes in brain structure, and here it does not look as if there are many structural alternations.[98] She adds that additional tests might provide a better understanding of what is going on, but at least in the filmed sequence, Melo does not refer Loizy for such tests. A few months later ANIS's researchers learn that Loizy gave birth to a daughter with severe CZS, became a full-time caregiver for her disabled child, and faces considerable financial and emotional hardship. Loizy strongly proclaims her love for her daughter but says that if she had had a choice when she was pregnant, she might have elected to have an abortion.[99]

Diniz's colleagues Anahi Guedes de Mello and Gabriela Rondon at the ANIS Institute present Amanda Loizy's story to argue that disability rights should not be pitted against abortion rights. People who perceive Loizy's views as contradictory confuse attitudes toward a fetus with those toward an already existing child and blame women who make difficult private decisions for existing discriminatory attitudes and unjust social conditions. "The only way to acknowledge women as beings worthy of the full protection of rights and not merely as beings who are means for biological and social reproduction," de Mello and Rondon argue, "is if they are guaranteed this power of choice. In other words, it is only possible to simultaneously protect all women and children if the right to legal abortion is guaranteed for those who cannot proceed with the pregnancy and if every social protection to childhood is guaranteed for children with disabilities, so that those women who wish to proceed can do so."[100]

Debora Diniz starts her moving book on experiences of women during the Zika epidemic with the story of an Italian woman who contracted Zika early in pregnancy during a stay in Brazil. She then returned to northern Italy and in the third trimester of pregnancy learned that the fetus displayed a severe brain anomaly. She then decided to go to Ljubljana, Slovenia, to a well-known center of tropical medicine. While she was in Ljubljana, her child died in the womb. The local doctors, with the help of American colleagues, isolated the Zika virus from the stillborn child's body.[101] A scientific article about this case tells a different story, one of a woman who requested, and obtained, the permission of the ethics committee of the Ljubljana hospital to terminate her pregnancy because of a severe fetal impairment. Ljubljana physicians confirmed that the woman came to Slovenia to seek an abortion because in Italy, especially in the conservative north, it was not possible to obtain a late termination of a pregnancy. Many Italian women who make the difficult decision to have a late abortion for fetal indication travel to neighboring Slovenia; there is no center of tropical medicine in Ljubljana. Italian journalists who reported this story wrote that an Italian woman who contracted Zika in Brazil had to travel to Slovenia for an abortion; some added that it was a shame that she was unable to end her pregnancy in Italy.

A young woman who went through an intensely traumatic experience found solace in the conviction that she was living a drama entirely independent of her will. This is highly understandable. Telling her version of the story in a bestselling book widely read in Brazil and abroad might, however, be interpreted as a statement that a woman whose child died in the womb following infection with ZIKV is entitled to our compassion—and, implicitly, that a woman who elected an abortion after learning that her child would be severely impaired might not have the same right to our sympathy. After the Brazilian Zika epidemic ended, public attention shifted to the fate of babies with CZS and their mothers. This identification of Zika with the important struggle for the rights of disabled children and their families and the somewhat more problematic diffusion of an idealized image of mothers whose whole life is dedicated to the care of their impaired children may lead to a further condemnation of the "selfish" women who elect a different path.[102]

Brave Women and the Absence of Choice

Between 2015 and 2017, Zika went from being a global menace to being a neglected disease. An official document published by the Brazilian Health Ministry in 2017, *Zika Virus in Brazil: The SUS Response*, is dedicated "to the greatness of the brave women Maria da Conceição Alcantara Oliveira Matias and Géssica Eduardo dos Santos of Paraíba."[103] These women, patients of Adriana Melo, learned that the fetuses they were carrying displayed severe brain malformations. They agreed to undergo amniocentesis; the analysis of their amniotic fluid was a decisive step in showing that Zika was the origin of the epidemic of microcephaly inn Northeastern Brazil. Maria's child was born with congenital Zika syndrome; Géssica's child died in the womb at the end of the pregnancy. These "Zika pioneers" were among the first women confronted with the dramatic consequences of the Zika epidemic. Their experience may have been especially distressing and frightening because at the time when they were diagnosed with fetal anomalies the cause of rapidly accumulating cases of severe malformations of fetuses and newborns was still imperfectly understood, and they may have feared that their bodies were deeply flawed or that something they had done during pregnancy harmed their future child. Maria and Géssica are certainly entitled to compassion and sympathy. But why were they lavishly praised for their greatness and courage?

A possible reason for dedicating the volume on the SUS response in Brazil to the "greatness of the brave women" might be the perception of pregnant women as a means, although a glorified one, to producing babies. The criminalization of abortion means that with very few exceptions woman cannot decide what the outcome of her pregnancy will be. In countries in which the diagnosis of fetal anomalies is part of routine monitoring of pregnancy, when a woman learns during an ultrasound examination that the fetus displays structural anomalies of unknown origin, her doctors frequently propose that she undergo amniocentesis. Through an analysis of the amniotic fluid and a study of the genetic makeup of fetal cells suspended in this fluid, the cause of the observed fetal anomaly can sometimes be discovered. Few women who learn that something is seriously wrong with their future child reject the doctor's suggestion of amniocentesis, above all because they are upset and worried and wish to know what is happening with the fetus and whether the problem might occur in subsequent pregnancies. They and their doctors believe that a woman is entitled to this knowledge, that it belongs above all to her, and that it will help her and, if applicable, her partner decide what the future of the pregnancy will be.[104]

The effusive praise of Maria da Conceição Alcantara Oliveira Matias and Géssica Eduardo dos Santos for agreeing to a search for the cause of a detected fetal anomaly can be read as a statement about the routine disempowerment of pregnant women in Brazil, especially those from lower social strata. Not infrequently, pregnant women are perceived as receptacles that sustain the growth of their future children, and passive receivers of knowledge transmitted by their doctors, not as active participants in medical decisions that concern them. Emotional support ("hug therapy") provided by compassionate physicians in SUS facilities is very important but does not replace detailed information about the existing medical options and the possibility of choosing among those options.

Debora Diniz and Luciana Brito narrate the story of Joselito and Maria Carolina, parents of Maria Gabriela, one of the first children born with CZS in Paraíba. In the first trimester of her pregnancy, Maria Carolina had a "viral disease," later recognized as Zika. During an ultrasound examination in a public clinic the doctor suspected that something was wrong and recommended additional tests. The results of these tests, which Joselito and Maria were obliged to pay for, with no reimbursement from the SUS, were "inconclusive." Later Joselito compared the ultrasound images of his daughter with the ones made during the pregnancy of his older son and became persuaded that either the specialists had made a mistake and failed to recognize microcephaly or they had deliberately hidden it because they suspected that the couple might elect to have an abortion. Joselito recalled that when their daughter was born with pronounced microcephaly, everybody in the hospital had come to look at her: "It was like the birth of an animal—she was my daughter." The couple decided to sue the state of Paraíba for failing to inform them about the problem with their future child. They were aware that at the time Maria Carolina was pregnant physicians had had a limited understanding of Zika and its consequences. Jose and Maria Carolina believed, nevertheless, that the physicians should have shared with them not only accurate information about their findings but also all they knew at the time about the potential consequences of the brain anomaly they had observed: in their words, "We want the knowledge that you have."[105]

Women Who Had a Choice: Zika in Martinique

The Brazilian debate on decriminalization of abortion in the context of the Zika epidemic carefully avoided the potential minefield of abortion for a confirmed fetal anomaly. In the Caribbean island of Martinique, this topic was integrated into a public health debate. Between January and November 2016, Martinique faced a massive outbreak of Zika. Although officially there were 36,500 cases, epidemiologists estimated that the number of people infected with ZIKV was considerably higher.[106] Martinique has a population of 370,000, mostly of mixed ethnic origin, with a strong predominance of individuals of African descent. It is a French *territoire d'outre mer*; its inhabitants are therefore French citizens.[107] The importance of religion on the island is attested by the great number of Catholic and evangelical churches.[108] In 2016 Martinique's health professionals, like their colleagues in France, received guidelines from the French Health Ministry for managing the Zika risk. These guidelines recommended intensive ultrasound surveillance of pregnant women in epidemic areas.[109] Martinican doctors who provided such surveillance discovered that performing routine ultrasound examinations during the second trimester of pregnancy was a highly effective way to identify ZIKV-induced changes in the fetal brain.[110] A pilot study conducted in another Caribbean island, Trinidad and Tobago, similarly had shown that a routine ultrasound examination using standard equipment could reliably detect the majority of Zika-induced brain impairments of the fetus.[111] Ultrasound findings were then confirmed by an MRI, while Zika infection of the fetus was confirmed by detection of ZIKV in the amniotic fluid. Ultrasound made possible the detection of major structural anomalies of the fetal brain. By contrast, measuring the head circumference of the fetus was not an effective screening tool: some fetuses with severe brain anomalies had heads of normal size.

The finding of the Martinique studies, their authors argued, demonstrated the feasibility of detecting Zika-induced anomalies during pregnancy. Testing all pregnant women for Zika is not an effective way to discover the risk of CZS. Diagnostic tests for ZIKV are expensive and not very reliable. Moreover, only in a small percentage of women does infection with Zika virus during pregnancy induce severe fetal anomalies. By contrast, a routine second-trimester ultrasound examination is a cost-effective tool for the detection of Zika-induced fetal impairment. Accordingly, a logical approach to the management of Zika during pregnancy should be the same as the approach to managing infections with cytomegalovirus or toxoplasmosis: testing for the presence of an infectious agent is proposed only after the identification of fetal anomalies by a routine ultrasound examination. Such an approach is suitable for screening for CZS in a resource-limited environment. A single ultrasound test conducted between 22 and 26 weeks of pregnancy should be able to identify the great majority of "suspicious" cases. Since infection with ZIKV is nearly always a benign event, and the main problem is the induction of fetal anomalies, second-trimester ultrasound screening makes perfect sense from a public health point of view.[112]

Ultrasound screening for Zika-induced fetal anomalies, the authors of the Martinique studies proposed, is feasible even in countries with a limited number of obstetrical ultrasound devices. It can be performed by midwives or nurses employing a mobile, handheld ultrasound instrument and then sending ultrasound images by cell phone to experts in a central facility. It is surely feasible in Brazil. Brazil has plenty of ultrasound machines and excellent ultrasound specialists.[113] Routine obstetrical ultrasound examinations, some conducted in inexpensive street-corner facilities, are very popular among pregnant women who wish to confirm the pregnancy and to find out what the fetus's sex is.[114] Facing a public health emergency, it might have been possible to harness the existing equipment and know-how and to propose to all pregnant women, or at least all those who lived in regions where Zika was widespread, a second-trimester ultrasound screening for brain anomalies. Such a screening might have been treated as "first-tier" testing in the existing ultrasound facilities, with all suspicious brain images sent for evaluation to specialized centers. However, despite the government's recommendation that pregnant women be tested for Zika and that the pregnancies of women who tested positive be closely monitored, such monitoring was offered only in a fraction of SUS facilities, and it did not include second-trimester diagnostic ultrasound examinations, which could detect relatively early anomalies of the fetal brain. Such diagnostic ultrasounds, if offered at all, were proposed only in the third trimester of pregnancy.[115] Moreover, since an abortion for a fetal indication is illegal, when they detect a major fetal malformation during an ultrasound examination, physicians who work in the public sector tend to emphasize the uncertainty of the prognosis, even when they know that the observed malformation will lead to severe impairment of the future child.[116] When Brazilian doctors diagnosed a Zika-induced severe brain anomaly of the fetus, they had only two lawful choices: to tell the mother to prepare herself for life as a caregiver of a severely disabled child or to keep the child's prognosis deliberately vague.

Martinican women had other options. Routine ultrasound examinations during the Zika epidemic on the island led to the identification of 15 women carrying fetuses with ZIKV-induced severe brain anomalies. Thirteen women elected to terminate the pregnancy. Nine had abortions in the middle of the second trimester (between 22 and 27 weeks); one, early in the second trimester, at 18 weeks; and three, in the third trimester, one at 33 weeks and two at 34 weeks of pregnancy. One fetus died in the womb, and one woman elected to continue her pregnancy and gave birth to a live child.[117] Speaking about woman's *choice* in the context of an abortion for a fetal anomaly may sound bitterly ironic. No pregnant woman chooses to receive a diagnosis of a severe fetal impairment, and none elects to face an agonizing decision about the fate of a wanted pregnancy. Still, in such traumatic circumstances women in Martinique who learned about brain anomalies of the fetus had the possibility of regaining some degree of control over their future.

CHAPTER SIX

Mães de Micro

Zika and Maternal Care

Becoming a Mãe de Micro

The discovery of microcephaly in a fetus or newborn was nearly always a shock. Adriana Melo explained in the documentary *Zika, the film* that in the hospital in Campina Grande distressed women who learned about the fetal anomaly received moral support and "hug therapy."[1] Not all health professionals provided such support. Not infrequently mothers of children with this condition learned about the "small head" of their child or future child from professionals they described as "cold" and "unfeeling." One mother was brutally asked by a physician just after she gave birth, "Do you know that your child has no brain?"[2] Women whose children were diagnosed with congenital Zika syndrome seldom received psychological help, even though such diagnosis was linked with a high frequency of postpartum depression.[3]

Here are some women's descriptions of their dramatic entry into the role of "Zika mother":

At the time of the ultrasound, the doctor said to his secretary: "There is something strange here," he said to her: "Call the other doctor there," she called the other doctor, he came, then when I looked, three doctors inside the room. I said, "My goodness!" I started to get scared and cry. Then he said: "You don't need to be scared, calm down!" And the other went and said: "There is no way out! You can put it there after the exam, it is microcephaly." Then he said: "Good luck!" And I left crying.

No one explained anything. And that's when the doctor came with a lot of academics there, the doctor there, right: "Look this child, probably congenital Zika, she has microcephaly. . . ." That's the way I heard it. They were there, talking to each other there, explaining each case for them to learn. Then she turned and said it like that. "This is a child with microcephaly, malformation, calcification, congenital Zika."

The doctor was the one who caused me a shock. The doctor said that she was not going to see, she was not going to walk, she was just going to be a vegetable child, that is, the rest of her life, and that she would need me.

At the moment of childbirth, when he was already born, right, the doctor said: "Look, the news is sad. But I have to tell you; the baby was born with a little head. We are going to investigate for Zika." . . . And it was, like this, I don't know, very ugly thing for a mother to see, I did not expect that. And it was very sad for me. I did not want to see it. I screamed and cried. . . . After the birth, I cried a lot.[4]

They took my baby girl away and they were in there with her for a long time. I thought she'd been born dead. I never imagined she'd been born with microcephaly. A long time afterward they came and talked to me about her.

I only found out at the time of the birth, in the worst possible way, when the doctor picked him up and said she needed to take him away because he "wasn't normal." So, we only received the diagnosis the following day.[5]

One woman said that at first she "became desperate, and thought of giving the child away" because she was not equipped financially or emotionally to care for a child with special needs. She did not tell her husband that she at first considered abandoning the child. Other women were very sad when they received the diagnosis of the child's microcephaly but then accepted it "I cried and cried," recalled one woman. "But then I thought that this was God's will, right, and then I was calmer. Because God willed this."[6]

These stories are at the same time familiar—learning that one's child or future child has a severe health problem is always distressing—and also specific to Zika, as CZS was not a random disaster that could strike any pregnant woman but the consequence of stratified reproduction in a highly unequal society.

Confirmed Zika Syndrome

In December 2015 the Brazilian Health Ministry introduced instructions for the coordination of medical and social aspects of care of children with CZS. This was followed in February 2016 by a complete protocol for monitoring children with this syndrome, together with detailed instructions for their care. These documents made it possible to effectively integrate services for children with microcephaly. Taken together, they provided a framework for implementing therapeutic, educational, and social interventions for CZS children, above all early stimulation, which was presented as essential if children with Zika syndrome were to reach their full potential. On the other hand, they were destined only for children with confirmed Zika syndrome, not for those initially classified as born with possible microcephaly but later excluded from the registry of confirmed Zika cases.[7] Pediatricians who cared for children with Zika syndrome hoped that the publicity around this syndrome would attract attention to the fate of children born with other severe neurological problems. This did happen, but on a limited scale only. In some localities children with other neurological impairments, such as cerebral palsy, were able to benefit from the wave of support for children with CZS, but this was far from the norm. ANIS's report on Zika in the northeastern state of Alagoas reproduces numerous testimonies of mothers of "excluded" children. These children had inborn neurological issues, but since they were not officially recognized as affected by CZS, their mothers did not receive any support from the state.[8]

The ANIS document exposed important differences between Brazilian states. The percentage of discarded cases in the state of Alagoas was twice as high as the percentage in another northeastern state, Bahia. It is possible that because Alagoas was poorer than Bahia and had fewer resources to help disabled children, the criteria for confirmation of CZS, and thus for giving public aid, were more stringent in that state. It is also possible that in Alagoas women had less access to diagnostic technologies (laboratory analyses, magnetic resonance imaging) and consultations with specialists necessary to confirm a CZS diagnosis. Mortality among children with "probable" or "possible" CZS who failed to obtain official recognition of this condition was found to be as high as among those officially recognized as having CZS. This may indicate that many of the children denied the state's help had CZS or a condition of a similar nature.[9] While official confirmation of a CZS diagnosis did help families of children with this condition, it did not automatically grant them access to essential services. According to the data provided by the Health Ministry, 35% of the children with a confirmed CZS diagnosis (often those who lived in or near major cities) benefited from regular early stimulation sessions provided by trained physiotherapists and educators; another 30% had partial access to such sessions; and 35% had very limited access to health and educational resources.[10]

In his introduction to the 2017 Brazilian Health Ministry document *Zika Virus in Brazil: The SUS Response*, Adeilson Cavalcante, of the ministry's Health Surveillance Department, praised the brave northeastern women, "who taught us a lesson of faith and hope, holding their babies in their arms and looking for assistance from public health services to ensure minimum comfort to their babies with microcephaly and other serious sequels. Just like the characters of Gracilliano Ramos's book, 'Vidas Secas' (Dry Lives), these women fight the adversities of the sertão, the shortage of resources, long distances, and still raise their children."[11] Cavalcante might have added that many women did this with very limited help from the Brazilian authorities.

Trajectories of Mothers of Children with CZS

Women often learned about the impairment of their child at the very end of their pregnancy or only after their child's birth. Before the link between microcephaly and Zika was recognized, some women believed that they had done something to harm their unborn child; others reported that their companions blamed them for their child's problems.[12] Many Zika mothers testified that they had not been told by their doctors what their child's health and cognitive problems would be, reported that they had often been treated in a condescending and paternalistic way, and complained of insufficient institutional support.[13] Thinking about their children, these mothers drew on the imagery developed by the international disability movement. A quotation from the testimony of Goreti, "I never expected this, it was a shock," is the title of Carneiro and Fleischer's article on *mães de micro* (mothers of children born with microcephaly, i.e., with a number of anomalies induced by the Zika virus) in Recife. Her full testimony reads: "I never expected this, it was a shock. It was as if you had planned to make a trip to Rio de Janeiro. But suddenly, the pilot announced that we would land in another city. Instead of Rio de Janeiro, the plane went to Maranhão. You had to change all the places you had planned to visit. You will have to plan what you want to visit in Maranhão."[14] Goreti's powerful parable was employed for many years by associations of parents of children with Down syndrome. It might have been interesting to learn where and when Goreti heard this parable and whether she or somebody else adapted the original story about a person who hopes to go to Italy, ends by landing in the Netherlands, is initially disappointed, and then learns to appreciate the beauty of windmills and tulip fields and transformed it into a story about a person who hopes to go to Rio de Janeiro and ends up in the northeastern state of Maranhão.[15] The Brazilian version of this parable may, however, convey a somewhat different meaning. Maranhão is not the Netherlands; it has beautiful landscapes but is also one of the poorest Brazilian states. In the Brazilian version, the focus might have been not on a different but equally rich and rewarding experience but on resilience and successful adaptation.

Caring for a child with severe CZS and multiple disabilities, mothers of these children explained, was extremely challenging. The children often had very complex medical trajectories, with frequent and severe setbacks. The difficulties of caring for children with CZS were amplified by poverty. Middle-class mothers of severely disabled children also faced a very difficult situation, but they could hire domestic help and deal with many logistic problems linked with the intensive care of their child. Poor women struggled not only with their children's multiple health problems and frequent emergency situations but also with endless mundane tasks, from shopping and cleaning to getting the right drugs to taking their child to numerous regular medical visits and stimulation sessions—by means of often rudimentary public transportation.[16]

The poverty of Zika mothers was frequently aggravated by the fact that nearly all were obliged to give up their jobs to become full-time caregivers. Only a few daycare centers are able to deal with the health problems of a child with Zika syndrome. A few mothers enrolled their children in nonmedical daycare centers but were obliged to remove them because the staff could not cope with the children's complicated needs and repeated medical crises. Unable to work, many mães de micro were obliged to rely on the state's very modest support for families of CZS children. Some children with Zika syndrome were enrolled for a few days a week in "regular" daycare centers, accompanied by a full-time caregiver. This arrangement, welcomed by their mothers, was available only to a fraction of the children with Zika syndrome.[17]

Debora Diniz and Ilana Ambrogi explained that in 2016 mães de micro in Campina Grande, Paraíba, a city frequently visited that year by foreign journalists interested in the microcephaly epidemic, received material help from these journalists, who were shocked by the mothers' abject poverty.[18] Many Zika mothers reported being abandoned by their male partners, in a few cases because the partner blamed the mother for the child's health problems but in the majority of cases because caring for the child took all the mother's time and energy, leaving them no time for a "normal" life as a couple. Men who stayed usually took little to no part in the daily care of their disabled child.

Those who did share some of the care duties received high praise for their help. By contrast, other women in the family—grandmothers, aunts, nieces—received no such praise for their help because it was taken for granted.[19]

Some mothers of CZS children reported negative attitudes of neighbors and acquittances toward their children, even a rumor that the children's microcephaly was the result of their mothers' trying to abort them.[20] That rumor might have been the result of a distortion of the information, widely propagated by the Brazilian media, that the use of the abortive pill misoprostol—in cases in which it did not lead to the termination of a pregnancy—induced fetal anomalies. Failed abortion with misoprostol was indeed linked with an increased risk of a neurological anomaly, the Moebius syndrome. However, this condition has very different manifestations from those of Zika syndrome; it is linked with difficulties in controlling facial muscles and occasionally with deformations of the limbs. Moreover, the risk of Moebius syndrome after uptake of misoprostol is very small. The largest Brazilian study of links between misoprostol and Moebius syndrome identified 38 such cases, while hundreds of thousands of Brazilian women employed illegally purchased misoprostol to terminate an unwanted pregnancy.[21] Still, widespread information linking visible anomalies with an abortive drug not only increased the plight of Brazilian women who could not afford a safe abortion but produced unintended and highly distressing "collateral damage": increased stigmatization and social isolation of mães de micro.

Zika Activism

To escape social isolation, cope with the difficulties of daily care of impaired children, and find camaraderie and support, mothers of children with CZS became engaged in a collective struggle for their and their children's rights.[22] Organizations such as the Recife-based União de Mães de Anjos (UMA), which started as a WhatsApp group and grew to become the most important organization of mothers of children with Zika syndrome, coordinate struggles for children's and families' rights.[23] In addition to their important practical achievement, these groups make it possible for mães de micro to develop social connections, collectively produce knowledge about the care of their children, and receive crucial psychological support from other women in a similar situation. Mothers' organizations also strive to imbue their members with a sense of purpose, often using a religious language, such as the following from UMA: "Our children are the mission God has given us and we are in this to the end. If our children can't walk, we will walk for them. If they can't hear, we will be their ears. If they can't interact, we will fight for them. If they can't speak, we will be the only voice declaring that microcephaly is not the end of the world."[24]

WhatsApp groups continue to be the backbone of mothers' self-organization and self-help. The use of cell phones for contact is especially important for women who live in remote areas and for those who have limited capacity to travel because of the round-the-clock care their children require. Mothers who actively participate in WhatsApp groups and Zika-centered organizations— an unknown proportion of all the mothers of children with Zika syndrome— constantly exchange information on practical issues, from how to cope with their children's medical and behavioral problems to how to negotiate with administrators and overcome bureaucratic hurdles. Occasionally WhatsApp groups also offered mothers humorous relief from their harrowing daily routine. Thus one can read on UMA's Facebook site a story about two Zika mothers who chatted on WhatsApp, but the connection was not very good. One remarked, "My cellphone seems to have convulsions," to which the other answered, "So give it Kypra [a drug widely used to control convulsions in CZS children]"; both burst out laughing.[25] In selected localities physiotherapists and educators who provide early stimulation for children with Zika syndrome collaborate with mothers' organizations. Among other things, they prepare, with the mothers' active input, educational materials, short videos that provide advice on the daily management of children with Zika syndrome—how to position them, feed them, and deal with problems such as convulsions or infections. These videos are then posted online by WhatsApp groups.

At first, organizations of mothers of children with Zika syndrome included only mothers of children with confirmed Zika syndrome, since only those children were entitled to the special stimulation and help specified in the Health Ministry protocol of February 2016. The rationale for distinguishing families of children with CZS, provided by both authorities and activists, was that because the Brazilian state had failed to control mosquitoes, it was directly responsible for the outbreak of Zika and its consequences. This argument was employed to legitimate the decision by the state of Pernambuco to give a "priority of priorities" to the care of children with CZS. Thanks to this policy, the state provides nonnegligible assistance to these children: medical and rehabilitation services, free medication, and help with lodging through Minha Casa, Minha Vida (a program that helps disadvantaged families to obtain state-supported lodging; it gives priority to families with disabled children).[26] Still, even in Pernambuco, the help provided by the state is far from being problem-free. It may vary between sites or even from one day to another. Anthropologists from the University of Brasília who followed a group of mothers of children with CZS in Pernambuco for four years recorded the significant practical difficulties and the occasional rupture of services some of these mothers faced. Thus one mother was stranded for more than 24 hours with her disabled child in the streets of Recife because the promised transportation service failed to materialize.[27]

The special help available to children with confirmed Zika syndrome became a source of tension between associations of mothers or parents of children with CZS and other advocacy groups. Thus activists of the Alianca de Mães e Familias Raras (AMAR) argued that the state should provide intensive therapy and stimulation to all children with inborn neurological impairments, whatever their cause. Some of these tensions attenuated thanks to the adoption of more inclusive policies by the associations of mães de micro. UMA fought for the inclusion of the anticonvulsive drug Kypra among the medications provided by the public health system, SUS. When the SUS accepted their demand, UMA's president, Germana Soares, declared it an important victory not only for parents of children with CZS but for parents of all children who might need the drug. However, Brazilian law continues to distinguish children with confirmed CZS, and the majority of the associations of mães de micro endorse this singularizing.

Professionals such as physiotherapists, nurses, and social workers (as a rule female) play an important role in the lives of mães de micro and their children, but as far as I know, their contribution has been investigated mainly through testimonies of mães de micro, not through studies focused on their tasks and attitudes.[28] When these health professionals were sympathetic and caring, regular contacts with mães de micro alleviated the mothers' plight. Even when a child made only minimal progress, regular physiotherapy sessions provided moral support to the mothers and gave them hope. One poignant narrative depicted a mother of a 2-year-old daughter with severe Zika syndrome who had a dream in which her child called her "mummy."[29] Not all health care providers were equally supportive. Some believed that women from lower socioeconomic strata had to earn the right to receive help from the state, for example by accepting experts' authority without question and regularly attending medical appointments and physiotherapy sessions. Mothers occasionally reported that when they were unable to take their children to all the therapy sessions, they were blamed by physiotherapists or physicians for the severity of the child's problems.[30]

Associations of mães de micro fulfill a very important role in maintaining the visibility of children with CZS in Brazil and spreading the message that the Zika epidemic might be over, but its long-term consequences are not. At the same time, the associations' activities are to an important extent legitimated by the Brazilian ideal of sacrificial motherhood. The ideology of maternal love is especially powerful in northeastern Brazil, the epicenter of the Brazilian Zika epidemic.[31] The centrality of Christianity in many women's lives and the rapid increase in the influence of socially and politically conservative (mainly evangelical) churches in Brazil bolster the value attributed to maternal devotion and suffering. Mães de micro stressed that they have a new mission, to show that they are able, "despite everything," to look after their children.[32] A group of mothers from Rio Grande do Norte created the WhatsApp group Mothers Elected by God (Mães Escolhidas por Deus, or MED). Its central slogan is "God selects only very special women to take care of an impaired child."[33] A conceptual framework that glorifies the maternal labor of love helps Zika mothers cope with a very difficult situation and achieve a higher level of societal value, earned through their sacrifice. Such valorization is, however, associated with extreme dependence on a disabled child and can hinder the acquisition of a different social identity.[34]

Zika Conspiracies

"Go viral" is what viruses do, but at least before the COVID-19 pandemic this expression was employed more frequently to describe the spread of information rather than the spread of infectious agents.[35] During the Zika epidemic in Brazil information spread mainly through WhatsApp. Not only did WhatsApp groups support the self-organization of Zika mothers but they were also the primary vehicle for the spread of information, accurate or not.[36] The rapid spread of imprecise, in some cases incorrect information was one of the reasons for the tensions between mães de micro and researchers studying children with CZS. From its first appearance, the mysterious new disease was accompanied by conspiracy theories. At first such theories were mainly linked with the suspicion that the epidemic had been induced by larvicides, or by genetically modified mosquitoes, released by the company Oxitec.[37] The latter rumor linked the genetic manipulation of mosquitoes with the Bill & Melinda Gates Foundation, often presented, especially in developing and middle-income countries, as shorthand for neocolonialist intervention. Thus in 2019 that Gates was directly involved in the spread of the Zika virus in Brazil was one of the most frequent claims of the antivaccination movement.[38]

In 2019 the *New York Times* reporters Amanda Taub and Max Fisher, who studied the role of fake news in Bolsonaro's victory in the presidential election of fall 2018, stumbled on an explanation of how such information became viral when they met Luciana Brito, an ANIS- affiliated clinical psychologist who worked with families affected by the Zika virus. Brito showed them, using the example of Zika, how WhatsApp and YouTube formed a powerful feedback loop of extremism and misinformation that spread conspiracy theories and political propaganda. While the internet is expensive in Brazil, sharing snippets of YouTube videos on WhatsApp is free, allowing the rapid diffusion of such snippets through networks of trusted correspondents. Parents of children with CZS reported to Brito rumors that blamed the disease on international conspiracies. Such rumors undermined the trust of mães de micro in activists who came to help them.[39]

The not entirely irrational perception of Western powers, international institutions, and pharmaceutical companies as uncaring, self-centered, and uninterested in helping poor populations facilitated the spread of conspiracy theories about Zika.[40] Rumors about the "doubtful" origins of Zika were rapidly linked with suspicions about the "manufacture" of this epidemic by secret power elites.[41] Such rumors often mix, in variable proportions, accurate, semiaccurate, and false statements and contain the predictable elements: genetically modified organisms, Bill Gates, greedy Big Pharma, and evil producers of pesticides such as Monsanto. The Zika epidemic added new elements to the list: the Rockefeller Foundation (RF), the eugenics movement, and feminists. Many people in Brazil were receptive to the argument that malevolent actors used the Zika virus to control population growth. The RF was targeted in this context because of its historical links with the Rockefeller-owned Standard Oil but above all, because of its close relations with the Population Council, which in its early years aspired to control population growth, especially in developing countries.[42]

Links between the RF and the Population Council might have been the reason for the claim that the RF had spread the Zika virus to persuade or force poor women in Latin America to have abortions. According to this argument, the Zika virus was the "property" of the RF, which spread it in targeted countries. The claim was so persistent that the foundation felt obliged to issue an official denial on its website that read: "Zika was first discovered at the Foundation-supported Virus Research Institute in Entebbe, Uganda in 1947, and a sample of the virus was given to ATCC (a nonprofit organization that authenticates and preserves microorganisms for research) by J. Casals of The Rockefeller Foundation in 1953. This appears to be the source of the rumor that the Rockefeller Foundation 'patented' the virus. There is no indication that the Rockefeller Foundation holds or has filed for any patent on the Zika virus or has received any royalties or payments."[43]

Another rumor, widespread in Brazil, was that Zika had been produced from an expired batch of measles, mumps, and rubella vaccine.[44] Thus Brito reported that mothers of children with CZS shared WhatsApp videos that linked their children's condition to childhood vaccination. The overall level of confidence in vaccines in Brazil is high. Nevertheless, when mães de micro repeatedly received antivaccination videos from other mothers through their WhatsApp group, some ended up believing the claims contained in these messages.[45] Not only parents but also some health professionals contributed to the propagation of this rumor.[46] In developing countries, anthropologists explain, conspiracy theories are frequently rooted in a legitimate mistrust of Western or scientific medicine and are an expression of complex issues that need to be confronted, not despised as an expression of ignorance.[47] On the other hand, in Brazil, Far Right organizations skillfully used the dramatic consequences of the Zika outbreak, especially for lower-class women, to promote their political agendas through the spread of misinformation that often hurt these women and their families. Alas, social scientists argued, there was no rapid and easy way to deal with this kind of misinformation. Supplying factually correct information, research had shown, could even make things worse by making the recipients of this information less sure what to believe.[48]

Trust can be built only through sustained, patient, long-term efforts, and those can be complicated by the attitudes of some health professionals. The anthropologists Rosamaria Carneiro and Soraya Fleischer report the following story, narrated by Eva, a mother of a child with CZS:

> When Eva took her son for a consultation with a neurologist, she was asked about the prenatal vaccines. She explained that, yes, she had been immunized for rubella, the flu. And in return she heard from the doctor:
>   Doctor: But now it is difficult to know if it was the vaccine or the virus.
>   Eva: What, doctor? A vaccine can also cause micro?
>   Doctor: My daughter, learn this. This is not a serious country, don't confide in vaccines. I, myself, never take a vaccine for anything.[49]

Overexposures

Mães de micro became the face of the Zika epidemic. They also became the guardians of valuable research material, their children. The future of research on ZIKV largely depends on the possibility of observing, studying, probing, testing, and retesting children with CZS. The vast majority of these children are cared for by the public health system.[50] In many localities, SUS institutions made a real effort to provide help to children with Zika syndrome, but this effort was hampered by the paucity of SUS resources. Children with congenital Zika were polyhandicapped and had to make frequent visits to numerous specialized services to treat their health problems. Such services were often fragmented and geographically distant, so that Zika mothers, who often relied on public transportation, had to make arduous trips to several locations. Moreover, in the majority of the sites health services provided to a given child were not coordinated by a single professional, such as a family doctor, nurse, or social worker. Primary health centers were not equipped to deal with children with complex health needs, while visits to specialized services focused on the medical problems of the child, not the holistic needs of the family or the specific difficulties of mothers as caregivers.[51] One interesting experiment attempted to train selected mothers as "experts" in the daily care of CZS children, then asked them to hold group sessions to teach other mothers how to feed, bathe, and stimulate their children. The experiment demonstrated the feasibility of this approach, but as far as I know, it did not lead to large-scale implementation of this model.[52]

Zika mothers' contacts with doctors and scientists, anthropologists who observed them attest, were frequently limited to exchanges about technical issues. Many mothers dealt on their own with very difficult practical problems, such as how to provide the physical stimulation prescribed by physiotherapists when the child had convulsions or very rigid muscles (arthrogryposis) and cried often. One mother testified, "I stretch her arm, but her arm is rigid like this, I also stimulate her legs . . . , she has a lot of strength. She also has many convulsions, we still didn't find the right medication to stop the convulsions." Another said, "I can't do it a lot . . . when I do it she cries. I do what the doctor tells me to do, I stretch as the doctor told me. His little legs too, I stretch, I'm able to, but he cries a lot." Yet another said that "I do what I can, what I can't, I feel afraid to do, that fear of hurting her, I'm afraid to break something or putting her little arm in a bad place, we get really afraid."[53]

Zika mothers whose children were enrolled in research protocols conducted in major research institutions had privileged access to medical and educational resources. However, they felt that this privilege depended on the goodwill of health professionals. Some mothers complained about doctors' patronizing attitude, their (presumed) tendency to see their children above all as "research objects," and their failure to inform the mothers about their children's diagnoses and prognoses.[54] Studies of children with CZS are conducted by researchers who, in order to publish their results, need to obtain signed consent forms from participants. All the mães de micro signed the required forms, but it is unclear whether they understood precisely what they signed and why they had to do it. With the intense interest in studying Zika, the physician's role as healer and caregiver was fused with his or her role as researcher. Zika mothers did not dare openly refuse to participate in research protocols because they feared that it might affect the quality of their children's care. Many also acceded to the experts' demands, including those they did not understand, because they shared the researchers' expectation that scientific progress would bring solutions to their child's problems.[55] In the early stages of the Zika epidemic, many mães de micro hoped that with the right stimulation and therapy their children would "catch up"—a powerful reason to maintain faith in health professionals despite the serious communication problems.[56] For many mothers, the hope of scientific advances gradually slipped away. Medications were not a miracle solution—they did not always help and they had side effects—while in many cases the progress of the child was slow and uneven, with periods of improvement followed by episodes of regression.[57]

Speaking in the third year of the epidemic, when it was clear that the majority of children with CZS would remain severely handicapped, Germana Soares was not optimistic about the achievements of children with CZS:

> We see wonderful images of a child with Down syndrome dancing classical ballet—it's great. But she can do it because she has a high cognitive level, supportive family, material advantages—but we cannot take such a case as a model of how a child with Down syndrome should look. Many are more severely impaired, as are many children with CZS, and . . . some people do not even want to look at such, a severely impaired child in a wheelchair. But we need to include those children too: she will not dance, she will not walk, she will be unable to do much, she will just stay like this—is this a reason not to include her? . . . We have to talk of people with disability, and their caretakers . . . we also need to stop blaming mothers, telling them "your child cannot walk because you did not stimulate her enough, she does not eat because . . ." Stop it. Which woman wants to have a disabled child? Not a single one! She did not ask to have a child with special problems. But people need to blame somebody, and this somebody is always a woman.[58]

Zika mothers who vacillated between hope and resignation became suspicious of the scientists who took care of their children. Sometimes physician-researchers organized groups of Zika mothers. Children whose mothers participated in such groups, especially if the group was organized around a clinical trial, benefited from better access to medical, educational, and social resources. On the other hand, not infrequently the presence of a physician, and the imposition of a hierarchy of knowledge, stifled spontaneous exchanges among mothers. Moreover, some of the physicians attempted to control the groups they structured: they recommended to mothers not to participate in competing groups or to share test results with other researchers.[59] Some mães de micro rebelled against what they perceived as overexposure to research and a loss of control over their and their children's bodies and actions. They were solicited by members of numerous professional groups: not only physicians and scientific researchers but also social scientists and journalists. All their interlocutors presented themselves as devoted to the well-being of their children, and all were suspected by the Zika mothers of having ulterior motifs, above all of profiting from their research on Zika.[60] In response to what they saw as the exploitation of their children, one WhatsApp group of Zika mothers in northeastern Brazil adopted the name "My child is not a guinea pig."[61]

The combination of a health emergency, great scientific and media interest, and the extreme social suffering of caregivers of Zika children could become a toxic brew. Anthropologists who followed closely interactions between Zika mothers and scientists became painfully aware of the tensions in exchanges between the two groups. Their interactions were infused with uncertainty, antagonism, and mistrust.[62] The mothers felt that they and their children were objectivized and instrumentalized. They resented that they were often asked the same questions repeatedly and in an uncoordinated way by different researchers. Mothers were often asked to explain their children's disability, as well as their own acts and decisions, to numerous strangers, and they were obliged to tell their stories again and again, an obligation described by the anthropologist Soraya Fleischer as a "purgatory narrative."[63] Mães de micro were also distressed by the focus on their poverty and their harsh living conditions, especially since the researchers who interrogated them were mainly middle-class whites, while most of the mothers were poor and non-white. Some of them also felt misled and exploited by researchers. For instance, there were reports of researchers who infiltrated the parent groups and WhatsApp networks to collect data for their studies.[64]

Zika mothers, especially in the "onlookers-saturated" northeastern localities, anthropologists reported, not infrequently became suspicious of anybody who might have had a hand in their objectification, journalists and anthropologists included.[65] But when dealing with health professionals—on whom the mothers and their children often depended—they could not express directly their distrust and anger. For example, during a session when blood samples were collected from CZS children, sometimes they had to be pricked with a needle several times, leading the children to cry and try to flee. When researchers failed multiple times to collect blood from a CZS child—according to them a more difficult task than collecting blood from a nonaffected child—the mothers were silent, but their body language revealed their anguish and distress. Later the mothers spoke about their fatigue and their difficult relationship with researchers, who "only ask questions" and do not always share with them the results of tests.[66]

Nevertheless, the mothers continued to submit their children and themselves to the research protocol. They rationally grasped that a better understanding of their children's condition could contribute to improved treatment. At the same time, they resented the asymmetry of their relationship with the researchers. As one of the mães de micro put it, "They [the researchers] gain money and fame from our suffering. We suffer, and they gain."[67] An additional difficulty was mothers' not entirely unjustified mistrust of international organizations heavily involved in studies of children with CZS. Mothers noted that many foreign researchers had become interested in the "exotic" Zika but had not shown interest in more frequently occurring pathologies, such as dengue fever. They interpreted this as evidence that foreign researchers and organizations wanted only to increase their prestige and status and were not interested in helping Brazilian people.[68]

One of the obstacles to trust between mothers and relatives of children with CZS and health care workers was the difficulty for the latter to balance giving truthful information about the child's prognosis with the mothers' wish to maintain a hopeful vision of their children's future. Mothers trusted caregivers (often physiotherapists) who provided a positive outlook for their children and were hurt by specialists (often doctors) who bluntly described their children as severely impaired, with little chance of significant improvement. Being told, for example, that the child would need a wheelchair might lead to despair but also distrust. Health workers risked losing the mothers' trust as bearers of bad news but also as promoters of false hopes. Some professionals were also disturbed by the fact that because of the media visibility of Zika, children with CZS received much more state help than children with similar neurological conditions, and by the fact that media-savvy associations of Zika mothers exploited their visibility in the media to get "unfair" advantages for them and their children.[69] Specialists who worked with CZS children might also have felt that anthropologists' descriptions of the tensions between mães de micro and the researchers who studied them were excessively bleak. One text on the experiences of families of CZS children ended with the testimony of a grateful mother who lavishly praised the treatment that she and her daughter received at a major research institution: "I find support here of people who care for her, with a lot of love and affection. . . . So, this is what I like to be here for. It is difficult, but I feel good here because I know that I am well accepted, and my daughter is well accepted."[70]

Complaints about the overexposure of children with CZS were expressed mainly by mothers of "protocolized" CZS children, those who were and are included in research cohorts. Only a small number of the more than 3,000 children officially diagnosed with inborn Zika syndrome are integrated into research cohorts and followed closely either from birth or from the moment of their diagnosis. "Protocolized" children are valuable research subjects. They are observed, measured, and studied intensively, and their physical and intellectual development are monitored frequently and regularly. They also have better access to medical resources. Researchers who study these children are persuaded that the help they provide to CZS children is a sincere expression of their care and compassion. Zika mothers may see the situation somewhat differently. While they do not deny that many professionals wish to improve the well-being of their children, they suspect that their actions may reflect mainly concern about a precious "property."

A "good" cohort of CZS children is valuable because with the end of the Zika epidemic it became extremely difficult to form new cohorts, especially prospective ones. "Ownership" of a good cohort secures the continuation of research and publications in high impact factor scientific journals. The Zika epidemic gave numerous Brazilian scientists international exposure, but for many that exposure decreased when Zika disappeared. Following an already established group of children with CZS prevented this from happening: a good cohort is a gift that continues to give. Mães de micro are conscious of the importance of their children for researchers. They might have encountered good and bad health professionals, wavered between a wish to trust experts and distrust of them, and heard positive and negative stories from other Zika mothers. Part of the problem may be the difficulty mothers have in trying to figure out how much of the experts' involvement with the study of CZS children can be attributed to a genuine wish to help them and how much stems from their desire to forward their professional goals.[71]

Debate Interrupted

In the summer of 2018 a group of mães de micro representing several associations were invited to participate, together with scientists, clinicians, and social scientists, in a special session on Zika during the ABRASCO meeting at Fiocruz. They were accompanied by their children with CZS, who were mostly between 2 and 3 years old. The children's presence made visible a seldom discussed issue: the great disparities in the physical and mental development of children with moderate and severe CZS. Some of the children looked "normal" for their age, lively and agile (which of course did not mean that they did not have serious developmental issues), while others looked strikingly "different." The latter children were also very quiet, perhaps partly because many were on high doses of anticonvulsive medication. The meeting had plenary sessions and smaller workshops. It aimed to produce a text that would articulate the demands of all the stakeholders in the Zika crisis in Brazil. The debates during this meeting led to the elaboration of the first draft. The draft was then circulated among participants in the meeting, and after a series of amendments it was approved a year later as a binding resolution by the Sixteenth National Conference on Health (16° Conferência Nacional de Saúde, CNS).[72]

The final text of the resolution might be described as a carefully crafted wish list. It asked for better state funding for the affected children and their families, especially those who belonged to vulnerable strata of society; more money for fundamental research on the Zika virus and on the clinical and social consequences of infection with this pathogen; increased investment in the control of mosquitoes; improved integration of health care and social interventions; the inclusion of users of health care in all the decisions that concern them; the provision of accurate information to the public about Zika-related risks; and the elaboration of rules of collection and circulation of data and biological samples. In a country in which numerous groups and individuals struggle for the "right to health" granted by the Brazilian constitution, a detailed list of demands addressed to the government can be a useful road map for future struggles.[73] On the other hand, the resolution carefully avoided contentious topics: it calls for improving access to contraception and prenatal testing but does not mention the termination of pregnancy; it describes the plight of parents of polyhandicapped children but does not mention "male abortion," the abandonment of severely handicapped children by their fathers;

it refers to "vulnerable populations" without speaking about the race or *cor* (skin color) of these populations; it mentions the need to educate the public about Zika but does not mention gender violence, which disempowers women and limits their ability to protect themselves from unwanted pregnancies and sexual transmission of ZIKV.

The organizers of the original meeting on Zika saw as its most important achievements the agreement of different groups of stakeholders to participate in this meeting, the lively exchanges during the meeting, and the active involvement of Zika mothers in the elaboration of a common text. The meeting's final resolution can be presented as a successful synthesis of divergent views, as a bland compromise that glossed over difficulties and minimalized contradictions, or both. As an external observer, more familiar with the point of view of researchers than with that of mães de micro, my initial impression was that all the participants, the Zika mothers included, were interested in the debates and satisfied with their result. Another external observer, a researcher who for several years worked closely with an association of Zika mothers and saw herself as being on the mothers' side, saw the event very differently. One of the mothers, she reported, participated in a working group on the diagnosis of Zika and was deeply offended by a scientist who mentioned "fantastic research opportunities" opened up by the study of Zika. This scientist probably assumed that people directly affected by the Zika outbreak would of course view the progress of research on this disease as a positive development. But the Zika mother who heard this discourse was deeply shocked by the scientist's discourse: "We are human beings, how can they speak about us like this? We are not objects!"[74]

One of the plenary sessions of the 2018 meeting was suddenly interrupted by sounds of shooting. The building in which the meeting took place, usually employed for teaching, was near the avenue that separates Fiocruz from the favela Manguinhos. On one side of this avenue are historical edifices, laboratories, workshops, animal houses, and an ultramodern, architecturally impressive building of Bio-Manguinhos, the Fiocruz production plant. On the other side is one of the most violent favelas in Rio, dubbed the Gaza Strip because of the frequent fierce conflicts between the official military police, paramilitary police-affiliated groups, and drug dealers. Fiocruz and the favela are separated by a busy road and a stretch of stagnant, foul-smelling water, a potential breeding ground for mosquitoes and pathogens. Foreign visitors who enter Fiocruz through the gate near the favela often find the contrast between these two entities disturbing. For people who work at Fiocruz, such a contrast is just another part of living in Rio, a city rich in dramatic disparities between poverty and opulence. The Manguinhos favela, it is important to add, is not entirely cut off from the research institute on the other side of the road. Some of the institute's lower-level workers live in that favela and neighboring ones, while Fiocruz's researchers conduct numerous sanitary and educational interventions in these favelas, usually in close collaboration with local activists. On the other hand, occasional exchanges of live fire in the immediate vicinity remind the institute's researchers' of the danger of being located so close to a favela that is often a battlefield.

The shooting started in the middle of the discussion on the meeting's final resolution. A representative of the institute's leadership who participated in the debates said at first that as far as she knew, the building in which the meeting was taking place had bullet-resistant windows. She then telephoned the institute's security services and learned that this was not the case. Leaving the room, we were told, would be more dangerous than staying inside. Finally, we all sat on the floor, far away from the windows, and tried to continue the debate. The Zika mothers sat in one corner. A few care workers who knew them well moved to sit near them. Less severely affected children with CZS were amused: finally there was an interesting activity. After approximately an hour, we were told that it was safe to leave the meeting room. Everybody rushed out to grab a coffee or a soft drink. The shooting incident seems to have been perceived as an unfortunate external event, entirely disconnected from the issues discussed in the Zika workshop, not as a brief incursion of the random violence that permeates the lives of many mães de micro into the sheltered universe of scientists and researchers.

Care and an Uncertain Future

Fetal medicine experts whom I interviewed in late 2015 and early 2016 were familiar with cerebral lesions similar to those observed in ultrasound images and MRI scans of fetuses diagnosed with Zika-induced brain anomalies. They predicted that the majority of children born with such anomalies would live but would display severe neurological problems. This was not, however, the usual early perception of Zika-induced inborn anomalies. On the one hand, mothers of children with CZS, as well as health professionals, affirmed that during the early stages of the microcephaly epidemic physicians believed that the great majority of the children with severe microcephaly would die in the first or second year of life. On the other hand, leaflets and booklets distributed to mothers of CZS children conveyed the opposite message. They did not distinguish between severe and moderate Zika syndrome, and they said that while a child with this syndrome would reach major developmental milestones at a slower rate than other children, with the right stimulation, patience, and love he or she would be able to thrive.

In the early days of the epidemic, Adriana Melo carried on her laptop computer images of a little girl born with microcephaly who, but thanks to the intensive efforts and ingenuity of her mother, a professional physiotherapist, at the age of fifteen months walked, talked, and looked like a "normal" child. This story is undoubtedly plausible. Microcephaly is a highly variable symptom. Scientists reported that about 10% of children diagnosed with microcephaly at birth suffered from minor impairments only. Intensive physiotherapy could significantly reduce the consequences of these impairments.[75] The majority of the children born with Zika-related microcephaly have, however, severe developmental problems. Many among them have convulsions that are difficult to control with standard drugs, especially in the first two years of life. More than half have severe posture problems, not only with walking but with sitting and rolling as well.[76] Around the age of 2.5 years, nearly all the children in one closely followed group of 121 infants with CZS demonstrated profound developmental delays in all areas of functioning. The level of functioning of the majority of these children was close to that of a 2- to 3-month-old infant. Because many among them had limited use of their hands and little ability to control the movements of their limbs, they were unable to demonstrate higher-order cognitive skills, such as object recognition or basic problem-solving. One exception was in receptive language: they recognized words and reacted to them. Given their significant motor and visual impairments, these children's primary means for interacting with their environment appears to have been through auditory input.[77] Several smaller studies reported similar findings. The main problems of CZS children, besides severe motor and developmental delays, are epilepsy, dysphagia (feeding difficulties), impaired hearing and sight, and sleep disorders.[78]

The "baby in the bucket," Jose Wesley Campos, of Bonito, Pernambuco, who in early 2016 became one of the faces of the Brazilian epidemic of microcephaly, is one of the children with severe developmental delays.[79] In June 2018 the Associated Press carried the article "From shrieks in bucket to laughs, Brazil Zika baby improves." It stated that Jose Wesley Campos was nearly 3 (he was born in September 2015), giggled frequently, could keep his head up, and could utter three words that are a mix of truncated Portuguese sounds: *goo*, *'gui*, and *ma*, for "oatmeal," "dad," and "mom," respectively. José's mother, Solange Ferreira, explained that José's evolution has been great and that her son had taught her so much about love, since "he will only develop if we love him a lot." When her son was born the doctors told her that he had little chance of staying alive.[80] His survival is therefore seen by his mother as an important victory, as is his steady progress. José does indeed have very severe health problems. He cannot eat and is fed with a tube that passes through the nose. He can move his arms and grab a pencil, but he cannot crawl or stand, and he can only sit up, propped up, for a short period. His mother received significant help from the municipality of Bonito. A driver paid by the city takes her and her son to medical visits and physical therapy in Recife, Pernambuco's capital, two hours away. Thanks to Pernambuco's policy of integrating severely impaired children in regular schools, José attends a "normal" daycare center two days a week, accompanied by a full-time caregiver. Despite doting teachers and socialization in an inclusive environment, José's schooling did not seem to have improved his skills. Ferreira also noted that she was frequently exhausted by the care of a child with very complex health needs. The Associated Press article ends, nevertheless, on a positive note: "Thanks to the devoted care and the unfailing affection of his family, the attention he gets in school, and the help of his doctors and therapists, José Wesley is thriving in his ways while touching people's lives along the way."[81]

Children with severe CZS frequently went through three stages: a stage of incessant crying, often calmed by drugs and occasionally by immersing the child in cold water or swaddling; a stage of convulsions, again treated by drugs, which, however, often made the child apathetic and nonreactive and led to developmental regression; and a stage of severe alimentary difficulties and the risk that food might enter the child's lungs, a complication that could lead to death. The latter problem was frequently solved by feeding the child through a nasal tube or a tube going directly into the stomach, a drastic intervention that not infrequently was resisted, initially at least, by the families.[82] Facing an accumulation of severe difficulties, some women fluctuated between acceptance and despair. In the words of one mother, "He was a gift, but as they say, I don't wish this for anyone. Eyeglasses, medication diapers, food. . . . It's very difficult, I don't wish this for even my worst enemy. My husband works, right, so I don't have to ask help from anyone."[83]

A *New York Times* article in August 2022 on the fate of children with congenital Zika syndrome seven years after the outbreak of the microcephaly epidemic presented a vivid picture of the difficulties faced by the affected families. Seven years after the epidemic, some among the affected children were nearly as big as their mothers—and all those born with severe CZS were profoundly disabled. They had implanted feeding tubes; the use of the arms and legs of many was stifled because of contracted muscles, and many needed hip surgeries for malformed joints; and above all, their motor and intellectual development had usually frozen at the age of six months. The *New York Times* article focused on the fate of one such child, João Guilherme, and his mother, Verônica Santos. Verônica Santos lives in Recife, where the municipality offered many services to children with CZS. Thus João Guilherme has physiotherapy and a session of audio and visual stimulation every day. On the other hand, João Guilherme's ability to communicate with others is very limited, and he needs constant care for changing his diapers, turning him over, attaching and cleaning his feeding tube, and suctioning his throat; he also wears a beeper that alerts his mother if he stops breathing at night. Verônica Santos cares for her son full time, and like many mothers of severely incapacitated children, she worries about what will happen to him if she becomes unable to fulfill this role.[84]

In a review in 2021 of 25 anthropological studies of the Zika outbreak in Brazil, Alessandra Santana Soares Barros, whose previous work was centered on disability activism in Brazil, criticized what she saw as an excessive "maternalism" of these studies. Their authors focused exclusively on the mothers' subjective experiences and their "militant maternity." They did not link their investigations with the existing sociological and anthropological literature on the care of children with severe brain damage and did not examine the intervention of other, mostly female actors who participated in these children's care—educators, physiotherapists, nurses, social workers. Moreover, the anthropologists who studied Zika mothers implicitly followed the social model of disability. Their research was focused almost exclusively on the role of social policies in the management of children with CZS, and they neglected to pay close attention to the material consequences of the child's severe disability and the adverse effects on their caregivers.[85] Their understandable wish to resist the definition of disability solely in terms of failing, breaking, and distorted physical bodies led in some cases to disembodied narratives of the experiences of these children and their caregivers. Anthropologists, Barros explains, seldom described "a baby who doesn't open his mouth wide enough to get the spoon in, who doesn't unlock his legs to be cleaned, who doesn't know how to cough up phlegm. A baby who was not a baby anymore; who was already three and would soon be four years old. A child for whom, in addition to providing for his or her hunger, thirst, and hygiene, one needs to take care of her or his choking, self-suffocation, pain in the joints from contractures of bent legs, the bedsores, the chilblains between the fingers of hands that won't open, diaper rash on the buttocks that will never be without diapers, the bandages on the belly through which tubes enter, the gums thickened by seizure medication."[86]

One of the key elements in narratives of mães de micro is their complex relationship with time. Mães de micro observed by the anthropologist Elisa Williamson lived in suspended time. They testified that they had to learn to live one day at a time and abandon long-term plans and projects, train themselves to "expect nothing" yet, at some level at least, maintain hope in the face of uncertainty.[87] Myriam, the mother of a CZS son, told Williamson:

> Everything is very uncertain. You never have a guarantee that he's going to be ok the whole week, without presenting something new. There's no such thing. There is always something new, good or bad. . . . Everything comes up very, for the parents, very sudden. . . . The children, I think, it's still very unknown [*incógnita*]. We don't know . . . I don't know if it's because for us everything is new, or if it's because of this condition of theirs that everything is very new, something is always coming up [*toda hora aparece uma coisa*]. . . . He's fine, he's not convulsing, in a little while he starts convulsing. He's not taking medication, [then] in a little while he starts taking it, and in a little while he does that, the boy is ok, then in a little while [you] put in a gastro [feeding tube], you put in a tráqueio [breathing tube]. It's insanity, insanity!

Treatment may help—sometimes. When her son Bruno developed convulsions at the age of 5 months, another mother told Williamson, he was given an anticonvulsive drug. The drug worked, but it also, his mother attested, arrested Bruno's development. According to his mother, "He stopped not only having seizures but, he stopped completely. Everything he did, held his head up, he looked, he fixed [his gaze], he laughed—everything that he had been doing he stopped doing. . . . It was very instantaneous, like, he just stopped doing everything. He stopped crying too. Stopped everything, stopped everything."[88]

Summing up their experiences several years after their children were born, mothers of children with CZS, especially those who had not benefitted from a support network, emphasized their persisting financial and emotional difficulties. Some mothers received help from members of their immediate family, nearly always female; others struggled alone. The majority obtained assistance from the state, but many considered the assistance grossly inadequate:

For me, the fact that she has microcephaly is not what hits me the most. . . . The only thing that is sad for us here at home is to know that she was born and she lives in a very difficult financial situation. We do not have decent living conditions.

I used to work, take care of myself, . . . now I don't eat, I quit doing everything, sometimes I don't even go to the bathroom. . . . Because she has these nervous breakdowns and she cries a lot. I am suffering a lot. I did not sleep this night.

I started to leave my son in the daycare, terrible daycare service. Wow, I would cry every time I left my son because they would not even shower him, they would not change diapers, and he got full of chafing.

And so, tiredness strikes, that routine, I don't go out, I don't do anything, I live inside this house, at night awake or going too much to the hospital, doctor, we just need to talk sometimes, we just need to cry, be heard.

Before we had the baby, everything was fine between us. But as the baby cried a lot, day and night because of microcephaly, he even had to move rooms so he would not hear him crying. He could not stand it and went away.

After I had him, I already had to take controlled medication, the doctor said that it was to give me more courage because there are days when it seems that I cannot stand or get up, so tired! . . . Goodness, there's been two months that I go to the capital every week for his treatment, and my other son is revolted, he said that he did not want to have a brother anymore, because he says that after his brother was born 'this house has no peace anymore, there is no peace,' he says that no one cares for him anymore, because the brother takes my whole time.[89]

Narratives about the Zika epidemic in Brazil were frequently framed as harrowing but ultimately uplifting stories about redemption through maternal love and care. But care, the anthropologist Carlo Caduff argues, is often difficult for those who require it, those who receive it, and those who provide it.[90] Care, Aryn Martin, Natasha Myers, and Ana Viseu propose, is complex, and while its descriptions tend to be romantic and laudatory, it has a darker side too. Care is a selective mode of attention: it circumscribes and cherishes some things, lives, or phenomena as its objects, but in the process it excludes others. Care organizes, classifies, and disciplines bodies.[91] In real life, the philosopher Anne Marie Mol explains, good care coexists with other logics, and with neglect and errors.[92] This may have been especially evident in the Zika crisis, during which, Paula Freitas and her colleagues stressed, Brazil's fragile policies on women's health failed to serve those affected.[93]

Zika Syndrome and the Law:
How Special Are the Children with CZS?

Mães de micro proudly described themselves as mothers of "special children."[94] In September and October 2019 the Brazilian parliament attempted to find a legal definition of these "special children." It discussed a law, Medida Provisória no. 895 (MP-895), that granted state support for children with CZS. At the very center of the debates was the question whether these children were entitled to special help from the state beyond the very limited support provided to children with severe inborn impairments. Children with neurological impairments akin to those of children with CZS were entitled only to that modest support. MP-895 proposed to grant to children with confirmed CZS—and only to those children—more substantial, although still limited, financial help: a lifelong monthly pension (*pensão vitalícia*). This monthly pension would replace earlier forms of support to children with CZS and their families established in 2016.[95]

The main issues discussed during the parliamentary debate on MP-895 were the specific responsibility of the state for the fate of children with CZS, the criteria for inclusion in this program, and the need to help children with other severe disabilities and their families.[96] Members of parliament and senators looked into the state's responsibility for the birth of children with CZS. Parliament member (PM) Ruy Carneiro claimed that the state had failed to protect pregnant women from mosquito bites. It should have determined which localities had high concentrations of mosquitoes and systematically sprayed insecticides in those localities. It should also have distributed mosquito repellent to all pregnant women. PM Bosco Costa disagreed, arguing that the main responsibility for the elimination of breeding sites of mosquitoes should be delegated to people living in the infested localities. He proposed making laws that would allow fines to be imposed on individuals who failed to eliminate the sites.

Parliament members interrogated the definition of CZS. PM Eduardo Barbosa raised the difficulties of establishing a correct diagnosis of CZS, especially in the early stages of the Zika epidemic. PM Natalia Bonavides evoked the slow pace of "official" recognition of CZS and said that a great number of children still awaited their diagnosis. PM Ruy Carneiro opined that since many children with probable CZS lived in regions where there was no access to advanced diagnostic techniques, the state should favor a broad definition of CZS that would include probable cases. PMs Tereza Nelma and Mara Rocha agreed: a focus on the size of the newborn's head, especially in the early stages of the epidemic, had led to the exclusion of many children who very likely had been infected with the Zika virus in the womb. Some advocacy groups, such as the National Association for the Right of People with Congenital Syndrome of Zika Virus also proposed to enlarge the definition of congenital Zika syndrome.

Several PMs and senators questioned the fairness of giving a state pension only to children with CZS. PMs Jaindra Faghali, Marcio Jerry, and Perpetua Almeida asked why a child with severe intellectual impairment or severe autism should not receive the state's help. Senator Telmário Mota similarly argued that the state should provide a pension to children with the same kinds of neurological problems as those induced by ZIKV. Senator Gabrilli proposed that before receiving compensation a disabled child be examined by an interdisciplinary commission of specialists to determine the child's level of impairment, instead of making the compensation dependent exclusively on a confirmed diagnosis of CZS. PM Edna Henrique contended that the state should provide a pension to all children with severe microcephaly, independently of its cause, while PM Daniel Coelho asked why children with other severe chronic conditions, such as cystic fibrosis, were not entitled to a state pension. Finally, PM Jorge Solla proposed adding to the law compensation for people with lifelong sequelae of Guillain-Barré syndrome, another severe pathology induced by the Zika virus.

Several parliament members argued that the proposed compensation was inadequate. PM Samia Bofim submitted a long document showing the skewed distribution of children with CZS among social classes and their concentration among the poorest strata of the Brazilian population. PM Ruy Carneiro explained that the great majority of these children lived outside important urban centers, so that it was often difficult for their mothers to take them to see health professionals. PM Assis Carvalho affirmed that the proposed allocation would cover only a small portion of a family's needs, especially because of the socioeconomic status of mothers of children with CZS: 77% of these mothers were Black or Brown, from a very poor background, and had a low education level, and many were in a situation of great social vulnerability. PM Marcelo Freixo produced similar statistics: 52% of the mothers had not completed elementary school, and because of their tasks as caregivers, only 27% were able to return to work, even part time. Senator Weverton pointed to the high cost of medical care for children with CZS and to the fact that only a fraction of the cost was covered by the state. During a public hearing for MP-895/2019, mothers of children with CZS, among them Germana Soares, representing UMA, stated that while this law was a step in the right direction, the proposed financial contribution was very modest.[97]

MP-895/2019 was passed by the parliament on December 17, 2019, and confirmed by the Senate on February 5, 2020.[98] It was definitively adopted in April 2020: MP-895/2019 became law number 13.985/2020.[99] The new law guaranteed a monthly pension for life, equal in value to one minimum wage (at that time R$1,045, approximately US$225), to all children with confirmed CZS. The Health Ministry estimated that 3,112 children born between January 1, 2015, and December 31, 2019, became entitled to this pension.[100] The new law did not include provisions for children born with other inborn impairments or for the "discarded" children, initially investigated for suspected CZS. Law number 13.985/2020 was celebrated by an official ceremony in Brasília in the presence of representatives of both the government and parents' associations. UMA activists held a prominent place in that ceremony.

Zika = Affect

In early March 2021 a small exhibition, *Zika: Affecting Lives*, was opened by Fiocruz's Museu da Vida (Life Museum), which was usually dedicated to educational activities. The exhibition was originally planned to take place in the museum's building, but because of the COVID-19 pandemic it was presented exclusively online. The exhibition exemplified the identification of the Zika outbreak with the care of children with CZS by their mothers. It displayed visually striking photographs of disabled children, their mothers, and their caregivers accompanied by short descriptions.[101] In the introduction to the exhibition Fiocruz's president, Nisia Trindade Lima, explained that the Zika epidemic invited viewers to rethink the relationship between scientific knowledge, public policies, and society. However, the exhibition itself did not discuss such relationships. Its title played on the multiple meanings of the word *affect*. The introduction affirmed that "relations built in life and in meetings can enhance the capacity to act. This is what happened to caregivers, managers, families, and researchers affected by Zika. If today we understand more about the congenital syndrome, if we have increased our capacity to act, it is because our lives have met and affected each other. We must continue to affect, to be affected, and, above all, to build affections."

The exhibition was divided into four sections. The first, "Zika: Suddenness in the World and Brazil," opened with the following statement: "The Brazilian experience resulted in an international recognition of our ability to face new health emergencies and global challenges." In March 2021, when Brazil grappled with the dramatic consequences of the COVID-19 outbreak, attributed partly at least to the incompetent management of the pandemic by the Bolsonaro government, a statement about the international recognition of "Brazil's ability to face new health emergencies" might have sounded ironic—or bitter. The second section, "Uncertainties and Emergencies," presented the difficulties of mothers and families of children with CZS. A panel explained that in 2017 the United Nations Development Programme had estimated that the costs associated with CZS were US$1,707 per month (circa R$9,745 in March 2021). A second panel stated, with no additional comment, that these children had been granted a lifelong monthly pension equivalent to one minimum wage, R$1,100 (circa US$192) in 2021. The third section, "Mobilization and Responses," pointed to the important volume of scientific studies of Zika and the prominent contribution of Brazilian researchers to these studies. It also emphasized the key role of associations of mothers of CZS children in the fight for the rights of their children. The final section of the exhibition, "What Needs to Be Done," explained that it was necessary to invest more in health care, follow-up studies of children with Zika syndrome, and the development of diagnostic tests, vaccines, and treatments. The exhibition ended with the following statement: "Zika showcased inequalities. Facing it properly depends on guaranteeing social rights, strengthening the health system, science, inclusive education, fighting poverty, basic sanitation, and accessible public transportation." These are undoubtedly important demands. They are also very broad, and not related to the unique traits of the Zika crisis.

The exhibition organizers explained that its main goal was to show the new pathways of collaboration between scientists, clinicians and activists developed during the Zika crisis. This collaboration had led in 2018 to the writing of a joint document, "Zika Epidemic in Brazil: Lessons Learned and Recommendations."[102] Between October 2018 and August 2020, members of the group involved in writing the joint document held three preparatory meetings, which culminated in the Fiocruz exhibition. The aim of the exhibition, its organizers explained, was to promote the articulation of education and research practices based on knowledge and strategies produced by users of the health system and by social movements in order to construct a roadmap for future actions. One of the main reasons the exhibition focused on "affect" was to highlight the key role of women during the Zika crisis—female scientists, physicians, members of paramedical professions, educators, social workers, and mothers of children with CZS. A strong feminine presence contributed to the innovative approaches that combine science with emotion.[103]

Two topics produced heated debates during the curation process that led to the construction and validation of the exhibition's project: the abandonment of children with CZS by their fathers and abortion for a fetal anomaly. The abandon of disabled children by their fathers ("male abortion") was at some point discussed publicly by activists, for example, in a TED talk by UMA's president, but some of the participants were concerned that mentioning this problem might lead to excessive generalizations.[104] The religiosity that underlined the discourse of some spokespersons of associations of families and their refusal to discuss termination of pregnancy together with disability made abortion for a fetal impairment a highly contentious topic. The exhibition's organizers decided that the exhibition should not mention controversial topics, because "their exercise in building the roadmap will be undermined by arousing irreconcilable interests."[105] They also did not mention another potentially contentious issue, the skewed class and race distribution of children with CZS, perhaps because of its almost total invisibility in the public space. The organizers explained that their main goal was the promotion of "environments and instruments that allow the Brazilian population to participate in a more democratic and citizen-oriented fashion in debates involving science and technology, particularly in the field of health."[106] Their focus on affect—that is, on shared humanity—could indeed promote compassion and solidarity. Such a focus, especially when coupled with broad and noncontroversial demands and the avoidance of potentially disturbing subjects, could also impede a democratic debate on science and technology and mask the specific reasons why the Zika outbreak in Brazil "showcased inequalities."[107]

CHAPTER SEVEN

After Zika

Open Questions, Complex Legacy

When an Epidemic Ends

An epidemic ends when people no longer perceive it as a frightening, unpredictable episode. "The social lives of epidemics," the historians Jeremy Greene and Dora Vargha proposed, "show them to be not just natural phenomena but also narrative ones: deeply shaped by the stories we tell about their beginnings, their middles, their ends."[1] Perceptions of what counts as an epidemic vary from one location to another. An outbreak of a given intensity can be seen as an epidemic in one geographic area and a continuation of an endemic pathogen in another.[2] This is even more true for pandemics because today the definition of an outbreak as a pandemic is decided by a handful of experts from international organizations.[3] A disease is no longer called a pandemic, the executive director of the Global Fund to Fight Tuberculosis, AIDS and Malaria, Peter Sands, explained, once it is not seen as putting people in affluent countries at risk. Pathologies that do not kill people in rich countries are usually called epidemics, and those that the world could have gotten rid of but hasn't are called endemic diseases.[4] Sands was most likely referring more specifically to the fate of AIDS. In the 1980s there was a widespread fear that the AIDS epidemic would affect everyone—that is, Western, heterosexual, middle-class, white people. The cover of the July 1983 issue of the ultraconservative magazine edited by Jerry Falwell, the *Moral Majority Report*, carried the heading "Homosexual diseases threaten American families" and a photograph of a white, middle-class family wearing surgical masks. In 1983 a photograph of a mask-wearing family aimed to project a terrifying vision of the future; it looked perfectly banal in 2023. More to the point, a rapid understanding, especially after blood transfusions and blood products were made safe, that HIV was not a major threat to mainstream Western families radically changed the perception of the AIDS pandemic. In 2017 the fear of middle-class Brazilians, especially women of reproductive age, of dramatic consequences of an infection with ZIKV during pregnancy was transformed into an implicit conclusion that "people like us" were not at high risk of giving birth to children with CZS. Zika became, as long as there was not another major outbreak, a neglected disease, one that affected silenced and marginalized populations.[5]

The Zika epidemic in Brazil officially ended with the end of the ESPIN in May 2017. While the Zika virus is endemic in Brazil, its reported frequency declined steadily, as did the frequency of CZS. In 2017 the Health Ministry investigated 2,646 suspected cases of congenital Zika syndrome, 304 of which were confirmed; in 2018 it investigated 1,018 suspected cases and confirmed 120; and in 2019 it investigated 480 suspected cases and confirmed 59.[6] With the declining threat of Zika, stories about the disease disappeared from the Brazilian media. From mid-2016 they were displaced by other topics, first the Olympic Games and then the economic crisis and the impeachment of the left-wing president Dilma Rousseff and her replacement by the conservative politician Michel Temer. During the latter process a little-known member of the National Congress, Jair Bolsonaro, dedicated his vote to the memory of Colonel Carlos Alberto Brilhante Ustra, seen as the man responsible for the torture of political opponents during the military dictatorship in Brazil (1964–85). The scandal that followed Bolsonaro's declaration brought him immediate notoriety and helped to jump-start his political ascent. During a period of severe political and economic turmoil, problems produced by the Zika virus quickly became invisible.

The Puzzle of Disappearing Zika

The rapid decline in the number of infections with the Zika virus in Brazil was unexpected. Experts assumed that the Zika epidemic in Brazil would end even without human intervention thanks to the development of herd immunity in the affected populations. Many believed, however, that this process would be gradual and take several years, especially since they presumed that the disease would move from one region in Brazil to the next. They did not predict the swift reduction in the number of infections not only in Brazil but in all Latin American countries.[7] Brazil reported 205,578 cases of Zika in 2016 and 13,253 cases for the period January–June 2017. It is doubtful that such a precipitous decline in the prevalence of Zika and CZS can be fully explained by the development of herd immunity. In the absence of reliable serological tests capable of detecting past infection with this virus, it is difficult to ascertain how many people were infected with the Zika virus.[8] Nevertheless, partial epidemiological data indicate that while a significant proportion of people living in the regions of Brazil with a very high incidence of Zika in 2015 and 2016 became immune to this virus, it was probably not the case in regions with a much lower incidence of Zika, such as the south of Brazil. The abrupt decline in infections with the Zika virus in all of Brazil is another "Zika puzzle."[9]

The World Health Organization declared the end of Zika's designation as a PHEIC (Public Health Emergency of International Concern) on November 18, 2016. The main reason for that declaration, experts that proclaimed this PHEIC explained, was that while there was not yet "definitive" proof that the Zika virus had been the source for severe malformations in newborn children, the similar results from studies of the effect of ZIKA in cultures of brain cells, research on Zika-infected laboratory animals, clinical observations of pregnant women and newborn babies, and prospective epidemiological investigations strongly indicated that the Zika virus had indeed produced inborn anomalies. Members of the WHO Emergency Committee on Zika argued that since the key uncertainty at the heart of the global emergency response had been successfully resolved, it was no longer necessary to define the ZIKA crisis as a public health emergency. The PHEIC had, however, other declared goals besides answering the question whether the Zika virus had induced neurological impairments in fetuses and newborns, including the rapid development of reliable tests for diagnosing Zika based on the presence of anti-Zika antibodies in the blood, the implementation of efficient anti-*Aedes* measures, and the elaboration of interventions that would allow pregnant women to protect themselves from the consequences of infection with Zika during pregnancy. These goals were not attained. The WHO Emergency Committee on Zika affirmed that the end of the PHEIC should not be interpreted as a reason to abandon intensive Zika studies. Just the opposite. The emergency research during the PHEIC period had created the conditions for sustained research to address the numerous aspects of the infection with the Zika virus that remained to be understood. The "sustained research" on Zika announced by WHO experts did not come into being. Key diagnostic and vaccine development efforts decreased dramatically after the lifting of the PHEIC, while the significant decrease in cases of infection with the Zika virus in Latin America had limited researchers' ability to conduct clinical trials of diagnostic tests and candidate vaccines. Despite the WHO's claim in November 2016 that Zika represented a highly significant long-term problem requiring a sustained research effort, it became increasingly evident that with the end of the international emergency, financial and scientific resources had been redirected elsewhere.

The Brazilian Ministry of Health, like the WHO, stated that the end of the ESPIN in May 2017 should not be interpreted as the end of epidemiological vigilance. It also affirmed that it continued to give high priority to efforts to control the mosquito *Aedes aegypti*, research on the Zika virus, and assistance to families of children with congenital Zika syndrome. In practice, for the Brazilian government too, the official declaration of the end of the Zika emergency meant a modulation of priorities in the distribution of funds for fundamental and clinical research, help to needy families, and public health interventions. With the sharp fall in the number of Zika cases, this disease became just one mosquito-borne infection among several others, and one among many causes of inborn impairments, especially among women from lower social strata. Solving the "Zika puzzles" was no longer a priority, especially when an economic crisis and a conservative shift in Brazilian politics led to severe cuts in funding for research, health care, and public health interventions.[10] It became an even lower priority with the advent of the COVID-19 pandemic.

The International Scientific Community and the Zika Crisis

The proclamation of Zika as a PHEIC in February 2016 produced an important flow of money to fundamental research on the Zika virus and a rapid expansion of studies. Brazilian researchers had already accumulated knowledge on the Zika epidemic and its consequences. They also had privileged access to "research materials," such as children affected by Zika syndrome and their mothers, and could collect samples of their tissues and body fluids. Brazilian scientists and physicians were thus quickly integrated into important and well-funded collaborative research programs financed by international organizations such as the European Community, the US National Institutes of Health, leading European and North American universities and research organizations, and private foundations. In the aftermath of the WHO's declaration of Zika as a PHEIC, one of its main authors, David Heymann, emphasized the key role of cooperation between Brazilian scientists and their colleagues in other countries in quickly finding solutions to the Zika crisis. International collaborations developed during the Ebola epidemic, Heymann and his colleagues added, had often been problematic. In 2013 and 2014, West

Africa had been a playground for researchers allegedly appropriating and transporting specimens and data to their home laboratories, sometimes without the knowledge or permission of the countries where these samples were collected. Similarly, the recent rapid spread of Middle East respiratory syndrome coronavirus (MERS-CoV) had been plagued by insufficient sharing of data between foreign researchers and those in countries where the epidemic took place. Local scientists had complained that Western researchers visited their countries for a short time only, collected data that they later used in prestigious publications, and entirely missed the opportunity to enhance the research capability of the host country scientists. It was important, Heymann concluded, to learn from experience and avoid such pitfalls during the Zika epidemic.[11]

Brazil has a long tradition of high-level biomedical research. Many among the scientists who studied Zika had solid international reputations, as did Brazilian research and teaching institutions and Brazilian biotechnology companies. The Zika epidemic further enhanced the reputation of Brazilian science. The Brazilian Health Ministry's official publication *Zika Virus in Brazil: The SUS Response* explained that the Zika epidemic allowed Brazilian scientists to publish numerous articles in top-ranking scientific journals, while close collaborations with well-known researchers from Western Europe and North America increased the prestige of Brazilian scientific and medical communities.[12] Zika also created new opportunities for young Brazilian scientists. They developed close links with investigators of prestigious research centers abroad, became firmly embedded in international networks, and found new sources of funding and new possibilities of training abroad, an especially welcome development in a period of a severe economic crisis and shrinking research budgets. The integration of Brazilian researchers into collaborative networks also strengthened inter-institutional collaborations within Brazil. In some cases, Brazilian scientists who worked in relative isolation discovered shared interests with colleagues in other parts of Brazil—and sometimes even in the same city—during a conference held abroad, or when they joined the same international program. Brazilian researchers' enlarged international and national cooperation networks became evident in the long lists of authors of key publications about the Zika epidemic in Brazil.[13] It is was also evident in the celebration of researchers such as Celina Turchi or Patricia Brasil as pioneers of Zika studies.

A more problematic aspect of contributions of international organizations to the study of the Zika epidemic was their reluctance to intervene in the thorny area of women's reproductive rights. Health authorities, the scientists interviewed by the New York Times journalist Donald McNeil explained, were fearful of offending religious conservatives and never seriously discussed abortion as an alternative to giving birth to a permanently deformed baby. Michael Osterholm, director of the University of Minnesota's Center for Infectious Disease Research and Policy, gave a blunter explanation of officials' reticence: "The C.D.C. [Centers for Disease Control and Prevention] always gets in trouble with Congress when it talks about contraception or bullets," he said. In reference to the latter he meant that CDC officials hesitated to point out that shootings were a major cause of American deaths because they did not want to offend the gun lobby. "And abortion?" he added. "You talk about third rails in politics? Abortion is the fifth rail. They can't touch it. If the C.D.C. had pushed the envelope any farther, its funding would have been at risk."[14] The failure to help women postpone pregnancies and protect themselves from sexual transmission of ZIKV and to allow those who contracted Zika during pregnancy and feared the consequences of this infection to have an abortion, Clare Wenham and her colleagues had persuasively shown, amplified the consequences of the health crisis produced by Zika, especially for the most vulnerable women.[15]

Another focus of critiques of international collaborations during the Zika crisis was the fact that international scientific organizations gave much higher priority to the safety of populations in industrialized countries than to the needs of those in developing and intermediary countries.[16] Until recently, the Brazilian political scientist Deisy Ventura explained, epidemic threats were managed mainly according to the rules of International Health Regulations, supervised by the WHO, but now they are increasingly managed according to the rules of the Global Health Security Agenda (GHSA), launched in 2014, an alliance of more than 50 countries, headed by the United States. This loosely structured alliance allocates resources that, Ventura argued, serve mainly to contain infectious diseases in the Global South. Not infrequently, research in global health has given relatively low priority to poverty-related diseases found only in developing countries and tended to focus on pathologies capable of spreading to the developed parts of the world, such as Ebola or Zika.[17]

International funding agencies also tend to prioritize funding of targeted interventions able to produce rapid results. An editorial in the *American Journal of Public Health* in April 2016 expressed the hope that international scientific cooperation on Zika would lead to the fast development of tools to control it—reliable and affordable diagnostic tests, a vaccine, a safe treatment, and better ways to control *Aedes*.[18] The Zika epidemic did not lead to the successful development of such control tools. Moreover, targeted interventions, especially vaccination campaigns, can reduce the burden of specific diseases but rarely produce structural changes that reduce inequalities in health care.[19] During the Zika outbreak, only a handful of international programs provided targeted help to children with Zika and their mothers. The public image of the Zika epidemic inside and outside Brazil was shaped by dramatic media stories about severely impaired children and the difficulties of their mothers, but international collaborative programs gave relatively low priority to the protection of rights and interests of women in epidemic areas or the care of children with CZS.[20]

In February 2016 the WHO, together with 23 partner organizations, launched a strategy designed mainly to prevent and manage the socioeconomic and medical problems caused by the epidemic and to coordinate research on these problems. The strategy aimed to provide women of childbearing age, especially pregnant women, along with their partners, households, and communities, with the information they needed to protect themselves from infection, as well as counseling on sexual and reproductive health and health education and care. However, over its first six months this strategy suffered a serious shortfall in funding: US$25 million was needed, but just over $4 million was received. In July 2016, Bruce Aylward, interim executive director of the WHO's Outbreaks and Health Emergencies Cluster, contrasted the impressive scientific progress in the understanding of the epidemiology and pathogenesis of the Zika virus with the shortfall in funding to help affected populations. "Why," Aylward asked, "is it so difficult to mobilize the funds needed to mitigate the consequences of such a horrific disease?"[21]

This trend continued in the second half of 2016 and in the next two years. Between 2015 and 2018, $3.8 million in research funds provided by international organizations was channeled to studies on the social aspects of the Zika outbreak broadly defined. By comparison, in 2016 alone the European Union contributed $51 million to scientific studies of Zika and the US National Institutes of Health contributed $81 million.[22] In mid-2016, the WHO and PAHO established a new, more ambitious program centered on preventing and managing medical complications of Zika virus infection and estimated that it would require $117 million before the end of 2017. This program too remained severely underfunded. Financed mainly by the UK Department for International Development (DFID) and USAID, it was able to obtain only $19 million by the end of December 2017, a far cry from its initial goal.[23]

The paucity of funds destined for the population directly affected by the Zika outbreak was matched by the lack of funding for research in social sciences. Studies aimed at improving the care of children with CZS and their families were given very low priority. The Zika Social Science Network estimated that between 2015 and 2018 only $3.8 million (approximately 2.9%) of the estimated $132 million provided by European Union and US funds to study Zika were dedicated to social sciences writ large.[24] Social science research on Zika was funded mainly by Brazilian research organizations. Since the funds allocated by these organizations were modest, excellent research was often conducted on a shoestring budget. One exception to the scarcity of international backing of social studies on Zika was support by the Wellcome Trust for studies of women and children affected by CZS, conducted by Debora Diniz and her colleagues at the ANIS Institute of Bioethics. Another exception was the joint funding by the Wellcome Trust, UKAID, and the European Union's Horizon 2020 program of a study conducted by a group of Brazilian and British social scientists, with the collaboration of an association of Zika mothers in Salvador, Bahia, "Abraço a microcephalic." That study aimed to provide critical insights into how communities cope in epidemics, uncover the voices of those suffering, identify unmet needs, and promote advocacy for the development of better services.[25]

The reason for the contrast between the impressive amount of international investment in the fundamental research on Zika and the paucity of funding for interventions aimed at alleviating the plight of children with CZS and their mothers, some Brazilian scholars proposed, was that the global health community's definition of *global* did not include zones of negligence, or rather of the neglected populations populating those zones.[26] The international response to the Zika crisis focused on preventing diseases from the Global South from threatening the countries of the Global North. As Deisy Ventura put it, "From the point of view of the PHEICs neither the existence of the disease nor its magnitude matters. What does matter is to prevent the disease from leaving the place where it should have stayed."[27]

The two contrasting views of the international scientific community's role during the Zika epidemic—that it enhanced the reputation of Brazilian researchers and favored the development of biomedical sciences in Brazil and that it made visible the indifference of Western scientists to the plight of vulnerable populations in Brazil—are probably both partly correct. Retrospective evaluations of the achievements of international collaborations on Zika vary greatly. Discussing the state of research on Zika in late 2017, David Morens and Anthony Fauci, of the US National Institutes of Health, pointed to the impressive achievements of fundamental studies of the Zika virus, the vast body of knowledge accumulated between 2013 and 2017 on this topic, and the fact that this was the first time an epidemic of fetal anomalies had been studied in real time.[28] Researchers from one of the European Union–funded collaborations on Zika, ZIKAlliance, in November 2018 proposed a more critical view. They pointed to the fragmentation of studies conducted in different countries, delays in regulatory and ethical approval of collaborative projects, difficulties of harmonizing research protocols and laboratory tests, and differences in rules for handling and shipping biological materials, such as blood and other body fluid samples, among participating countries.[29]

Summing up the detailed history of the emergence of global health, George Weisz and Noémi Tousignant explained that the sphere of global health was characterized by a high level of disagreement on key issues—"about how much emphasis should be placed on biomedical technologies versus underlying social and environmental conditions; about the role of cost-effectiveness analysis versus other criteria; about which diseases should be prioritized; about the balance between local capacity building in low-income countries and research in the developed world to produce immediate biomedical solutions; and about reinvigorating old institutions as opposed to creating new ones." Yet, they added, "what is striking is how, for the most part, potential conflicts were often muted, buried in committee discussions, technical reports, or debates about appropriate metrics. Faith in 'science' and the drive to provide rational, seemingly apolitical foundations for action in the expanding, heterogeneous, often chaotic world of global health did not so much blur these points of disagreement as suspend them from time to time in pursuit of a single overarching goal that everyone could rally behind: producing more and better research."[30] Important international investment in research on Zika undoubtedly produced "more and better research," but the question remains, better for whom?

Vulnerable Populations and Endemic Zika

The rapid increase in Zika's media coverage was followed by its equally rapid disappearance from the news. The last time Zika was amply discussed in the media outside Brazil was in the summer of 2016, in the context of the Rio de Janeiro Olympic Games. From 2017 on, the infrequent media reports about Zika, published mainly in Brazil, have focused on the fate of children with CZS and their mothers. Other questions raised by the Zika epidemic, above all how to prepare for future outbreaks of this or similar pathologies, have received very little public attention. However, despite significant investment in research on Zika between 2016 and 2018, Brazil's capability of preventing another outbreak is probably not very different in 2023 than it was in 2015. Factors that have made it difficult to control the *Aedes aegypti* mosquito in urban areas for the last 40 years are still around: rapid and often chaotic urbanization, increases in urban poverty, intensification of population movements, growth in the volume of air travel, and, increasingly, the consequences of climate change. ZIKV, like the dengue and chikungunya viruses, became endemic in Brazil, and it is reasonable to assume that Zika will be able to sporadically induce larger outbreaks. The COVID-19 pandemic may have complicated Brazil's efforts to contain arboviruses. According to official Brazilian data, the prevalence of dengue, chikungunya, and Zika decreased in 2020. Some experts argued, however, that the decrease was a consequence of a significant reduction in testing for these pathologies. The mobilization of available laboratory resources to detect SARS-CoV-2 infections led to serious delays and underreporting of infections with other viruses.[31] Moreover, COVID-19 produces highly variable symptoms that may be confounded with those of diseases such as dengue, chikungunya, or Zika, while a co-infection with SARS-CoV-2 and an arbovirus may aggravate the patient's sickness.[32]

In 2015–16 the high density of *Aedes* mosquitoes in Brazil, the presence of an immunologically naïve population, and probably also the sexual transmission of this pathogen produced a perfect storm: an unchecked and very rapid spread of Zika in Brazil, especially in the northeast. An additional aggravating element was the economic crisis in Brazil, which coincided with the Zika epidemic.[33] Since the mid-1970s no Brazilian government, right, center, or left, has perceived the control of *Aedes* mosquitoes as a high priority. Politicians pledged before each election to invest in infrastructure and improved sanitation to reduce the circulation of mosquitoes; once elected, they failed to fulfill these promises. And inhabitants of mosquito-infested areas frequently saw other problems, such as poverty and high levels of violence, as more urgent than *Aedes*-propagated diseases.[34] The growing prevalence of such diseases in Brazil is seen as regrettable but inescapable. But the acceptance of mosquito-borne diseases as a part of life, especially in poorer neighborhoods, has a price. These diseases, experts stated in the spring of 2020, continue to impose a great health burden on the population in Brazil and are a constant challenge for health authorities.[35]

An increase in the problems produced by arboviruses was not limited to

Brazil. The Global Burden of Disease Study, which collects data on diseases worldwide, noted a significant increase in the number of people who died from dengue fever in 2017.[36] Nearly all these people lived in the Global South, and the great majority of them were poor. Since effective control of *Aedes* in Brazil through social measures and progressive urban policies has increasingly been perceived as an impossible task, many experts have turned to a search for technical solutions to the mosquito problem: sterilization of mosquitoes by X-rays, their genetic modification, or their infection by the bacterium *Wolbachia*, which prevents them from disseminating viruses. Such technical solutions, if they work, are expected to be considerably less expensive than investments in sanitation and infrastructure. However, despite successful localized experiments, these approaches have failed to produce a large-scale decline in the prevalence of mosquito-borne pathologies, and it is not certain whether on their own they will be able to control the spread of such pathologies.

The development of an efficient anti-Zika vaccine—and eventually anti-dengue and anti-chikungunya vaccines as well—is seen as a more promising technical solution. Vaccines, as the recent example of the Ebola outbreak in the Central Republic of Congo in 2018 showed again, can play an important role in the containment of transmissible diseases. The elaboration of a vaccine is not easy or predictable. The yellow fever vaccine, 17D, developed circa 1937, continues to be a highly efficient tool for limiting the spread of this pathology, and the rapid development of anti-SARS-CoV-2 vaccines in 2020 was hailed as an unprecedented success. By contrast, despite the intensive efforts of scientists and pharmaceutical companies, there is still no efficient and widely accepted vaccine against dengue fever, a failure underscored in 2017 by the problematic fate of an anti-dengue vaccine developed by the pharmaceutical firm Sanofi. The vaccine, presented as highly promising, was tested on a large scale in the Philippines, where it was linked with several suspected deaths; its testing was then halted.[37] The disappearance of Zika from the Americas considerably slowed down the initial intensive efforts to produce a vaccine against this pathology. On the other hand, some of the vaccines against COVID-19, such as the Astra-Zeneca vaccine developed in collaboration with the Jenner Institute at Oxford University, relied on earlier efforts to elaborate an anti-Zika vaccine. That the success of anti-COVID vaccines will boost the efforts to develop vaccines against Zika and other arboviruses cannot be ruled out.

In 2023 the Zika virus represents a threat of an unknown magnitude. In the states of Parana and Pernambuco, antibodies against the Zika virus were found in capuchin monkeys. The observation that jungle monkeys with known contact with humans could carry the Zika virus and potentially serve as a permanent reservoir of this virus increased the fear of a cyclical return of Zika to Brazil. Experts tend to agree that at some point Brazil will face another Zika epidemic, but their estimates of how soon it may happen vary widely. Some researchers believe that thanks to the widespread immunity to ZIKV in Brazil developed during the 2015–16 outbreak and maintained through a continuous low-level circulation of this virus, Brazil is safe from a major Zika epidemic for a half-century at least. Other researchers are more pessimistic. They believe that without an effective vaccine, Zika may establish itself as a disease with periodical eruptions of variable severity and may become a "new normal" in many parts of the world, and a pathology that continues to selectively harm vulnerable women.[38]

Still Risky, but Not for All: Endemic CZS

Since the Zika virus did not entirely disappear from Brazil, it is reasonable to assume that sporadic cases of Zika syndrome in newborns will continue to occur there. On the other hand, as long as such cases are relatively rare, CZS will probably be perceived as one among the many fetal anomalies induced by an infection of a pregnant woman. It is also reasonable to assume that as during the Zika pandemic, the risk of Zika-induced inborn impairments will be unevenly distributed, transforming CZS into a "neglected pathology" that selectively affects children of women from lower social strata. The risk of CZS shares many traits with the risk of fetal anomalies induced by cytomegalovirus (CMV). In numerous cases, an infection with this virus leads to pregnancy loss. However, not all pregnant women infected with CMV miscarry. In those who do not, this virus can induce fetal anomalies. CMV, like ZIKV, is neurotropic. Experts estimate that about 20% of the fetuses infected with CMV develop inborn impairments such as microcephaly, intellectual delays, seizures, and hearing and vision problems. CMV was among the main causes of microcephaly in Brazil before the Zika epidemic. CMV-induced brain anomalies are quite similar to those induced by ZIKV, although the latter are often more severe.

CMV is one of the most frequent among the TORCH infections, but in absolute numbers infections with this pathogen during pregnancy are relatively rare. Therefore, health authorities in Western Europe and North America do not recommend screening all pregnant women for CMV infection but integrate surveillance of CMV-induced harm into routine monitoring of pregnancy. In Brazil too, the infection of the fetus by CMV, which is not strongly associated with social class, is seen as an accidental misfortune. The main difference is that while in Western countries the majority of pregnant women undergo during the second trimester a diagnostic ultrasound that facilitates a prenatal diagnosis of CMV-induced anomalies of the fetus, in Brazil women who use SUS services do not have routine access to this examination. During the Zika epidemic, SUS facilities that did offer diagnostic ultrasounds to women offered it between 30 and 35 weeks of pregnancy, that is, well past the point of fetal viablity.[39] One can speculate that surveillance of sporadic, Zika-induced impairment in Brazil will follow the CMV model: replacement of a systematic screening of pregnant women for infection with ZIKV by selective testing for the presence of this pathogen following the detection of fetal anomalies during routine ultrasound surveillance of pregnancy. Such a model entails, however, access to a quality ultrasound surveillance of pregnancy, follow-up of abnormal findings, and, implicitly, the possibility for a woman who learns about a severe fetal impairment to elect to terminate the pregnancy. It may thus be accessible only or mainly to middle-class women.

Not all the anomalies induced by ZIKV can be detected during pregnancy or immediately after birth. Children born with a normal-size head and no detectable brain lesions can still develop serious neurological problems and hearing and sight anomalies later in life. Such problems were found in up to 20% of children born to women with a confirmed diagnosis of Zika during the early stages of pregnancy and classified as "normal" at birth.[40] Since a significant proportion of infections with ZIKV are asymptomatic, it might have been desirable to closely follow the development of all the children born during the Zika epidemic, including those with no visible signs of neurological impairment at birth. In practice, only a small fraction of these children have been followed, those whose mothers entered a prospective clinical trial.[41]

Experts who follow cohorts of Brazilian children born to mothers infected with Zika during pregnancy plan to continue their investigations until the children reach the age of seven. It is not sure, however, that all the problems linked to maternal infection with Zika will be visible before the child's seventh year. North American specialists followed for 40 years a cohort of children whose mothers contracted rubella in the first trimester of pregnancy during the 1962–63 epidemics in Western Europe and North American and who were classified as "normal" at birth and during their first years of life. They discovered that about a third of the initially symptom-free "rubella children" had learning difficulties. Such difficulties frequently increased with age. Even more distressing, approximately 20% of them developed schizophrenia-spectrum disorders as young adults; others developed psychiatric disorders, such as major depressive or bipolar disorder. Only 41% of individuals in this group were defined as totally free from cognitive or psychiatric complications at the age of 40.[42] It cannot be ruled out that some of the children born to women infected with ZIKV early in pregnancy and initially classified as "normal" will develop learning, behavioral ,or psychiatric difficulties later in life. However, it is also possible that since the great majority of these children were born to lower-class mothers, their potential cognitive and psychiatric problems will be attributed to other causes, such as deprivation, "unhealthy" habits, life in a violent environment, or substance abuse. It is not certain whether scientists will ever learn the full extent of the harm produced by the 2015–16 Zika outbreak in Brazil.

A Never-Ending Story?

The history of public health in Brazil, the historian Maria Alice Rosa Ribeiro proposed, is a never-ending story. Problems are treated in a fragmentary way, and the great majority never reaches a final resolution: "they are not confronted, nor eliminated—they just go on and on."[43] Another way to speak about the persistence of public health problems in Brazil is to describe the country as "on the brink." As in a game of Snakes and Ladders, Brazil "nearly gets there"— "there" being the level of development of industrialized countries—then slides back into periods of regression in many areas. Brazilians rightly point to important achievements of Brazilian biomedical sciences and significant progress in many public health domains. Public health progress is, however, often fragile, easily destabilized by the persistence of drastic inequalities, and shaped by changing political circumstances.[44] This may be especially true in the fraught domain of women's reproductive health.

In 1916, when one of the leaders of the Brazilian sanitary movement, the physician Miguel Pereira, described Brazil as an "immense hospital," he was referring above all to the dramatic health situation in rural areas.[45] The main goal of the Sanitary Movement, active in the early twentieth century, was to end the severe neglect of Brazil's interior by physicians and scientists. Some of the activists of the Sanitary Movement disagreed with the claim that Brazil's principal problem was the neglect of the health and well-being of the populations in the country's interior and argued that the main dividing line in Brazil was not the one between the littoral and the interior but the one separating the affluent classes from the poor. In a comment on Pereira's statement, the physician and writer Alfrânio Peixoto explained in 1918 that in Brazil numerous people suffer from two pathologies or more. He saw children in primary school shivering from malaria. And, he added, this was not just in some distant provinces but in Rio de Janeiro too. "Do not have any illusions— our hinterland (sertão) starts at the end of Avenida (the central avenue of Rio de Janeiro)."[46]

The Zika outbreak and then the COVID-19 pandemic dramatically illustrated the persistence of the *sertão* behind the Avenida and the great difficulty of promoting collective health in a country in which impressive achievements in some areas of public health coexist with extremes of economic and social inequality. During and after the Zika outbreak, Brazilian social scientists produced two kinds of narratives about this epidemic, affirmative and critical. The affirmative narratives highlighted positive elements, such as the achievements of Brazilian scientists and public health experts or the exemplary struggles of associations of mães de micro. The critical narratives emphasized the systemic failures of the Brazilian state: the neglect of sanitation in poor areas, facilitating the proliferation of *Aedes* mosquitoes; chronic underfunding of the SUS, hampering the surveillance of pregnant women; the deterioration of the national health system following the severe political and economic crisis that started in 2013; and the shortcoming of social policies destined to help children with CZS and their mothers. Both narratives are essentially noncontroversial. The majority of Brazil's citizens, it is reasonable to assume, are proud of the successes of Brazilian scientists and public health experts, and important segments of the public do not question, in principle at least, the necessity of improving sanitation and health care in poor areas and providing support to children with disabilities and their families. While opinions about priorities and the efficacy of the existing governmental interventions vary greatly, there is a widespread although not general recognition of the need to do more and better.

The plight of vulnerable populations is a relatively safe topic, as is their courage and resilience. "In the time of such immense despair," the anthropologist Rosamaria Carneiro wrote in 2020, alluding to the grave political and economic problems of Brazil at the time, "I am inspired by the example of these women [mães de micro], brave but also exhausted and socially unappreciated, who reinvented practically everything in the name of their children."[47] Justified indignation at the suffering of the poor and legitimate admiration of their courage may, however, deflect attention from less comfortable matters. Zika arrived in Brazil during a period of acute political turmoil, and the microcephaly epidemic was followed by a period of growing despair among progressive scholars. Understandably, they looked for inspirational narratives. In the long run, however, a reluctance to tackle unsettling issues may hinder the progressives from achieving their aims. Epidemics are revealing episodes that, in the words of the French anthropologist Claude Lévi-Strauss, are "good to think with," but, one might add, only if one is willing to reject simplified narratives, engage with complex and confusing subjects, acknowledge the presence of unsettling elements, and as the feminist scholar Michelle Murphy explained, accept working through the discomfort, messiness, worry, anger, and pain.[48] Especially if the goal is to put an end to a never-ending story.

Embodied Inequality

An Epidemic of Signification

The Zika outbreak in Brazil can be seen as an *epidemic of signification*. This expression, coined by the social critic Paula Treichler, who wrote about AIDS, aptly describes how the latter pathology was linked to sex, drugs, blood, and death and reveals the discrimination and stigmatization of groups such as homosexuals, Haitians, drug users, sex workers, and African migrants.[1] The visibility of all these topics produced a climate in which AIDS was perceived not as one infectious disease among many others but as a pathology endowed with a strong emotional charge. Zika can be similarly seen as epidemic of signification. It connected mosquitoes, poverty, race, sexuality, fertility, and harm to the unborn (the fear of "monstrous births" can be traced to antiquity). It also exposed the plight of previously invisible groups, such as children with neurological impairments and struggling mothers of disabled children, and produced, mainly through striking photographs of affected babies, an emotionally charged image of Zika that was quite different from the image of a closely related pathology, dengue fever. On the other hand, the Zika epidemic was also shaped by "public secrets," elements known to many people but perceived as disturbing and therefore seldom presented in public debates about this disease.[2] One such public secret was the role of stratified reproduction in Zika times. Women from higher social strata (mostly white) had much greater opportunities than those from lower strata (mostly non-white) to evade contamination by disease-carrying mosquitoes; avoid sexually transmitted diseases, including Zika; control their fertility; obtain a reliable diagnosis of exposure to the Zika virus during pregnancy; get access to quality monitoring of fetal development and, if applicable, safe termination of pregnancy—and therefore avoid the birth of a child with congenital Zika syndrome.

Brazilian public health authorities treated the Zika epidemic mainly as a "contamination" and concentrated their attention on viruses and mosquitoes.[3] Social scientists who studied the Zika epidemic, aware of the disproportional suffering ZIKV infection brought to neglected populations, saw it as a complex "configuration" produced by a unique alignment of interconnected biological, environmental, socioeconomic, and political variables. Their studies documented how the Zika outbreak was shaped by poverty, exclusion, and neglect. They focused, however, nearly exclusively on the consequences of ZIKV infection on women from lower social strata: the configuration they studied disregarded important segments of Brazilian society. Speaking about inequality, the anthropologist Didier Fassin contends, should involve analyzing the whole of society, not merely its lower sectors. An exclusive focus on the poor, even when it is done with the best possible intentions, may be tricky and misleading. The point is, Fassin explains, not to isolate the oppressed and the exploited but "to insert them into social relations whose fundamental injustice resides precisely in an implicitly established or explicitly acknowledged hierarchy of lives. It's this hierarchy that allows them to be interiorized, stigmatized, and brutalized while other lives are privileged."[4] Privilege of the affluent extends also to their future children. The signification of the Zika outbreak in Brazil was constructed not only thorough the increased visibility of some elements but also through the exclusion of other elements, such as middle-class advantages and stratified reproduction, from the collective social imagery. Epidemics question the existing global health governance and invite us to develop different ways to study the interdependence of local and global, domestic and transnational, chronic and infectious, human and nonhuman.[5] One place to start might be to carefully examine the of sites of production of situated, embodied injustice.

Seeing Injustice

The Brazilian environmental activist Chico Mendes (1944–1988) stated that ecology without class struggle was gardening. Mendes's claim, which is relevant to many other areas of activism, was that it was not sufficient to tinker with ad hoc solutions; one had to confront the roots of major social problems. In 1970s and 1980s Brazil, *class struggle* was a common term. With the waning of Marxist influence, it was often replaced by *striving for more social justice*, a term that occasionally masks the violence of social relations in neo-liberal societies. This is especially true when, as it is sometimes the case, this goal becomes a vague demand to better the lot of the downtrodden, a discursive equivalent of focusing the debates on ecology on planting trees and recycling domestic trash. Instead of speaking of loosely defined justice, it might be more fruitful, the political philosopher Nancy Fraser proposes, to focus on injustice. She draws on the philosophy of Plato and John Rawls and above all Kazuo Ishiguro's novel *Never Let Me Go* to investigate why certain kinds of social arrangements are intolerable and how their intolerability is neutralized and "normalized" by those in positions of power.[6]

Ishiguro's novel is written from the point of view of clones, children educated in a pleasant and enlightened boarding school who gradually learn that they are collections of "spare organs" destined to be "sacrificed" so that their "originals" can live longer and better. Fraser does not see Ishiguro's powerful narrative as other critics did—as futuristic dystopia, bildungsroman, a story about friendship and fidelity, or a parable of human mortality—but above all as a meditation on an unjust world and the profound suffering inflicted on its inhabitants. To understand the abstract concept of justice, Fraser proposes, one should contemplate what it would take to overcome injustice. The clones in Ishiguro's novel do not count as subjects of justice. Their distinct and inferior moral status is achieved through rigid segregation from their "originals." Such segregation is, however, a fiction. The two groups participate in a single, shared bio-economy because the originals rely on the clones for their survival, yet they deny them the status of partners in their interaction. The clones, socialized in a highly exploitative order, fail to perceive its immense injustice. Society does not provide them with the language or the means to do so. The extreme violence of social arrangements to which they are born is hidden behind a neutral language: robbing them of vital organs is called "donation," and their final killing "completion."

The clones, Fraser explains, speak "for all those whom our social order simultaneously interpellated as individuals and treats as spare parts—as sweatshop labor, as breeders, as disposable workers; as providers of organs, babies and sex; as performers of menial service, as cleaners and disposers of waste; as raw material to be used up, ground down and spat out, when the system has got from them all that it wants." In a society in which one group depends on another group for such vital necessities as domestic work, childcare, eldercare, cleaning, or waste disposal—the member of both inhabit the same moral universe and deserve equal consideration in matters of justice—which those perceived as providers of services fail to receive. Fraser concludes that one should not treat formal citizenship as the principal determinant of who counts. It is important to carefully examine the broader patterns of stratification, the causal mechanisms that produce hierarchy, and the ideological strategies that obscure them, such as an exclusive focus on private emotions and individual achievements.

In Ishiguro's novel, the clones believe that their "donations" and their final demise can be deferred for several years if they display true feelings, such as love or passion for art. This belief helps them to accept their fate. Ishiguro's heroine, Kathy, makes a stubborn claim to a measure of dignity in the face of a social order that disrespects her at every turn and persists in the effort to make meaning even when the basic structure of her society has granted her nothing from which to fashion it except debris. Emotional identification with the aspirations of those made powerless by an unjust society—the "affect" at the center of Fiocruz's Zika exhibition—however important, is not a substitution for honest and careful examination of the mechanisms that keep some individuals powerless. One such mechanism is situated privilege. Some privileges—money, status, in some societies birthright or caste—are displayed openly. Others are so efficiently minimized, masked, or naturalized that in some cases at least the privileged can forget the gulf that separates them from the less fortunate.

The two kinds of health citizenship in Brazil studied by the anthropologist Emilia Sanabria illustrate the naturalization of embodied privilege.[7] Comparing the standardized contraceptive services provided to lower-class women in SUS clinics with the individualized care available to middle-class women of gynecologists in private practice, Sanabria argues, following the sociologist Roberto da Matta, that there is a central tension in Brazil between a formal embracing of the principles of equality and individualism and a tacit hierarchical mode or relationality. Affluent women who have access to safe and moral-reprimand-free abortion live in a different material and moral environment than do poor women, who lack such possibilities. The abortion experience of an upper-middle-class woman who ends an unwanted pregnancy in a private clinic where she is treated with respect, receives anesthesia, and benefits from appropriate postabortion follow-up is radically different from that of a poor woman, which is marked by pain, fear, and not infrequently, if she seeks medical assistance in a public facility, disparaging and humiliating treatment.

The difference between the embodied experiences of poor and affluent women is, however, seldom made visible, because the majority of studies focus exclusively on low-income groups, without giving due consideration to developments at the other end of the social spectrum. In Brazil individuals who have private insurance (approximately 25% of the population), and especially those who have a quality health plan, belong to a very different social category (super-citizens) than those who rely exclusively on SUS services (sub-citizens). Although the health system is supposed to be universal, in practice the state systematically collects data only on patients in the public sector, effectively, Sanabria argues, rendering a whole segment of the population beyond, or above, public policy. Consequently, "the emerging public domain—via the policy landscape—is characterized by a notable absence: that of the elites and middle classes who rely on private services." There has been "a welcome academic and policy focus on the exclusion of the most marginal from health services, but no interest in another exclusion: that of the elites."[8] Privilege has become invisible.

Ambivalence of Protest

The strategy of approaching justice negatively, through injustice, Nancy Fraser suggests, is powerful and productive. One of the key messages of Ishiguro's description of injustice is that a focus on the individual's feelings and acts can efficiently hide the existence of structural problems and impede collective action. "Individuality is a double-edged sword," writes Fraser. "On the one hand, it is the mark of personhood and intrinsic value, the admission ticket for moral consideration. On the other hand, it is easily made into a ruse of power, an instrument of domination. When divorced from a structural understanding of an exploitative social order, individuality can become a cult object, a substitute for critical thinking, and an impediment to overcoming injustice. . . . As 'individuals' we are exhorted to assume responsibility for our own lives, encouraged to fulfill our deepest longings by purchasing and owning commodities, and steered away from collective action toward 'personal solutions.'"[9]

Fraser provides a fine-grained analysis of how a focus on individual achievements and responsibility deflects attention from the basic structures of oppression. The underlying assumption is, however, that a better understanding of the community of fate and the rise of collective struggle is an effective antidote to an exclusive focus on individuals' actions. The Brazilian example may complicate this view. It indicates that when collective struggles are not accompanied by the questioning of privileges, they may not be sufficient to put an end to oppression and injustice. For historical reasons, above all the recent history of the SUS and the inclusion of the right to health in the Brazilian constitution, Brazilians who rely exclusively on the SUS are allowed, and sometimes actively encouraged, to protest against the insufficiency of means accorded to government-sponsored health and social services. Many users of public health services fight for their rights, whether through individual but collectively sustained actions—such as suing the state to demand medical interventions not accessible to them via the SUS—or through the actions of organized groups, such as those of associations of mothers of children with CZS.[10] These are important actions. On the other hand, their success is often insufficient and fragile.

Mães de micro successfully fought to obtain better care for their children. They were able to gain a minimum wage (1,100 reais, approximately US$190 in 2021) for their children for life. This is undoubtedly important for families at the lower end of the social scale, especially when added to the maximum support for poor families, the Bolsa Família (205 reais, approximately US$35). It is, however, woefully inadequate given the monthly costs of care for a child with CZS in Brazil, estimated by the United Nations to be more than nine times the minimum wage.[11] In a society ruled by an "excluding universalization," even when legal struggles succeed in obtaining better health and social services from the state, their success is only partial. In such a society, Poliana Cardoso Martins and her colleagues explain, a significant portion of the population has access to only limited health services, those provided by the SUS, while the well-remunerated social groups "self-exclude" themselves through their use of a private health system, a move that may resonate with their self-exclusion in high-rise buildings that have adequate hygienic arrangements and are guarded 24 hours a day by a busy staff of doormen–cum–sanitation agents.[12]

In theory, calls for "more social justice" and for "the elimination of social injustice" are symmetrical. In practice, this is often not the case. Not infrequently a desire for *more* social justice implicitly involves a reluctance to question the privileges of the upper social strata. Protests against injustice are often a gut reaction to the fundamental immorality of many such privileges, especially those that undermine human dignity. It is also one of the fundaments of a "decent society," one that does not humiliate its members.[13] Fraser is right: "a searing vision of an unjust world and the profound suffering inflicted on its inhabitants" is a powerful moving force for social change. The key term here is *searing vision*. It is not sufficient to note the presence of suffering and to be compassionate; one must have a clear vision of injustice and rebel against it.

A Divided World

The "universal right to health" bestowed by the Brazilian constitution is in practice used by those who cannot afford the advantages provided by private health services. Private and public health sectors coexist in numerous countries, but the situation in Brazil may provide an especially sharp contrast between the image of the national health system as a key motor of social progress and solidarity and the reality in which an exclusive dependence on the SUS is an important marker of the difference between the haves and the have-nots. Western European national health services are (mostly) seen as providers of services for all the citizens, not just for those who cannot afford alternative solutions.[14] This is not the case in Brazil. Almost all the Brazilian progressive health experts adhere to the Latin American concept of collective health (*saúde coletiva*), which sees health as inseparable from other determinants of human well-being. They also enthusiastically back the SUS, are proud of its achievements, and actively defend them. On the other hand, since they usually have private health insurance, they do not need to "earn" their right to health or fight for it.[15] The problem is emphatically not the choice of private health services by middle-class people, including those who earnestly support the National Health Service. The SUS has severe shortcomings, and understandably, people wish to protect their own and their family members' health. The knotty issue is the low visibility of consequences of the chasm between health services available to higher and to lower classes. To follow Fraser—and Roberto da Matta—Brazilian society, including in the health care arena, is characterized by a dual social order, with one set of rights for "us" and another for "them" and in which the rights for "us" frequently evade detailed scrutiny.

Progressive Brazilian and international health experts protested vigorously against putting the onus of avoiding Zika and CZS on individuals, above all women, rather than assigning responsibility for the proliferation of mosquitoes and mosquito-borne diseases to the state. They strongly denounced a policy that told women to clean their houses and avoid getting pregnant and indirectly blamed women who "failed" to protect themselves and gave birth to a child with CZS.[16] Structural changes necessary to reduce the *Aedes* threat were, however, a long-term goal, while an epidemic that specifically affected pregnant women was an emergency that called for rapid solutions. With the declaration of Zika as an ESPIN, all Brazilian women urgently needed to gain access to interventions capable of reducing their risk of having an impaired child, which would decrease their fear and feelings of helplessness.[17] At the peak of the Zika/CZS epidemic in Brazil, neither the government nor, with a few notable exceptions, nongovernmental organizations promoted making such interventions available to lower-class women. One of the elements that might have impeded interventions in the area of women's sexual and reproductive rights was the glorification of maternity and the criticism of "anti-*mãe*" attitudes. Universal acclaim of mothers who care for their disabled children may resonate with the applaud of the clones' emotional and artistic achievements in Ishiguro's book, a posture that may help to mask structural injustice. Poor women are depicted as brave, resilient, and guided by admirable moral principles. Upper-class women are free to make choices that reduce their need to be brave and resilient, but they may wish to divert attention from disturbing questions. Focusing the researchers' attention on the struggles and the courage of mothers of impaired children might have been a way to avoid such questions.[18]

The Zika epidemic exposed structural weaknesses of the Brazilian public health system but also the persistence of dramatic social inequalities and middle-class privilege. Reproduction is one of the principal sites of the unfolding of such privilege. Tensions between mothers of children with CZS and the researchers who studied them were attributed to the researchers' blunders, their lack of sensitivity to the mothers' plight, the mothers' feeling of powerlessness in dealing with health professionals, or the absence of "translators" able to mediate between mothers and researchers. They may also have reflected a shared awareness of a "family secret"—that mães de micro and the scientists studying their children live in radically different worlds. In the first minutes of the ANIS documentary feature *Zika, the film*, the gynecologist Adriana Melo talks to Amanda Loizy, who has just received confirmation of the diagnosis of microcephaly for her future child. Melo, visibly distressed at being the bearer of bad news, asks Loizy, "It is difficult, right?," and Loizy answers that it is "very difficult. One always hopes that the test will be negative." Melo then says, "I understand. But now we face another struggle, right? This struggle starts now, and let's see what we have to do."[19] The "we" links a white professional who, one may assume, has a comfortable lifestyle and a poor, non-white woman who after the birth of a daughter with a severe CZS was obliged to leave her job to become a full-time caregiver for her daughter and struggled to survive with her three children on a minimum wage.[20] Some mães de micro might have resented such inclusive language.

Disadvantaged women who have little control over their fertility and are afraid that they might die as a consequence of an illegal abortion have no access to quality prenatal tests. Those who learn about their future child's impairment are entitled, if they are lucky, to hug therapy; if they do not receive it, they may face disparaging and sometimes brutal treatment from health professionals. Lower-class women that rely exclusively on SUS services have dramatically different experiences from women who can decide more easily whether and when they will have a child, have access to high-quality prenatal testing and safe abortions, and are treated with respect by health providers. They inhabit a different world than less privileged women. The Zika epidemic made visible the deep chasm between the different worlds of these women.

From One Epidemic of Signification to the Next

The Zika outbreak was followed by the COVID-19 pandemic, another pathology that made visible the inscription of social injustice on bodies. The mechanisms of inscription by Zika and COVID-19 were not identical—women's sexual and reproductive functions in the case of Zika; occupational risks, living in crowded quarters, and the presence of chronic pathologies in the case of COVID-19—but the targets were the same: vulnerable populations living in precarious conditions. The lockdown that followed the COVID-19 eruption suddenly made visible the previously invisible work of service workers, cleaning personnel, delivery service workers, and shop assistants. It also highlighted the key role of care workers. In all the societies hit hard by COVID-19, the mortality rate among those who provided these services was much higher than the rate among upper-class people who benefited from their services— a telling illustration of Fraser's claim that the clones in *Never Let Me Go* are a metaphor for members of the "service classes," who "donate" their bodies to dominant groups.[21] During a short time in late 2015 and early 2016, the shocking photographs of babies with CZS and their mothers attracted attention to the injustice and violence in the lives of poor, non-white women who often worked in service and care jobs or provided unremunerated care for other family members. The Zika epidemic, perhaps more than other recent outbreaks of infectious diseases before COVID-19—such as H1N5 influenza, SARS, MERS, H1N1 influenza—made visible the links between the consequences of an outbreak of transmissible disease and social status.[22] The Zika epidemic may thus be perceived as a forerunner of the staggering inequalities, societal failings, and vulnerabilities made visible by the COVID-19 pandemic.

COVID-19 reached Brazil in April 2020. The outbreak had a chaotic trajectory but predictable consequences: those affected most by the new pathology were the poor. While Zika and COVID-19 were very different diseases, they shared one common trait: the central role of inequality in exacerbating epidemic-related risks. The Zika epidemic, the anthropologist Soraya Fleischer suggested, "reveals—as perverse contemporary photography—the decadent Brazilian welfare state, where minorities, diversity, and social rights are being drastically destroyed."[23] The trajectory of COVID-19 in Brazil can be seen as a further intensification of this trend. The paucity of solutions to social problems revealed by Zika prefigured developments during the next, major pandemic that "nobody predicted." While there were numerous warnings about the "next plague," in the exhaustive scenario of "preparedness" for a major outbreak of infectious disease—usually modeled on influenza pandemics—the possibility that one of the main consequences of such an outbreak would be the aggravation of social inequality and women's plight was seldom discussed.[24] This was especially true in Brazil. The "Brazilian," or gamma, variant of SARS-CoV-2 was found to be especially dangerous to pregnant women with comorbidities such as malnutrition, overweight, diabetes, and cardiovascular disease, that is, mostly women from lower social strata. In April 2021, Brazilian women were advised again by a Health Ministry official, Raphael Perente, to delay pregnancies until the worst of the epidemic had passed.[25] Indeed, many women—those who could—decided again to put their reproductive plans on hold, as they had in 2016. They also reported, as they had during the Zika outbreak, being stressed and scared.[26]

In early 2016, when Debora Diniz wrote her pioneering book *Zika: From the Brazilian Backlands to Global Threat*, she could not know that by the time it was published the Zika epidemic in Brazil would already be on the wane. Nor could she predict that in the second half of 2020 a different global threat would emerge in Brazil: the gamma variant of SARS-CoV-2. Epidemics are biosocial entities, shaped by the specific biological traits of the pathogens that induce them. Because of its unique pattern of spread and induction, Zika affected mainly lower-class women. Such restriction of harm induced by a pathogen to specific socioeconomic strata is less likely in the case of a respiratory virus. No social group was fully protected from COVID-19, but some groups, such as people with disabilities, especially underprivileged people with disabilities, were much more vulnerable to its effects than others.[27] The combination of the sequelae of Zika with COVID-19 created especially harrowing situations.

The difficulties of mothers of children with CZS were magnified by the COVID-19 epidemic. Individuals with severe respiratory problems, such as children with congenital Zika syndrome, were at very high risk for COVID-19, but because of their multiple health problems and lesser probability of survival, they were less likely to be admitted to overcrowded hospitals. During a sanitary emergency children with CZS also were unable to obtain adequate treatment for their persisting health problems. Medical services were not available, and the pandemic led to shortages in the stock of essential medications, such as anticonvulsive drugs. Although there were no precise data, mães de micro reported on their WhatsApp networks the deaths of children with congenital Zika syndrome. Some of these children might have died from COVID-19, and others because they failed to obtain appropriate treatment for their other ailments.[28] It also became very difficult to continue to provide physiotherapy and reeducation to children with CZS. Mães de micro testified that the COVID-19 pandemic seemed to have erased the modest achievements of their children. At the same time, the material condition of their own lives often deteriorated, while lockdown and social-distancing rules decreased the mothers' ability to rely on the help of family members and friends and increased their isolation, stress, and psychological anguish.[29] Moreover, during periods of lockdown, some mães de micro were exposed to increased domestic violence, another element that put their mental health in danger.[30]

Epidemics often make visible the mechanisms that shield some individuals from the harm produced by an encounter with a pathogen and expose others to it.[31] Explanations for epidemics are contextual.[32] The interactive context that shaped the COVID-19 epidemic in Brazil, like the context that shaped the 2015–16 Zika epidemic, was a dramatically unequal society in which the outbreak of an infectious disease amplified the existing social trends. Zika intensified the vulnerabilities inscribed on the bodies of disadvantaged Brazilian women and their disabled children but also the privileges inscribed on the bodies of well-off women and their offspring. The Zika outbreak in Brazil may be described as an epidemic that signified above all the omnipresence of reproductive injustice.

Control of Aedes Mosquitoes

The history of efforts to control *Aedes* mosquitoes is closely tied to the history of yellow fever. Numerous studies have examined the history of this disease in Latin America, among them Nancy Stepan's "The interplay between socio-economic factors and medical science: Yellow fever research, Cuba and the United States," *Social Studies of Sciences* 8 (1978): 397–423, and Mariola Espinola's, *Epidemic Invasions: Yellow Fever and the Limits of Cuban Independence, 1878–1930* (Chicago: University of Chicago Press, 2009). Rodrigo César da Silva Magalhaes's *A erradicação do Aedes aegypti: Febre amarela, Fred Soper e saúde pública nas Américas, 1918–1968* (Rio de Janeiro: Editora Fiocruz, 2016) provides a detailed background on Aedes eradication policies in Latin America from the 1920s to the 1970s. The efforts to control *Aedes aegypti* in Brazil are summarized in my book *Virus, moustiques et modernité: La fièvre jaune au Brésil, entre science et politique* (Paris: Editions des archives contemporaines, 2001), translated by Ernest Dias into Portuguese as *Virus, mosquitos e modernidade: A febre amarela no Brasil entre ciência e política* (Rio de Janeiro: Editora Fiocruz, 2005). The book examines mainly the efforts to get rid of this insect that culminated in the 1950s in its successful, although temporary, eradication. The collective volume on the control of *Aedes* and yellow fever in Brazil, *Febre amarela: A doença e a vacina, uma história inacabada*, edited by Jaime Larry Benchimol (Rio de Janeiro: Editora Fiocruz, 2001), covers roughly the same period. My article "Leaking containers: Success and failure in controlling the mosquito *Aedes aegypti* in Brazil," in *American Journal of Public Health* 107, no. 4 (2017): 517–24, examines the reasons for the reinfestation of Brazil by *Aedes aegypti* in the 1960s and the gradual abandonment of the plans to eradicate it. The same story is told from a different angle by Gabriel Lopez and Luisa Reis Castro in "A vector in the (re)making: A history of Aedes aegypti as mosquitoes that transmit diseases in Brazil," in, *Framing Animals as Villains: Histories of Non-Human Disease Vectors*, ed. Christos Lynteris (London: Palgrave, Macmillan, 2019), 147–75.

Abortion and Reproductive Rights

There is a rich literature on the abortion debate in the United States. I find especially useful Kirsten Luker's classic study, *Abortion and the Politics of Motherhood* (Berkeley: University of California Press, 1985), and, among more recent works, Katie Watson's *Scarlet A: The Ethics, Law, and Politics of Ordinary Abortion* (New York: Oxford University Press, 2018). Laura Briggs's book *How All Politics Became Reproductive Politics* (Berkeley: University of California Press, 2018) examines the key political role of interventions in the area of reproduction. Briggs's argument is especially important in countries such as Brazil, where politicians frequently present dramatic restrictions of women's reproductive rights as a "niche" issue, disconnected from major political questions and at best marginally relevant to the striving for social justice. Leslie Reagan's *Dangerous Pregnancies: Mothers, Disability and Abortion in Modern America* (Berkeley: University of California Press, 2012) is a fine-grained history of the role of rubella outbreaks in shaping attitudes toward diagnoses of severe fetal impairment or of risk of such an impairment. My book *Tangled Diagnoses: Prenatal Testing, Women and Risk* (Chicago: University of Chicago Press, 2018) compares attitudes toward the detection of a severe fetal anomaly in France, where abortion for a fetal anomaly is legal, with those in Brazil, where it is illegal, and examines the far-reaching consequences of criminalizing abortion.

Cassia Roth's study *A Miscarriage of Justice: Women, Reproductive Lives and the Law in Twentieth-Century Brazil* (Stanford: Stanford University Press, 2020) provides the historical background for the repression of women's reproductive rights in Brazil today. There are numerous studies of the status of abortion in Brazil in the twenty-first century, for example, Debora Diniz and Marilena Correa, eds., *Aborto e saúde pública: 20 anos de Pesquisas no Brasil* (Brasilia: Ministério de Saúde, 2008); and Debora Diniz, Marcelo Medeiros, and Alberto Madeiro, "Pesquisa nacional de aborto 2016, "*Ciência e Saúde Coletiva* 22, no 2 (2017): 653–60. On the use of the drug misoprostol in Brazil to terminate unwanted pregnancies see, e.g., Sylvia de Zordo, "The biomedicalisation of illegal abortion: The double life of misoprostol in Brazil," *História, Ciências, Saúde—Manguinhos* 23, no. 1 (2016): 19–35; and Ilana Löwy and Marilena Correa, "The 'abortion pill' misoprostol in Brazil: Women's empowerment in a conservative and repressive political environment," *American Journal of Public Health* 110, no. 5 (2020): 677–84.

Wendel Ferrari's book *Entre o segredo e a solidão: Aborto illegal na adolescência* (Rio de Janeiro: Editora Fiocruz, 2021) contains detailed testimonies of young women who underwent an illegal abortion. On the frequently traumatic experiences of women who were treated in public hospitals for complications from a presumably self-induced abortion see Maria das Dores Nunes, Alberto Madeiro, and Debora Diniz, "Histórias de aborto provocado entre adolescentes em Teresina, Piauí, Brasil," *Ciência e Saúde Coletiva* 18, no. 8 (2013): 2311–18; and Cecilia McCallum, Greice Mendez, and Ana Paula dos Reis, "The dilemma of a practice: Experiences of abortion in a public maternity hospital in the city of Salvador, Bahia, " *História, Ciências, Saúde—Manguinhos* 23, no. 1 (2016): 37–56.

The History of the Zika Epidemic in Brazil

Two books published in 2016 tell the story of the Zika epidemic in Brazil. Donald McNeil Jr.'s *Zika. The Emerging Epidemic* (New York: Norton, 2016) is a well-researched journalistic account of the early stage of the epidemic. Debora Diniz's *Zika: Do sertão nordestino ã ameaça global* (Rio de Janeiro: Editora de Civilização Brasileira, 2016), translated into English by Diane Grosklaus Whitty as *Zika: From the Brazilian Backlands to Global Threat* (Chicago: University of Chicago Press, 2017), provides a detailed and moving picture of the unfolding of the Zika epidemic in Brazil through testimonies of pregnant women, mothers or parents of children with CZS, and health professionals. Both authors described the Zika epidemic when it was perceived as a global threat. They had no way of knowing that by the time their books were published the epidemic would already be weakening. The Brazilian government's official position on the Zika outbreak of 2015–16 is summarized in Marcia Turcato, ed., *Zika Virus in Brazil: The SUS Response* (Brasilia: Ministry of Health of Brazil, Health Surveillance Department, 2017).

Flavio Coehlo and his colleagues argued that although Brazilian health authorities focused exclusively on the role of the mosquito in the propagation of the Zika virus, sexual transmission played an important role in the spread of this pathogen. See Flavio Codeco Coelho, Betina Durovni, Valeria Saraceni, et al., "Higher incidence of Zika in adult women than adult men in Rio de Janeiro suggests a significant contribution of sexual transmission from men to women," *Journal of Infectious Diseases* 51 (2016): 128–32. Their argument was consolidated later by epidemiological investigations of Tereza Magalhaes and her collaborators. See Tereza Magalhaes, Clarice Morais, Iracema Jacques, et al., "Follow-up household serosurvey in northeast Brazil for Zika virus: Sexual contacts of index patients have the highest risk for seropositivity," *Journal of Infectious Diseases* 223, no. 4 (2021): 673–85.

On the management of uncertainty in Zika times see Ann H. Kelly, Javier Lezaun, Ilana Löwy, et al., "Uncertainty in times of medical emergency: Knowledge gaps and structural ignorance during the Brazilian Zika crisis," *Social Science and Medicine* 246 (2020): 112787; and Koichi Kameda, Ann H. Kelly, Javier Lezaun, and Ilana Löwy, "Imperfect diagnosis: The truncated legacies of Zika testing," *Social Studies of Science* 51, no. 5 (2021): 683–706.

The journalist Donald McNeil Jr. pointed to major failures of the international response to the Zika crisis in "How the response to Zika failed millions," *New York Times*, January 16, 2017. Maria Joana Passos, Gustavo Matta, Tereza Maciel Lyra, et al., called attention to the paucity of means dedicated to studying the social aspects of the Zika epidemic in "The promise and pitfalls of social science research in an emergency: Lessons from studying the Zika epidemic in Brazil, 2015–2016," *BMJ Global Health* 5, no. 4 (2020): e002307, while Barbara Ribeiro, Sarah Hartley, Brigitte Nerlich, and Rusi Jaspald examined the role of the media in masking the centrality of social inequality during the Zika epidemic in "Media coverage of the Zika crisis in Brazil: The construction of a 'war' frame that masked social and gender inequalities," *Social Science and Medicine* 200 (2018): 137–44.

Class, Race, and Congenital Zika Syndrome

On the problematic attitudes toward women's reproductive health during the Zika epidemic in Brazil see, e.g., Deisy Ventura, Danielle Rached, Jameson Martins, et al., "A rights-based approach to public health emergencies: The case of the 'More Rights, Less Zika' campaign in Brazil," *Global Public Health* 16, no. 10 (2021): 1–14; Abigail Aiken, Catherine Aiken, and James Trussell, " In the midst of Zika pregnancy advisories, termination of pregnancy is the elephant in the room," *BJOG* 124 (2017): 546–48; and Luísa Reis-Castro and Carolina de Oliveira Nogueira, "Uma antropologia da transmissão: Mosquitos, mulheres e a epidemia de Zika no Brasil," *Ilha* 22, no. 2 (2020): 21–63. On women's often limited reproductive choices during the Zika epidemic see Letícia Martello, Abigail Weitzman, Raquel Zanata Coutinho, and Sandra Valongueiro Alvez, "Women's reproductive intentions and behaviors during the Zika epidemic in Brazil," *Population and Development Review* 43, no. 2 (2017): 199–227. And for a synthetic overview of the failure to grant reproductive rights to women during the epidemic see Clare Wenham, *Feminist Global Health Security* (Oxford: Oxford University Press, 2021).

Two Brazilian social sciences journals, *Interface* and *Revista Antropológicas*, published special issues dedicated to the difficulties of *mães de micro*, mothers of children with CZS: *Interface* (Botucatu) 22, no. 66 (2018), and *Revista Antropológicas* 29, no. 2 (2018). Similarly, in late 2019 and early 2020 the online journal *Somatosphere* published a series of articles titled "Zika histories," edited by Luiza Reis Castro, http://somatosphere.net/2019/historias-of-zika.html/, focused mainly on the experiences of mothers of children with CZS. More recently, studies on the experience of *mães de micro* were gathered in the volume *Micro-histórias para pensar macropolíticas,* ed. Barbara Marques, Raquel Lustosa, Thais Valim, and Soraya Fleischer (São Carlos: Áporo Editorial, 2021).

A document produced by the human rights organization ANIS in 2017, "Zika in Brazil: Women and children at the center of the epidemic," http://anis.org.br/wp-content/uploads/2017/06/Zika-in-Brazil_Anis_2017.pdf, describes the distressed mothers of children born with CZS in the resource-poor northeastern state of Alagoas, who have only limited access, if any, to medical and educational help. In the same year, Human Rights Watch published a document on Zika in northeastern Brazil based on interviews with multiple actors: Human Rights Watch, *Neglected and Unprotected: The Impact of the Zika Outbreak on Women and Girls in North-*

eastern Brazil, https://www.hrw.org/report/2017/07/13/neglected-and-unprotected/impact-zika
-outbreak-women-and-girls-northeastern. In the summer of 2022 a *New York Times* article poignantly described the ongoing difficulties of Brazilian women and families who continue to
care for severely disabled children with CZS. See Stephanie Nolen, "The forgotten virus: Zika
families and researchers struggle for support," *New York Times*, August 16, 2022.

On the difficult relationships between mães de micro and the scientists who studied children with CZS see Luciana Lira and Helena Prado, "Les effets collatéraux de la recherche sur
l'épidémie de Zika au Brésil," *Anthropologie et Santé* 21 (2020); and, by the same authors, " 'Nossos filhos não são cobaias': Objetificação dos sujeitos de pesquisa e saturação do campo durante
a epidemia de Zika," *Ilha* 22, no. 2 (December 2020): 96–131. Alessandra Santana Soares Barros
persuasively argues in "Deficiência, sindrome congênita do zika e produção de conhecimento
pela antropologia," *Revista Scientia* (Salvador) 6, no. 1 (2021): 142–63, that Brazilian scholars'
almost exclusive focus on mothers of children with CZS may have led to the neglect of the existential difficulties of the children themselves.

Zika, COVID-19, and Embodied Injustice

My reflections on embodied reproductive injustice were inspired by Avishai Margalit's definition of a decent society in *The Decent Society* (Cambridge, MA: Harvard University Press, 1996)
and by Nancy Fraser's description of the naturalization of injustice in "On justice: Lessons from
Plato, Rawls, and Ishiguro," *New Left Review* 74 (2012): 41–51, while my understanding of the
multiple meanings of the gap between the haves and the have-nots in health care in Brazil was
based on Poliana Cardoso Martins, Rosangela Minardi Mitre Cotta, Fabio Farias Mendes, et
al., "Conselhos de saúde e a participação social no Brasil: Matizes da utopia," *Physis* 18, no. 1
(2008):105–21; and Emilia Sanabria, "From sub- to super-citizenship: Sex hormones and the
body politic in Brazil," *Ethnos* 75, no. 4 (2010): 377–401.

On the ways the Zika crisis and then the COVID-19 pandemic amplified the already dramatic inequalities in health care in Brazil see, e.g., Letícia Marteleto and Molly Dondero, "Navigating women's reproductive health and childbearing during public health crises: Covid-19
and Zika in Brazil," *World Development* 139 (2021): 105305; and Claudia Fonseca and Soraya
Fleischer, "Vulnerabilities within and beyond the pandemic: Disability in Covid-19 Brazil," in
Viral Loads: Anthropologies of Urgency in the Time of COVID-19, ed. Lenore Manderson, Nancy J.
Burke, and Ayo Wahlberg (London: UCL Press, 2021), 243–60.

And a final suggestion. The 2016 documentary film *Zika, the Film*, made by Debora Diniz and
her colleagues from the Institute of Bioethics, Human Rights and Gender (ANIS), https://www
.youtube.com/watch?v=j9tqtojaoGo, records the reactions to the diagnosis of a severe fetal
anomaly late in pregnancy of physicians, of women directly affected by the Zika threat, of those
who discovered that they were carrying an affected fetus, and one woman who lost a child to
the infection. It poignantly recaptures the strong emotions of that time and an impending sense
of doom. The film makes the story of Zika in Brazil concrete and immediate. It shows what was
difficult to deal with in an emergency and makes one think about what might have been done
differently to reduce Zika's harm. It also makes one think about interventions that might mitigate the danger of a new eruption of Zika or related pathogens. Such a danger is far from hypothetical. The Zika virus is on the short list of pathogens listed by the WHO in 2022 that could
cause future outbreaks and pandemics. Climate change increases the risk of mosquito-borne
diseases, including in geographic areas previously immune from this risk, while few people believe in 2023 that the existing sexual and reproductive rights cannot be upturned. Humanity was
(relatively) lucky during the 2015–16 Zika outbreak, just as it had been during the first major
coronavirus outbreak, the SARS epidemic of 2003. Alas, such luck may not hold forever.

Preface · *A Forgotten Virus and Expunged Memories*

1. Stephanie Nolen, "The forgotten virus: Zika families and researchers struggle for support," *New York Times*, August 16, 2022.

2. On the US Army commission to study yellow fever in Cuba, see, e.g., Nancy Stepan, "The interplay between socio-economic factors and medical science: Yellow fever research, Cuba and the United States," *Social Studies of Sciences* 8 (1978): 397–423; and Mariola Espinola, *Epidemic Invasions: Yellow Fever and the Limits of Cuban Independence, 1878–1930* (Chicago: University of Chicago Press, 2009).

3. Decree 2240 of the parliamentary session of March 7, 1901, established the Yellow Fever Mission, with a budget of 150,000 francs (approximately 660,000 euros in 2022).

4. David Arnold, ed., *Warm Climates and Western Medicine* (London: Clio Medica, 1996); Mark Harrison, *Disease and the Modern World: 1500 to the Present Day* (London: Polity Press, 2004).

5. Fiocruz, the short name of the Fundação Oswaldo Cruz, is a scientific institution for research, development, and teaching in the biological sciences and biomedicine. Its main campus is located in Rio de Janeiro, and it has 10 satellite campuses in other Brazilian states.

6. Ilana Löwy, *Virus, moustiques et modernité: La fièvre jaune au Brésil, entre science et politique* (Paris: Éditions des archives contemporaines, 2001), translated into Portuguese as *Virus, mosquitos e modernidade: A febre amarela no Brasil entre ciência e política* (Rio de Janeiro: Editora Fiocruz, 2005).

7. Jaime Larry Benchimol, ed., *Febre amarela: A doença e a vacina, uma história inacabada* (Rio de Janeiro: Editora Fiocruz, 2001); Rodrigo César da Silva Magalhães, *A erradicação do Aedes aegypti: Febre amarela, Fred Soper e saúde pública nas Américas, 1918–1968* (Rio de Janeiro: Editora Fiocruz, 2016).

8. Löwy, *Virus, moustiques et modernité*, 349.

9. Ilana Löwy, *Tangled Diagnoses: Prenatal Testing, Women, and Risk* (Chicago: University of Chicago Press, 2018).

10. Still active in 2023, the network Rede Zika e Ciências Sociais has an English-language bulletin that summarizes its participants' main findings (https://fiocruz.tghn.org/zikanetwork/), an excellent resource for learning about new scholarship on Zika, and an active Facebook site: https://www.facebook.com/groups/1141151722607356.

11. See, e.g., Emily Oster, "Let's declare a pandemic amnesty," *Atlantic*, October 22, 2022, https://www.theatlantic.com/ideas/archive/2022/10/covid-response-forgiveness/671879/. On the social conditions that lead to decisions about the end of epidemics see Jeremy Greene and

Dora Vargha, "How epidemics end," *Boston Review*, June 20, 2020, https://www.bostonreview
.net/special_project/thinking-pandemic-project-page/.

12. The equation of Zika with care of children with congenital Zika syndrome and of their mothers was at the center of the March 2021 Fiocruz exhibition on the Zika epidemic in Brazil, *Zika: Affecting Lives*. See http://expozika.fiocruz.br/en/.

13. The expression "acting in an uncertain world," the title of a research program dedicated to Zika financed by the Newton Fund, is borrowed from Yannick Barthe, Michel Callon, and Pierre Lascumes, *Agir dans un monde incertain: Essai sur la démocratie technique* (Paris: Seuil, 2001), translated into English by Graham Burchell as *Acting in an Uncertain World: An Essay on Technical Democracy* (Cambridge, MA: MIT Press, 2009).

14. Nolen, "Forgotten virus."

15. Peter Burke, "History as social memory," in *Varieties of Cultural History* (Ithaca, NY: Cornell University Press, 1997), 59.

16. Ilana Löwy, "Zika ghosts," in *Uma história brasileira das doenças*, vol. l7, ed. Sebastião Pimentel Franco, Dilene Raimundo do Nacimento, and Anny Jackeline Torres (Belo Horizonte: Fino Traço Editora, 2017), 84–97. The text is based on a talk I presented at a conference on the history of diseases in Vitória, Espírito Santo, October 16–17, 2016.

17. I borrow the "ghost" theme from Banu Subramaniam, *Ghost Stories for Darwin: The Science of Variation and the Politics of Diversity* (Urbana: University of Illinois Press, 2014).

Introduction

The title of this chapter is inspired by Charles Rosenberg's "Disease in history: Frames and framers," *Milbank Quarterly* 67, suppl. 1 (1989): 1–15.

1. Many children with congenital Zika syndrome suffer from severe convulsions. Anticonvulsant drugs can control the convulsions and alleviate the child's distress, but in some cases they also make the child apathic and nonresponsive. Eliza Williamson, "Care in the time of Zika: Notes on the 'afterlife' of the epidemic in Salvador (Bahia), Brazil," *Interface* (Botucatu) 22, no. 66 (2018): 685–96.

2. See https://www.bbc.com/news/av/world-latin-america-35643345/the-story-of-the
-brazil-s-zika-bucket-baby. The short film was made in February 2016.

3. See https://globalnews.ca/news/2497368/in-photos-photographer-reflects-on-bucket
-baby-brazil-child-born-with-zika-virus-linked-microcephaly/.

4. Three out of four mothers of children with CZS in Pernambuco reported that they had been abandoned by their male partners after the birth of an affected child. Germana Soares, "Como transformar a superação em uma missão?," TED video, accessed January 10, 2022, https://www.youtube.com/watch?v=u-iOwWGs8gA.

5. Dana's presentation of Ferreira's state of mind contradicts Ferreira's statement in the BBC short video that she sees her son as "normal." It is probably not surprising that a mother of a severely affected child might vacillate between different states of mind.

6. WHO, "Zika, 4th Emergency Committee Press Conference," September 2, 2016, https://
extranet.who.int/pagnet/?q=es/node/674.

7. Ludwik Fleck, "On the crisis of 'reality,' " in *Cognition and Fact: Materials on Ludwik Fleck*, ed. Robert Cohen and Thomas Schnelle (1929; reprint, Dordrecht: Reidel, 1986), 47–58.

8. Charles Rosenberg, "Explaining epidemics," in *Explaining Epidemics, and Other Studies in the History of Medicine* (Cambridge: Cambridge University Press, 1992), 293–304.

9. Janina Kehr, "Messianic medicine: Treating disease in the time that is left," Somatosphere, June 25, 2016, http://somatosphere.net/2016/messianic-medicine-treating-disease-in
-the-time-that-is-left.html/.

10. «O véu foi levantado. O microscópio falou.» Monteiro Lobato, *Urupe* (São Paulo: Editora da Revista do Brasil, 1919).

11. Dora Vargha, "After the end of disease: Rethinking the epidemic narrative," Somatosphere, May 17, 2016, http://somatosphere.net/2016/after-the-end-of-disease-rethinking-the -epidemic-narrative.html/.

12. Bharat Jayram Venkat, "Awakenings," Somatosphere, May 25, 2016, http://somatosphere .net/2016/awakenings.html/.

13. Tine Gammeltoft, "Toward an anthropology of the imaginary: Specters of disability in Vietnam," *Ethos* 42, no. 2 (2014): 153–74.

14. Charles Rosenberg, "What is disease? In memory of Owsei Temkin," *Bulletin of the History of Medicine* 77 (2003): 491–505; Stefan Timmermans and Steven Hass, "Towards a sociology of disease," *Sociology of Health and Illness* 30, no. 5 (2008): 659–76.

15. Paula de Souza Freitas, Gabriella Barreto Soares, Helaine Jacinta Mocelin, et al., "Síndrome congênita do vírus Zika: Perfil sociodemográfico das mães," *Revista Panamericana de Salud Pública* 43 (2019): e24, https://doi.org/10.26633/RPSP.2019.24.

16. The link between dengue fever and low socioeconomic status is not always clear. Kate Mulligan, Jenna Dixon, Chi-Ling Joanna Sinn, and Susan J. Elliott, "Is dengue a disease of poverty? A systematic review," *Pathogens and Global Health* 109, no. 1 (2015): 10–18.

17. Oliver Brady, Aaron Osgood-Zimmerman, Nicholas Kassebaum, et al., "The association between Zika virus infection and microcephaly in Brazil 2015–2017: An observational analysis of over 4 million births," *PLOS Medicine* 16, no. 3 (2019): e1002755, https://doi.org /10.1371/journal.pmed.1002755.

18. On the nonselective distribution of inborn impairments induced by the rubella virus before the generalization of vaccination for this condition see Leslie Reagan, *Dangerous Pregnancies: Mothers, Disability and Abortion in Modern America* (Berkeley: University of California Press, 2012).

19. Keith Wailoo, "Spectacles of difference: The racial scripting of epidemics disparities," *Bulletin of the History of Medicine* 94 (2020): 602–26.

20. Ann Laura Stoler, introduction to *Duress: Imperial Durabilities in Our Times* (Durham, NC: Duke University Press, 2016).

21. Paul Wenzel Geissler, Guillaume Lachenal, John Manton, and Noémi Tousignant, eds., *Traces of the Future: Archeology of Medical Science in Africa* (Chicago: University of Chicago Press, 2016).

22. My book *Virus, moustiques et modernité: La fièvre jaune au Brésil, entre science et politique* (Paris: Éditions des archives contemporaines, 2001) traces the history of Brazilian efforts to control yellow fever in the first half of the twentieth century. See also Jaime Larry Benchimol, ed., *Febre amarela: A doença e a vacina, uma história inacabada* (Rio de Janeiro: Editora Fiocruz, 2001).

23. Nancy Stepan, *The Beginning of Brazilian Science: Oswaldo Cruz, Medical Research and Policy, 1890–1920* (New York: Science History Publications, 1976), 84–91; Lukas Engelmann and Christos Lynteris, *Sulphuric Utopias: A History of Maritime Fumigation* (Cambridge, MA: MIT Press, 2020).

24. Fred L. Soper, D. Bruce Wilson, Servulo Lima, and Waldemar Sa Antunes, *The Organization of Permanent, Nation-Wide Anti Aedes aegypti Measures in Brazil* (New York: Rockefeller Foundation, 1943); Rodrigo Cesar da Silva Magalhães, *A erradicação do Aedes aegypti: Febre amarela, Fred Soper e saúde pública nas Américas, 1918–1968* (Rio de Janeiro: Editora Fiocruz, 2016).

25. Cristina Oliveira Fonseca, "Interlúdio: As campanhas sanitárias e o Ministério da Saúde, 1953–1990," in Benchimol, *Febre amarela*, 299–305.

26. Ilana Löwy, "Leaking containers: Success and failure in controlling the mosquito *Aedes aegypti* in Brazil," *American Journal of Public Health* 107, no. 4 (2017): 517–24.

27. Maria Glória Teixeira, Maria da Conceição Costa, Florisnei de Barreto, and Maurício Lima Barreto, "Dengue: Vinte e cinco anos da reemergência no Brasil," *Cadernos de Saúde*

Pública 25, suppl. 1 (2009): S7–S18; Mauricio Barreto, Gloria Teixeira, Francisco Bastos, et al., "Successes and failures in the control of infectious diseases in Brazil: Social and environmental context, policies, interventions, and research needs," *Lancet* 377 (2011): 1877–89.

28. Cristina Possas, Ricardo Lourenço-de-Oliveira, Pedro Luiz Tauil, et al., "Yellow fever outbreak in Brazil: The puzzle of rapid viral spread and challenges for immunization," *Memorias do Instituto Oswaldo Cruz, Rio de Janeiro* 113, no. 10 (2018): e180278; Gabriel Lopes and Andre Felipe Candido da Silva, "O *Aedes aegypti* e os mosquitos na historiografia: Reflexões e controvérsias," *Tempo e Argumento* 11, no. 26 (2019): 67–113.

29. Leon Eisenberg, "Rudolf Ludwig Karl Virchow, where are you now that we need you?," *American Journal of Medicine* 77 (1984): 524–32.

30. Laura Briggs, *How All Politics Became Reproductive Politics* (Berkeley: University of California Press, 2018).

31. The expression "To be a mother is suffering in paradise," from the poem "Ser mãe," by the Brazilian poet Henrique Maximiliano Coelho Neto (1864–1934), is a common one in Brazil. The last strophe of Coelho's poem is, "Ser mãe é andar chorando num sorriso, / Ser mãe é ter um mundo e não ter nada, / Ser mãe é padecer num paraíso" (To be a mother is to walk crying with a smile, / To be a mother is to have a world and to have nothing, / To be a mother is to suffer in a paradise).

32. Pope Francis, "Abortion is evil, not the solution to Zika virus," Catholic News Agency, February 18, 2016, https://www.catholicnewsagency.com/news/33451/pope-francis-abortion-is-evil-not-the-solution-to-zika-virus.

33. Ilana Löwy, *Tangled Diagnosis: Prenatal Testing, Women and Risk* (Chicago: University of Chicago Press, 2018), chap. 4.

34. Bruno Mayerfeld, "Au Brésil, l'inquiétude du camp Lula, pour qui la campagne présidentielle s'est transformée en chemin de croix," *Le Monde*, October 11, 2022.

35. The French philosopher Sandra Laugier writes that "theories of care, like many radical feminist theories, suffer from misrecognition . . . because contrary to general gender approaches, a veritable ethics of care cannot exist without social transformation." Quoted by Carol Gilligan in introduction to *Joining the Resistance* (London: Polity Press, 2018), 11. See also Sandra Laugier, "The ethics of care as a politics of the ordinary," *New Literary History* 46 (2015): 217–40.

36. Jutta Schickore, "Mess in science and wicked problems," *Perspectives on Science* 28, no. 4 (2020): 482–504.

37. J. Paim, C. Travassos, C. Almeida, L. Bahia, and J. Macinko, "The Brazilian health system: History, advances, and challenges," *Lancet* 377 (2011): 1778–97.

38. Leo Heller, "Melhoramento dos serviços de água e saneamento é a resposta ao Zika vírus," ABRASCO, March 8, 2016, https://www.abrasco.org.br/site/noticias/ecologia-e-meio-ambiente/zika_saneamento_leo_heller/16639/.

39. Comissão de Epidemiologia da Abrasco, "Zika virus: Challenges of public health in Brazil," *Revista Brasileira de Epidemiologia* 19, no. 2 (2016): 225–28, https://doi.org/10.1590/1980-5497201600020001.

40. The Brazilian government's focus on the responsibility of individual women is discussed in, for example, Clare Wenham's *Feminist Global Health Security* (Oxford: Oxford University Press, 2021).

41. Charles Rosenberg, "Explaining epidemics," in *Explaining Epidemics, and Other Studies in the History of Medicine* (Cambridge: Cambridge University Press, 1992), 293–304.

42. Collective health, a concept developed in Latin America, is broader and more inclusive than public health: it includes attention to the effects of sociocultural, economic, political and environmental variables on health and well-being.

43. Mino Carta, "A culpa pelas 300.000 mortes deve ser dividida equitativamente," *Carta Capital*, March 24, 2021.

44. Brazil is one of the most unequal countries in the world. Lucas Chancel, Thomas Piketty, Emanuel Saez, and Gabriel Zucman, *World Inequality Report* (Cambridge, MA: Harvard University Press, 2022). However, while the country's utra-rich are very rich indeed, the country's middle class is far from opulent. Professionals in Brazil have a roughly similar income level to that of their peers in Western Europe, and some, especially at the lower levels of their profession, struggle to make ends meet. The main difference in the income levels of Brazilians and their Western European peers is among the lower social classes. In 2021 the minimum wage (net) in France was 1,230 euros ($1,465), while in Brazil it was 1,100 reais, or 187 euros ($222), with a significant proportion of the population living on much less. There are no big differences between the cost of living in Brazil and that in France (food, lodging, transportation, access to the internet, etc.). On the rarified world of the Brazilian ultra-rich see Alex Cuadros, *Brazillionaires: Wealth, Power, Decadence, and Hope in an American Country* (New York: Spiegel & Grau, 2016).

45. There is no linear correlation between an objective level of risk and an individual's perception of this risk. It is reasonable to assume that some middle-class women, especially those who found themselves pregnant in the midst of the Zika epidemic and wished to continue the pregnancy, were very much afraid even though they knew that even in the worst-case scenario it was likely that they would be able to decide whether to give birth to a child with severe CZS. But it is also reasonable to assume that women who felt powerless when facing the Zika threat to their future child were, on average, even more afraid.

46. Debora Diniz, *Zika: From the Brazilian Backlands to Global Threat*, trans. Diane Grosklaus Whitty (Chicago: University of Chicago Press, 2017), originally published as *Zika: Do sertão nordestino à ameaça global* (Rio de Janeiro: Editora Civilização Brasileira, 2016). The Portuguese edition reflected an early view of the Zika outbreak.

47. Jorge Lyra, in Human Rights Watch, *Neglected and Unprotected: The Impact of the Zika Outbreak on Women and Girls in Northeastern Brazil*, 2017, p. 90, https://www.hrw.org /report/2017/07/13/neglected-and-unprotected/impact-zika-outbreak-women-and-girls -northeastern.

48. Nancy Fraser, "On justice: Lessons from Plato, Rawls, and Ishiguro," *New Left Review* 74 (2012): 41–51; Avishai Margalit, *The Decent Society* (Cambridge, MA: Harvard University Press, 1996).

49. Didier Eribon's *Réflexions sur la question gay* (Paris: Flammarion 1999), translated into English by Michael Lucey as *Insult and the Making of the Gay Self* (Durham, NC: Duke University Press, 2004), provides a fine-grained account of a life dominated by apprehension, in Eribon's case of being insulted and attacked for being a homosexual.

50. The collaborative work of the latter project led to two publications: Ann H. Kelly, Javier Lezaun, Ilana Löwy, et al., "Uncertainty in times of medical emergency: Knowledge gaps and structural ignorance during the Brazilian Zika crisis," *Social Science and Medicine* 246 (February 2020): 112787, https://doi.org/10.1016/j.socscimed.2020.112787; and Koichi Kameda, Ann H. Kelly, Javier Lezaun, and Ilana Löwy, "Imperfect diagnosis: The truncated legacy of Zika testing," *Social Studies of Science* 51, no. 5 (2021): 683–706.

51. João Biehl, "The pharmaceuticalization and judicialization of health: On the interface of medical capitalism and magical legalism in Brazil," *Osiris* 36 (2021): 325–26.

Chapter 1 · Viruses and Mosquitoes

1. See Brazilian Yellow Fever Service photographs, 1930s, nos. 30–63, Archives of Casa Oswaldo Cruz, Fiocruz, Rio de Janeiro (ACOC).

2. Odair Franco, *História da febre amarela no Brasil* (Rio de Janeiro: Ministério da Saúde, 1969), 110–12.

3. Elmer Rickard, "The organization of the visceroctomy service of the Brazilian Cooperative Yellow Fever Service," *American Journal of Tropical Medicine* 17 (1937): 163–90.

4. See, e.g., Patrick Petitjean, Anne Marie Moulin, and Catherine Jami, *Science and Empires*, Historical Studies about Scientific Development and European Expansion (Dordrecht: Kluwer, 1994); David Arnold, *Colonizing the Body: State Medicine and Epidemic Disease in Nineteenth-Century India* (Berkeley: University of California Press, 1993); Warwick Anderson, *Colonial Pathologies: American Tropical Medicine, Race, and Hygiene in the Philippines* (Durham, NC: Duke University Press, 2006); and Michael Osborne, *The Emergence of Tropical Medicine in France* (Chicago: University of Chicago Press, 2014).

5. William Coleman, *Yellow Fever in the North: The Methods of Epidemiology* (Madison: University of Wisconsin Press, 1987).

6. Paul Wenzel Geissler, "Public secrets in public health: Knowing not to know while making scientific knowledge," *American Ethnologist* 40, no. 1 (2013): 13–34.

7. On the Reed mission see, e.g., Nancy Stepan, "The interplay between socio-economic factors and medical science: Yellow fever research, Cuba and the United States," *Social Studies of Science* 8 (1978): 397–423; Francois Delaporte, *The History of Yellow Fever: An Essay on the Birth of Tropical Medicine* (Cambridge, MA: MIT Press, 1991); and Mariola Espinosa, *Epidemic Invasions: Yellow Fever and the Limits of Cuban Independence, 1878–1930* (Chicago: University of Chicago Press, 2009).On the role of yellow fever in producing racialized "immunocapital" in New Orleans, see Kathryn Olivarius, *Necropolis: Disease, Power, and Capitalism in the Cotton Kingdom* (Cambridge, MA: Harvard University Press, 2022).

8. William Bean, "Walter Reed and the ordeal of human experiments," *Bulletin of the History of Medicine* 51, no. 1 (1977): 75–91; Bean, *Walter Reed: A Biography* (Charlottesville: University Press of Virginia, 1982).

9. William C. Gorgas, "Recent experiences of the United States Army with regard to sanitation of yellow fever in the tropics," *Journal of Tropical Medicine* 6 (1903): 50.

10. Juan Guiteras, "Experimental yellow fever at the inoculation station of the sanitary department of Havana, with a view of producing immunization," *American Medicine*, November 23, 1901, 809–17; William B. Bean, "Water Reed and yellow fever," *JAMA* 250, no. 5 (1983): 659–62.

11. As noted earlier, decree 2240 of the French parliamentary session of March 7, 1901, established the Yellow Fever Mission with a budget of 150,000 francs. Chambre des Députés, 1901, National Archives, Paris, doc. F-17-13052.

12. Pierre Louis Simond, notebook, Simond Papers, SIM/9, Pasteur Institute Archives, Paris, http://www.pasteur.fr/infosci/archives/sim1.html; Carlos Seidl, "Renascença: A missão Pasteur," *Revista Brasil Médico*, April 1905, 166–72.

13. Simond to Pierre Charin, September 9, 1902, Simond Papers, SIM/9, http://www.pasteur.fr/infosci/archives/sim1.html.

14. The Pasteur experts communicated their decision to experiment on humans to Roux, who supervised the Yellow Fever Mission's work. Roux replied that "it is really a pity you cannot make experiments on 'men of good will,'" as had been done in Cuba. Emile Roux to (probably) Antonio Salimbeni, March 28, 1902, Simond Papers, SIM/4.

15. Emile Marchoux, Albert Taurelli Salimbeni, and Paul Louis Simond, "La fievre jaune: Rapport de la mission française," *Annales de l'Institut Pasteur* 17 (1903): 665–80.

16. Simond, notebook, Simond Papers, SIM/9, .

17. Roux to Simond, May 5, 1903, Simond Papers, SIM/4.

18. Simond, notebook, April–June 1903, Simond Papers, SIM/10.

19. Letter to Etienne Clémentel, French Minister of Colonies, November 23, 1905, Simond Papers, SIM/9.

20. Nancy Stepan, *The Beginning of Brazilian Science: Oswaldo Cruz, Medical Research and Policy, 1890–1920* (New York: Science History Publications, 1976), 84–91.

21. Sidney Chalhoub, "The politics of disease control: Yellow fever and race in nineteenth-century Rio de Janeiro," *Journal of Latin American Studies* 25, no. 3 (1993): 441–63. Other historians, such as Marcos Chor Maio, have argued that racial politics played a more limited role in efforts to control yellow fever in Brazil. Marcos Chor Maio, "Raça, doença e saúde publica no Brasil: Um debate sobre o pensamento higienista do século XIX," in *Raça como questão: História, ciência e identidades no Brasil*, ed. Marcos Chor Maio and Ricardo Ventura Santos (Rio de Janeiro: Editora Fiocruz, 2010), 51–82.

22. Chalhoub, "Politics of disease control."

23. Nicolau Sevtchenko, *A revolta da vacina: Mentes insanas em corpos rebeldes* (São Paolo: Editora Brasiliense, 1984).

24. Sidney Chalhoub, *Cidade febril: Cortiços e epidemias na corte imperial* (São Paolo: Companhia das Letras, 1996).

25. On fumigations see Lukas Engelmann and Christos Lynteris, *Sulphuric Utopias: A History of Maritime Fumigation* (Cambridge, MA: MIT Press, 2020).

26. Nara Apud Britto, *Oswaldo Cruz: A construção de um mito na ciência brasileira* (Rio de Janeiro: Editora Fiocruz, 1995).

27. Nisia Trinidade Lima and Gilberto Hochman, "Condenado pela raça, absolvido pela medicina: O Brasil descoberto pelo movimento sanitarista da primeira república," in Chor Maio and Ventura Santos, *Raça como questão*, 23–40.

28. Dominichi Miranda de Sa, "A voz do Brasil: Miguel Pereira e o discurso sobre o 'imenso hospital,'" *História, Ciências, Saúde—Manguinhos* 16, no. 1 (2009): 333–48.

29. Gilberto Hochman, *O era de sanamento* (Rio de Janeiro: Editora Hucitec, 1998).

30. Michael Connor and William Monroe, "*Stegomyia* indices and their value in yellow fever control," *American Journal of Tropical Medicine* 3 (1923): 9–19.

31. Joseph White, "General report of the yellow fever campaign in Brazil," November 6, 1924, Rockefeller Archive Center, Sleepy Holllow, NY (henceforth RAC), Record Group (RG) 5, series 2, box 23, file 138; White, "Memorandum on the principle of yellow ever control," RAC, RG 5, series 2, box 25, file 155.

32. Michael Connor, director of the RF's Brazilian bureau, to Frederick Russell, head of the RF's international division, March 6, 1927, RAC, RG 1.1, series 30, box 20, file 155.

33. Franco, *História da febre amarela no Brasil*, 97–104.

34. Fred Lowe Soper, *Ventures in World Health: The Memoirs of Fred Lowe Soper*, ed. John Duffy (Washington, DC: Pan American Health Organization, 1977).

35. Fred Soper to Russell, November 30, 1931, RAC, RG 1.1, series 305, box 21, file 168.

36. Fred Soper, Henrique Penna, Ernesto Cardoso, et al., "Yellow fever without *Aedes aegypti*: Study of a rural epidemic in the Valle do Chanaan, Espírito Santo, 1932," *American Journal of Hygiene* 18 (1933): 555–87.

37. Wilbur Sawyer to Soper, January 4, 1932, RAC, RG 1.1, series 305, box 21, file 169. Sawyer, a yellow fever expert, became the head of the RF's international division in 1935.

38. Boris Fausto, *A Revolução de 1930: Historiografia e história* (São Paulo: Companhia das Letras, 1970); Italo Tronca, *Revolução de 30: A dominação oculta* (São Paulo: Editore Brasiliense, 1982); Valentina de Rocha Lima, ed., *Getúlio, uma história oral* (Rio de Janeiro: Editora Record, 1980); Simon Schwartzmann, *Bases do autoritarismo brasileiro* (Rio de Janeiro: Editore Campus, 1982).

39. Franco, *História da febre amarela no Brasil*, 104–8.

40. The organization of anti-larval activities by the Brazilian Yellow Fever Service in the 1930s is summed up in Fred L. Soper, D. Bruce Wilson, Servulo Lima, and Waldemar Sa Antunes, *The Organization of Permanent, Nation-Wide Anti Aedes aegypti Measures in Brazil* (New York: Rockefeller Foundation, 1943).

41. Soper diary, April 24, 1932, RAC, RG 1.1, series 305, box 28, file 208A.

42. Soper, Wilson, Lima and Sa Antunes, *Organization of Permanent, Nation-Wide Anti Aedes aegypti Measures in Brazil.*

43. Maria Da Penha Vasconcellos, ed., *Memória da saúde pública* (São Paolo: Editora Huitec, 1995), 48–50; Maria Alice Rosa Ribeiro, *Historia sem fim: Inventário da saúde pública, São Paulo, 1880–1930* (São Paolo: Editora UNESP, 1993), 255–61.

44. Porter Crawford journal,1932, RAC, RG 1.1, series 305, box 27, file 208B.

45. Soper journal, 1931, RAC, RG 1.1, series 305, box 27, file 207A.

46. Soper later popularized the eradication of disease vectors in the context of worldwide efforts to eradicate malaria. Nancy Leys Stepan, *Eradication: Ridding the World of Diseases Forever* (Ithaca, NY: Cornell University Press, 2011).

47. Henrique da Rocha Lima, "O diagnostico post-mortem da febre amarela," *Folha Medica* 7 (1926): 169–75; Oskar Klotz and T. H. Belt, "The pathology of liver in yellow fever," *American Journal of Pathology* 6 (1930): 663–87.

48. Emilie Marchoux and Pierre Luis Simond, "Études sur la fièvre jaune: Troisième mémoire," *Annales de l'Institut Pasteur* 20 (1906):104–48.

49. Hideyo Noguchi, "Etiology of yellow fever: II. Transmission experiments of yellow fever," *Journal of Experimental Medicine* 29 (1919): 565–84, 401–10; Noguchi, "Etiology of yellow fever: XI. Serum treatment of animals infected with *Leptospira ictéroides*," *Journal of Experimental Medicine* 31 (1920): 159–68; Noguchi, "Yellow fever research, 1918–1924: A summary," *Journal of Tropical Medicine and Hygiene* 28 (1925):185–95. For Noguchi's biography see Isabel R. Plesser, *Noguchi and His Patrons* (London: Associated University Press, 1980).

50. Hideyo Noguchi, Henry Muller, Octavio Torres, Flaviano Silva, Horacio Martins, Alvaro Ribeiro dos Santos, Godofredo Vianna, and Mario Biao, *Experimental Studies of Yellow Fever in Northern Brazil* (New York: Rockefeller Institute for Medical Research, 1924).

51. Max Theiler and Andrew Watson Sellards, "The relations of L. icterohaemorrhagiae et L. icteroides as determined by the Pfeiffer phenomenon in guinea pigs," *American Journal of Tropical Medicine* 6, no. 6 (1926): 383–402; Douglas Merrill Gay and Andrew Watson Sellards, "The fate of Leptospira icteroides and Leptospira icterohaemorrhagiae in the mosquito Aedes aegypti," *American Journal of Tropical Medicine* 21 (1927): 321–42.

52. Adrian Stokes, Johannes Bauer, and Paul Hudson, "Transmission of yellow fever to *Macaccus rhesus*: A preliminary note," *JAMA* 90 (1928): 253–54; Andrew J. Warren, "Landmarks in the conquest of yellow fever," In *Yellow Fever*, ed. George Strode (New York: McGraw Hill, 1951). Stokes died in 1928 from yellow fever acquired during his studies of that disease. Noguchi, who continued to defend his *Leptospira* theory, died from yellow fever the same year, during an expedition to study the disease in East Africa.

53. Soper, *Ventures in World Health*, 167.

54. J. Gordon Fierson, "The yellow fever vaccine: A history," *Yale Journal of History of Medicine* 83 (2010): 77–85; Deborah Doroshow, Scott Podolsky, and Justin Barr, "Biomedical research in times of emergency: Lessons from history," *Annals of Internal Medicine* 173, no. 4 (2020): 297–99.

55. Journal of the yellow fever laboratory, Rio de Janeiro, for 1936–37, RAC, RG 1.1, series 305, box 44.

56. Fred Soper and Hugh Smith, "Yellow fever vaccination with immune and hyperimmune serum," *American Journal of Tropical Medicine* 18 (1938): 111–34.

57. Max Theiler and Hugh Smith, "The use of yellow fever modified by in vitro cultivation for human immunization," *Journal of Experimental Medicine* 65 (1937): 765–800.

58. For detailed studies of the history of yellow fever vaccination in Brazil see Jaime Larry Benchimol, ed., *Febre amarela: A doença e a vacina, uma história inacabada* (Rio de Janeiro: Editora Fiocruz, 2001); and Ilana Löwy, *Virus, moustiques et modernité: La fievre jaune au Brésil, entre science et politique* (Paris: Éditions des archives contemporaines, 2001).

59. Hugh Smith journal, May 25, June 8, July 10, and August 22, 1937, RAC, RG 1.1, series 305, box 36, folder 223; H. H. Smith, H. A. Penna, and A. Paoliello, "Yellow fever vaccination with cultured virus (17D) without immune serum," *American Journal of Tropical Medicine* 18 (1938): 437–68.

60. F. L. Soper, H. H. Smith, and H. A. Penna, "Yellow fever vaccination: Field results as measured by the mouse protection test and epidemiological observations," *Third International Congress for Microbiology, New York, 2–9 September 1939 (Report of the Proceedings)* (New York, 1940), 351–53; Jaime Benchimol, "Yellow fever vaccine in Brazil: Fighting a tropical scourge, modernising the nation," in *The Politics of Vaccination: A Global History,* ed. Christine Holmberg and J. Hillis Miller (Manchester: Manchester University Press, 2017), 174–208.

61. Fred Soper, *Summary of Activities of the Yellow Fever Service of Ministry of Education of Brazil* (Rio de Janeiro: Imprensa Nacional, 1939).

62. Angelo Moreira da Costa Lima, "Consideraçes sobre a propagação da febre amarela e a vacinaço contra esta doença," *Revista Médico-Cirurgica do Brasil* 46 (1938): 371–82, quoted in Benchimol, "Yellow fever vaccine in Brazil," 187.

63. J. P. Fox, E. H. Lenette, C. Manso, and J. R. S. Aguiar, "Encephalitis in man following vaccination with 17D yellow fever virus," *American Journal of Hygiene* 36 (1942): 140.

64. Soper journal, January 22 and June 17,1940, RAC, RG 1.1, series 305, box 32, folder 216.

65. Fox, Lenette, Manso, and Aguiar, "Encephalitis in man following vaccination with 17D yellow fever virus."

66. John Fox journal, May 15, 1940, RAC, RG 1.1, series 305, box 32, folder 215; September 3, 1940, RAC, RG 1.1, series 305, box 32, folder 216.

67. Soper journal, November 13, 1940, RAC, RG 1.1, series 305, box 32, folder 216; Fox journal, August 28, September 30, and December 10, 1940, RG 1.1, series 305, box 32, folder 216; J. P. Fox, C. Manso, H. Penna, and M. Para, "Observations on the occurrence of icterus in Brazil following vaccination against yellow fever," *American Journal of Hygiene* 36 (1942): 68–116.

68. Arnold Theiler, "Acute liver atrophy and parenchymatous hepatitis in horses," in *5th and 6th Reports of the Director of Veterinary Research, Department of Agriculture, Union of South Africa* (Pretoria: Government Printing and Stationery Office, 1918), 7–164.

69. G. M. Findlay and F. O. MacCallum, "Note on acute hepatitis and yellow fever immunization," *Transactions of the Royal Society of Tropical Medicine and Hygiene* 31, no. 3 (1937): 297–308.

70. W. A. Sawyer, K. F. Meyer, M. D. Eaton, et al., "Jaundice in army personnel in the western region of the United States and its relation to vaccination against yellow fever: Part I," *American Journal of Hygiene* 39, no. 3 (1944): 341.

71. Sawyer, Meyer, Eaton, et al., "Jaundice in army personnel in the western region of the United States . . . Part I."

72. Editorial, "Jaundice following vaccination against yellow fever," *JAMA* 125, no. 17 (1944): 1190–91; W. A. Sawyer, K. F. Meyer, M. D. Eaton, et al., "Jaundice in army personnel in the western region of the United States and its relation to vaccination against yellow fever: Parts II, III, and IV," *American Journal of Hygiene* 40, no. 1 (1944): 35–107.

73. Leonard Seef, Gilbert Beebe, Jay Hoofnagle, et al., "A serological follow up of the 1942

epidemics of post-vaccination hepatitis in the United States Army," *New England Journal of Medicine* 316, no. 1 (1987): 965–70; James Norman, Gilbert Beebe, Jay Hoofnagle, and Leonard Seef, "Mortality follow-up of the 1942 epidemics of hepatitis in the US army," *Hepatology* 18 (1993): 790–97; John Marr and John Cathey, "The yellow fever misadventure of 1942," *Journal of Public Health Management and Practice* 23, no. 6 (2017): 651–57.

74. Sawyer, Meyer, Eaton, et al., "Jaundice in army personnel in the western region of the United States . . . Part I."

75. Ilana Löwy, "The 1942 massive contamination of yellow fever vaccine: A public health consequence of scientific arrogance," *American Journal of Public Health* 111, no. 9 (2021): 1654–60; Scott Podolsky, "Puncturing hubris . . . and insularity: The 1942 yellow fever vaccine disaster and Covid-19," *American Journal of Public Health* 111, no. 9 (2021): 1565–66.

76. Soper, Wilson, Lima, and Sa Antunes, *Organization of Permanent, Nation-Wide Anti Aedes aegypti Measures in Brazil.*

77. Archives of National Yellow Fever Service, notes for 1940–50, ACOC.

78. See, e.g., report of Dr. Eduardo Cotta on the case of Maria Helena Martin, who died in Patrocinio, Minas Gerais, April 21, 1954; and report of Dr. Luis Pereira Tavares Lessa on the case of Cenelita Terezinha Costa, 2 years old, who died in Esmeraldas, Minas Gerais. Archives of National Yellow Fever Service, notes for 1940–50, ACOC.

79. This was still true in 2018. Cristina Possas, Ricardo Lourenço-de-Oliveira, Pedro Luiz Tauil, et al., "Yellow fever outbreak in Brazil: The puzzle of rapid viral spread and challenges for immunization," *Memorias do Instituto Oswaldo Cruz, Rio de Janeiro* 113, no. 10 (2018): e180278.

80. Fred Soper, "The 1964 status of *Aedes aegypti* eradication and yellow fever in the Americas," *American Journal of Tropical Medicine and Hygiene* 14, no. 6 (1964): 887–91; Soper, "Rehabilitation of the eradication concept in prevention of communicable diseases," *Public Health Report* 80 (1965): 855–69.

81. Soper, *Ventures in World Health,* 343; Rodrigo Cesar da Silva Magalhães, *A erradicação do Aedes aegypti: Febre amarela, Fred Soper e saúde pública nas Américas 1918–1968* (Rio de Janeiro: Editora Fiocruz, 2016).

82. Soper, *Ventures in World Health,* 351–57; Magalhães, *A erradicação do Aedes aegypti,* 292–315.

83. George Shidrawi, "Laboratory tests on mosquito tolerance to insecticides and development of resistance by *Aedes aegypti,*" *Bulletin of the World Health Organization* 17 (1957): 377–411; Soper, *Ventures in World Health,* 340–43.

84. Soper,"1964 status of *Aedes aegypti* eradication," 888; Soper, *Ventures in World Health,* 342–43.

85. Magalhães, *A erradicação do Aedes aegypti,* 276–86.

86. Soper, *Ventures in World Health,* 342–43; Francisco Pinheiro and Michael Nelson, "Re-emergence of dengue and emergence of dengue haemorrhagic fever in the Americas," *Dengue Bulletin* 21 (1997): 16–24.

87. William Reeves, "Recrudescence of arthropod-borne virus diseases in the Americas," and J. Ralph Audy, "Aspects of human behavior interfering with vector control," in *Vector Control and the Recrudescence of Vector-Borne Diseases: Proceedings of a Symposium Held during the Tenth Meeting of the PAHO Advisory Committee on Medical Research,15 June 1971* (Washington, DC: Pan American Sanitary Bureau, 1972.

88. Cristina Oliveira Fonseca, "Interlúdio: As campanhas sanitárias e o Ministério da Saúde, 1953–1990," in Benchimol, *Febre amarela,* 299–305.

89. Amilcar Tavarez da Silva, interview in *Memória de Manguinhos: Acervo de depoimento,* ed. Nara Britto Rose, Ingrid Goldschmidt, and Wanda Hamilton (Rio de Janeiro:

Editora Fiocruz, 1991); Randall Packard and Paulo Gadelha, "A land filled with mosquitoes: Fred L. Soper, the Rockefeller Foundation and the *Anopheles gambiae* invasion in Brazil," *Parasitologia* 36 (1993): 197–213.

90. Memoires of SUCAM agents are reproduced in Helbio Fernandez Moraes, ed., *Sucam: Sua origem, sua história*, vol. 2 (Brasilia: Editora Ministério da Saúde, 1988), 23–76.

91. Odair Franco, "A erradicação do *Aedes aegypti*," in *História da febre amarela no Brasil* (Rio de Janeiro: Ministério da Saúde, 1969), 135–56.

92. Oliveira Fonseca, "Interlúdio."

93. Magalhães, *A erradicação do Aedes aegypti*.

94. Fernando Antônio Pires-Alves, Carlos Henrique Assunção Paiva, and Nísia Trindade Lima, "Baixada Fluminense in the shadow of the 'Sphinx of Rio': Popular movements and health policies in the wake of the SUS," *Ciência e Saúde Coletiva* 23, no. 6 (2018): 1849–58; Gabriel Lopes and Andre Felipe Candido da Silva, "O *Aedes aegypti* e os mosquitos na historiografia: Reflexões e controvérsias," *Tempo e Argumento* 11, no. 26 (2019): 67–113.

95. See, e.g., *Jornal do Brasil*, April 24 and 27, 1986. The narrative of dengue epidemics in Baixa Fluminense is mainly based on materials collected by Eduardo Costa, at that time vice director of sanitary services for the state of Rio de Janeiro. File on dengue, ACOC, Fundo FSESP, Seção Assistencia medico sanitaria, TMP/CD/70, 71, 72.

96. Editorial, "Return of quarantines," *O Globo*, April 29, 1986.

97. Pires-Alves, Paiva, and Lima, "Baixada Fluminense."

98. "A sanitarian criticized public health," *Jornal do Brasil*, April 29, 1986.

99. "Health ministry follows closely the dengue epidemics," *Jornal do Brasil*, April 27, 1986.

100. "The state uses students to fight dengue," *O Globo*, May 25, 1986.

101. "The decline of dengue," *O Globo*, July 1, 1986.

102. "Inhabitants of Baixada block Doutra to ask for better health," *Jornal do Brasil*, May 28, 1986; Pires-Alves, Paiva, and Lima, "Baixada Fluminense."

103. "Soldiers participate in fight against dengue," *Ultima Hora*, June 4, 1986; "Decline of dengue." Brazil purchased Leco fumigation machines in June of 1985.

104. "Retrograde sanitation," *Jornal do Brasil*, June 3, 1986.

105. "Decline of dengue."

106. Pires-Alves, Paiva, and Lima, "Baixada Fluminense," 1857.

107. Maria Glória Teixeira, Maria da Conceição Costa, Florisnei de Barreto, and Maurício Lima Barreto, "Dengue: Vinte e cinco anos da reemergência no Brasil," *Cadernos de Saúde Pública* 25, suppl. 1 (2009): S7–S18; Jorge Tibilletti de Lara, "As impressões da primeira grande epidemia de dengue do Brasil entre os jornais O Globo, O Fluminense e Jornal do Brasil," *Revista Trilhas da História* 8, no. 16 (2019): 177–94; Gabriel Lopes and Jorge Tibilletti de Lara, "Entre a arma biológica e o 'mosquito estadual': Cooperação Brasil-Cuba e as epidemias de dengue, 1981–1988," *Revista Nupem* (Campo Mourao) 13, no. 29 (2021): 72–92.PEM,/ago.021

108. Keyla Belizia Feldman Marzochi, "Dengue in Brazil—situation, transmission and control," *Memorias do Instituto Oswaldo Cruz* 89, no. 2 (1994): 235–45.

109. Janice Perlman, *Favela: Four Decades of Living on the Edge in Rio de Janeiro* (Oxford: Oxford University Press, 2010); Erica Robb Larkins, *The Spectacular Favela: Violence in Modern Brazil* (Berkeley: University of California Press, 2015).

110. Teixeira, Costa, Barreto, and Barreto, "Dengue: Vinte e cinco anos da reemergência no Brasil."

111. Mauricio Barreto, Gloria Teixeira, Francisco Bastos, et al., "Successes and failures in the control of infectious diseases in Brazil: Social and environmental context, policies, interventions, and research needs," *Lancet* 377 (2011): 1877–89.

112. João Bosco Siqueira, Celina Maria Turchi Martelli, Giovanini Evelim Coelho, et al., "Dengue and dengue hemorrhagic fever, Brazil, 1981–2002," *Emerging Infectious Diseases* 11, no. 1 (2005): 48–53; Teixeira, Costa, Barreto, and Barreto, "Dengue: Vinte e cinco anos da reemergência no Brasil"; Lopes and Felipe Candido da Silva, "O *Aedes aegypti* e os mosquitos na historiografía."

113. Packard and Gadelha, "Land filled with mosquitoes."

114. Mac Margolis, "The bug is back," *Newsweek International*, June 17, 2002, 60.

115. Jean Segata, Elisa Obrest Varga, and Nathalia de Santos Silva, "Um vetor de ciência, tecnologia e governo da vida: O mosquito *Aedes aegypti* e constituição insecto-viral das políticas públicas de saúde," *Passo Fundo* 21, no. 3 (2021): 190–209.

116. Ricardo Lourenço-de-Oliveira, "Editorial: Rio de Janeiro against *Aedes aegypti*: Yellow fever in 1908 and dengue in 2008," *Memorias do Instituto Oswaldo Cruz* 103, no. 7 (2008): 627–28.

117. In 2021 too, the focus is on technical solutions to the mosquito problem that do not involve costly investment in infrastructure or changing people's habits. See, e.g., James Gallagher, "Miraculous mosquito hack cuts dengue by 77%," *BBC News*, October 6, 2020, https://www.bbc.com/news/health-57417219. Gallagher commented on an article that reported the successful release of *Wolbachia*-infected mosquitoes in Indonesia. A. Utarini, C. Indriani, R. A. Ahmad, et al., "Efficacy of Wolbachia-infected mosquito deployments for the control of dengue," *New England Journal of Medicine* 384, no. 23 (2021): 2177–86.

118. Denise Valle, Denise Nacif Pimenta, and Rivaldo Venâncio da Cunha, eds., *Dengue: Teorias e práticas* (Rio de Janeiro: Editora Fiocruz, 2015).

119. Barreto, Teixeira, Bastos, et al., "Successes and failures in the control of infectious diseases in Brazil."

120. Denise Nacif Pimenta, "Determinação social, determinantes sociais da saúde e a dengue: Caminhos possíveis?," in Valle, Pimenta, and da Cunha, *Dengue: Teorias e práticas*, 407–47.

121. Jorge Tibilletti de Lara, "A emergência da dengue como desafio virológico: De doença fantasma à endemia 'de estimação,' 1986–1987" (MSc thesis, Casa Oswaldo Cruz, Fiocruz, 2020). Another important center of studies of the dengue virus and, later, the Zika virus was the virology laboratory of Fiocruz in Recife.

122. Natalia Ingrid Oliveira Silva, Lívia Sacchetto, and Izabela Maurício de Rezende, "Recent sylvatic yellow fever virus transmission in Brazil: The news from an old disease," *Virology Journal* 17, no. 9 (2020), https://doi.org/10.1186/s12985-019-1277-7; PAHO, "Brazil works to control yellow fever outbreak, with PAHO/WHO support," March 28, 2017, https://reliefweb.int/report/brazil/brazil-works-control-yellow-fever-outbreak-pahowho-support; Possas, Lourenço-de-Oliveira, Tauil, et al., "Yellow fever outbreak in Brazil"; Poliana de Oliveira Figueiredo, Ana Gabriella Stoffella-Dutra, Galileu Barbosa Costa, et al., "Review: Re-emergence of yellow fever in Brazil during 2016–2019: Challenges, lessons learned, and perspectives," *Viruses* 12, no. 11 (2020):1233, https://doi.org/10.3390/v12111233.

123. Shasta Darlington and Donald G. McNeil, "Yellow fever circles Brazil's huge cities," *New York Times*, March 5, 2018.

124. Figueiredo, Stoffella-Dutra, Barbosa Costa, et al., "Review: Re-emergence of yellow fever."

125. Dom Phillips, "'We didn't expect this': A historic yellow fever outbreak spreads in Brazil," *STAT*, April, 13, 2017, https://www.statnews.com/2017/04/13/yellow-fever-brazil-outbreak/.

126. Darlington and McNeil, "Yellow fever circles Brazil's huge cities."

127. Possas, Lourenço-de-Oliveira, Tauil, et al., "Yellow fever outbreak in Brazil."

128. Phillips. "'We didn't expect this.'"

Chapter 2 · Fetuses

1. Ana Claudia Costa, Gustavo Goulart, and Rafael Nascimento, "Os doutores do aborto," *O Globo*, October 10, 2014.

2. Elisa Clavery, "Médico de hospital público no Rio e assessor parlamentar são presos em clínica de aborto," *O Globo*, April, 5, 2016.

3. Lucila Scavone, "Politicas feministas do aborto," *Estudos Feministas* (Florianópolis) 16, no. 2 (2008): 675–80; Cassia Roth, *A Miscarriage of Justice: Women, Reproductive Lives and the Law in Twentieth Century Brazil* (Stanford: Stanford University Press, 2020).

4. The women's rights activist Debora Diniz notes that imprisoning all the women who have abortions in Brazil would quadruple the already very high number of incarcerated people. Debora Diniz, "The Brazilian litigation on abortion: Zika epidemics and beyond," *NYU Law Review*, March 2017, http://www.law.nyu.edu/sites/default/files/upload_documents /Diniz_March.pdf.

5. Debora Diniz, "Conscientious objection and abortion: Rights and duties of public sector physicians," *Revista de Saúde Pública* 45, no. 5 (2011): 981–85.

6. Resolution 1.989, May 10, 2012, "Dispoe sobre diagnostico de anencefalia para a antecipacão terapeutica do parto da outras providencias," *Diario oficial da união [da Republica Federativa do Brasil]* 149, no. 92 (2012): 308–9; Debora Diniz, "Selective abortion in Brazil: The anencephaly case," *Developing World Bioethics* 7, no. 2 (2007): 64–67.

7. Sandra Costa Fonseca, Rosa Maria Domingues, Maria do Carmo Leal, Estela Aquino, and Greice Menezes, "Aborto legal no Brasil: Revisão sistemática da produção científica, 2008–2018," *Cadernos de Saúde Pública* 36, suppl. 1 (2020): e00189718.

8. Fabíola Rohden, *A arte de enganar a natureza: Contracepção, aborto e infanticídio no início do século XX* (Rio de Janeiro: Editora Fiocruz, 2003); Joana Maria Pedro, ed., *Práticas proibidas: Práticas costumeiras de aborto e infanticídio no século XX* (Florianópolis: Cidade Futura, 2003); Cassia Roth, "Policing pregnancy: Reproduction, poverty, and the law in early twentieth-century Rio de Janeiro," *Journal of Women's History* 29, no. 4 (2017): 85–108; Roth, *Miscarriage of Justice*.

9. Alberto Madeiro and Debora Diniz, "Serviços de aborto legal no Brasil: Um estudo nacional," *Ciência e Saúde Coletiva* 21, no. 2 (2016): 563–72.

10. Clarice Novaes de Mota, "A prática do aborto provocado no Rio de Janeiro: A perspectiva da clientes e professionais de saúde," final research report, UFRJ, 1995, Archivio Oswaldo Cruz, Fiocruz, Rio de Janeiro (ACOC), fond Sarah Hawker, file SH-19, quotations on 32–33.

11. Kirsten Luker, *Abortion and the Politics of Motherhood* (Berkeley: University of California Press, 1985); Katie Watson, "The unacknowledged consensus on abortion," *American Journal of Bioethics* 10, no. 12 (2010): 57–59; Watson, *Scarlet A: The Ethics, Law, and Politics of Ordinary Abortion* (New York: Oxford University Press, 2018), 213. Luker persuasively argued that the US "fetus wars" mirror above all incommensurable views about women's role in society.

12. Drauzio Varella, "'Aborto já é livre no Brasil: Proibir é punir quem não tem dinheiro,' diz Drauzio Varella," interview by Ricardo Senra, *BBC Brazil*, February 2, 2018, https://www .bbc.com/portuguese/noticias/2016/02/160201_drauzio_aborto_rs.

13. Wendell Ferrari, Simone Peres, and Marcos Nascimento, "Experiment and learning in the affective and sexual life of young women from a favela in Rio de Janeiro, Brazil, with experience of clandestine abortion," *Ciência e Saúde Coletiva* 23, no. 9 (2018): 2937–50.

14. Wendell Ferrari, "Foi a melhor coisa que eu fiz: Aborto induzido entre adolescentes de uma favela da Zona Sul de Rio de Janeiro" (master's thesis, Federal University of Rio de Janeiro, 2016), published with slight modifications as *Entre o segredo e a solidão: Aborto ilegal*

na adolescência (Rio de Janeiro: Editora Fiocruz, 2021); Wendell Ferrari and Simone Peres, "Itinerários de solidão: Aborto clandestino de adolescentes de uma favela da Zona Sul do Rio de Janeiro, Brasil," *Cadernos de Saúde Pública* 36, suppl. 1 (2020), https://doi.org/10.1590 /0102-311X00198318 .

15. The rule that misoprostol could only be purchased by men might have been specific to this favela. Debora Diniz and Alberto Madeiro, who studied the circulation of misoprostol in Brazil, reported that it was diffused by male-dominated networks that also diffused illegal drugs, but this was not the only way to obtain the abortive drug. It was also possible to obtain it (illegally) in some pharmacies and on the internet. Debora Diniz and Alberto Madeiro, "Cytotec e aborto: A polícia, os vendedores e as mulheres," *Ciência e Saúde Coletiva* 17, no. 7 (2012): 1795–1804. The majority of the teenaged women from Teresina, Piauí, in the south of Brazil, who used misoprostol to terminate a pregnancy purchased the drug themselves in a pharmacy. Maria das Dores Nunes, Alberto Madeiro, and Debora Diniz, "Histórias de aborto provocado entre adolescentes em Teresina, Piauí, Brasil," *Ciência e Saúde Coletiva* 18, no. 8 (2013): 2311–18.

16. Ferrari, *Entre o segredo e a solidão*, 97–98.

17. Ferrari, *Entre o segredo e a solidão*, 171–72.

18. Researchers who have studied illegal abortion in Brazil provide ample evidence of the frequent mistreatment of women in need of an abortion in public hospitals and clinics. See, e.g., Sylvia de Zordo, "The biomedicalisation of illegal abortion: The double life of misoprostol in Brazil," *História, Ciências, Saúde—Manguinhos* 23, no. 1 (2016): 19–35; Cecilia McCallum, Greice Mendez, and Ana Paula dos Reis, "The dilemma of a practice: Experiences of abortion in a public maternity hospital in the city of Salvador, Bahia," *História, Ciências, Saúde— Manguinhos* 23, no. 1 (2016): 37–56.

19. Ferrari, *Entre o segredo e a solidão*, 119.

20. The configuration described by Ferrari, with a predominance of surgical abortions, may be atypical and specific to the favela he described. In the study of abortion of teenaged girls in Teresina, Piauí, the interviewed girls had all undergone curettage for a partial abortion in a public hospital. Nearly all these girls had used misoprostol to terminate a pregnancy, and 3 of the 30 girls interviewed had suffered severe complications following their abortions. Nunes, Madeiro, and Diniz, "Histórias de aborto provocado."

21. Ferrari, *Entre o segredo e a solidão*, 166.

22. In the 1960s and early 1970s, lay women from the Chicago feminist collective Jane learned how to perform surgical abortion by observing doctors. They did not have a higher level of complications than professionals. Laura Kaplan, *The Story of Jane: The Legendary Feminist Abortion Service* (Chicago: University of Chicago Press, 1997).

23. Caitlin Moran, *How to Be a Woman* (London: Ebury Press, 2011), translated into Portuguese as *Como ser mulher* (São Paolo: Editora Paralela—Companhia das Lettras, 2012). Simone de Beauvoir's *The Second Sex* was available in Portuguese from the 1960s.

24. Ferrari, *Entre o segredo e a solidão*, 184.

25. *Atenção humanisada au abortamento: Norma technica de aborto*, 2nd ed. (Brasília: Ministério da Saúde, 2011).

26. Leila Adesse, "Aborto no Brasil—Estudos de suas complicações, estigma e impactos na saúde" (PhD thesis, Instituto Fernandes Figueira, Fiocruz, 2011); Nunes, Madeiro, and Diniz, "Histórias de aborto provocado"; McCallum, Mendez, and Dos Reis, "Dilemma of a practice."

27. Mariana Ramos Pitta Lima, Cecilia Anne McCallum, and Greice Maria de Souza. Menezes, "The ultrasound scene in abortion care: Practices and meanings in a public maternity hospital in Salvador, Bahia State, Brazil," *Cadernos de Saúde Pública* 36, suppl. 1 (2020): e00035618; Mariana Ramos Pitta Lima, Cecilia Anne McCallum, and Greice Maria de Souza Menezes, "Violences gynécoloqiques et obstétricales, technologies biomédicales est avorte-

ment dans une maternité publique du nord-est du Brésil," *S.P.S.P. Santé Publique* 33, no. 5 (2021): 675–83.

28. Hospitais Universitarios Federais, *Protocolo do programa Atenas, programa de atençào extra hospitalar a mulheres em situaçàe de abortamento* (Salvador, Bahia, 2017), http://www2 .ebserh.gov.br/documents/215335/4407336/Protocolo+Programa+Atenas.pdf/dd73a5df -3a01-4cd9-a8f6-45a7d8226e96.

29. Ana Gabriela Lima Bispo de Victa, Adriana Monteiro dos Santos Lopes, and Luci Laura Almeida Brandão, "Mulheres e abortamento, um relato de experiência," delivered at the 13th Women's World Congress and Doing Gender 11 Seminar, Florianópolis, 2017, https:// www.en.wwc2017.eventos.dype.com.br/simposio/view?ID_SIMPOSIO=49&impressao. I am grateful to Ana Gabriela Bispo de Victa for sharing with me additional results of her unpublished study "Uma etnografia de um servicio extra hospitalar a mulheres em situaçàe de abortamento em uma maternidade publica do Nordeste brasileiro," conducted at the Federal University of Bahia.

30. Hospitais Universitarios Federais, *Protocolo do programa Atenas*, 26.

31. Victa, Lopes, and Brandão, "Mulheres e abortamento." Among the 34 professionals who participated in the Atenas project—doctors, nurses, nurse's aides, technicians, administrative assistants—only two did not have private health insurance and relied exclusively on SUS services.

32. During the COVID-19 pandemic, some women in the United States who did not have access to a hospital abortion because of the lockdown and were obliged to end their pregnancy using misoprostol—without mefipristone and without professional assistance—had a distressing experience, described by one woman as a "twisted purgatory." Nathalie Lampert, "During the pandemic, more women must miscarry at home," *New York Times*, July 29, 2020.

33. Victa, Lopes, and Brandão, "Mulheres e abortamento."

34. Dominique Béhague, Cesar Victora, and Fernando Barros, "Consumer demand for caesarean sections in Brazil: Informed decision making, patient choice, or social inequality?," *British Medical Journal* 324 (2002): 942–48.

35. Simone Diniz and Alessandra Chacham, "The 'cut above' and the 'cut below': The abuse of caesareans and episiotomy in São Paulo, Brazil," *Reproductive Health Matters* 12, no. 23 (2004): 100–110.

36. Maria do Carmo Leal and Silvana Granado Nogueira da Gama, "Nascer no Brasil," *Cadernos de Saúde Pública* 30, suppl. 1 (August 2014).

37. An educational film made as part of the Nascer no Brasil project juxtaposes testimonies of distressed women who gave birth in hospital wards, where they were alone and suffered obstetrical violence, with testimonies of satisfied women who gave birth in a "humanized" maternity environment, in the presence of their partner or a family member. Some women testified that while the childbirth itself was long and very painful, they were grateful for the help and encouragement of the hospital staff. Gabriella Dias de Oliveira, "Nascer no Brasil: O retrato do nascimento na voz das mulheres," *RECIIS—Revista Eletrônica de Comunicação, Informação e Inovação em Saúde* 9, no. 2 (April–June 2015), https://www.reciis.icict.fiocruz .br/index.php/reciis/article/view/97 .

38. For a dissenting view see José Guilherme Cecatti, "Beliefs and misbeliefs about current interventions during labor and delivery in Brazil," *Cadernos de Saúde Pública* 30, suppl. 1 (2014): S17–S19.

39. Maria do Carmo Leal, Ana Paula Esteves Pereira, Rosa Maria Soares, et al., "The authors reply," *Cadernos de Saúde Pública* 30, suppl. 1 (2014): S27–S31.

40. Victa, Lopes, and Brandão, "Mulheres e abortamento."

41. Walter Fonseca, Ana Julia Cauto Alencar, Francisco Sullivan Bastos Mota, and Helena Lutescia Luna Coelho, "Misoprostol and congenital malformations," *Lancet* 338 (1991): 56–57;

Ilana Löwy and Marilena Correa, "The 'abortion pill' misoprostol in Brazil: Women's empowerment in a conservative and repressive political environment," *American Journal of Public Health* 110, no. 5 (2020): 677–84.

42. Mariana Ramos Pitta Lima documented the failure of health professionals to provide accurate information to women in a situation of abortion, and the active production of ignorance on this topic, in "Tecnologias biomédicas a aborto em uma maternidade pública de Salvador: Estudo etnográfico" (PhD thesis, Universidade Federal da Bahia, 2022). I am thankful to her for sharing with me additional results of her research.

43. On the collaboration between professionals and feminists in reducing risks of illegal abortions in Argentina see Lucila Szwarc, "Les services d'accueil et de conseils en avortement sûr à Buenos Aires et en banlieue: De la réduction des risques à l'avortement populaire" (MSc thesis, EHESS, Paris, 2013).

44. Susan Mayor, "Abortion requests increase in Latin America after Zika warning, figures show," *British Medical Journal* 353 (2016): 3492–94, https://doi.org/10.1136/bmj.i3492; Abigail Aiken, James Scott, Rebecca Gomperts, et al., "Requests for abortion in Latin America related to concern about Zika virus exposure," *New England Journal of Medicine* 375, no. 4 (2016): 396–98. On the very limited use of the services of Women on the Web in Brazil see Nanda Isele Gallas Duarte, "O dispositivo da maternidade em tensão: A poliphonia das narrativas sobre aborto provocado em uma comunidade on line" (master's thesis, Escola Nacional de Saúde Pública, Rio de Janeiro, 2019), esp. 53–57, and for an estimate of the number of illegal abortions in Brazil see Debora Diniz, Marcelo Medeiros, and Alberto Madeiro, "Pesquisa nacional de aborto 2016," *Ciência e Saúde Coletiva* 22, no. 2 (2017): 653–60.

45. "Elas não têm gosto ou vontade / Nem defeito, nem qualidade / Têm medo apenas / Não tem sonhos, só tem presságios" (They have no taste or will / No flaws, no qualities / No dreams, only omens / They are only scared).

46. M. F. G. Monteiro, L. Adesse, and J. Drezett, "Atualização das estimativas da magnitude do aborto induzido, taxas por mil mulheres e razões por 100 nascimentos vivos do aborto induzido por faixa etária e grandes regiões: Brasil, 1995 a 2013," *Reproducão e Climatério* 30 (2015): 11–18.

47. Thália Velho Barreto de Araújo, Estela Aquino, Greice Menezes, et al., "Delays in access to care for abortion-related complications: The experience of women in Northeast Brazil," *Cadernos de Saúde Pública* 34, no. 6 (2018): e00168116.

48. Diniz, "Selective abortion in Brazil."

49. Emanualle Pelizzari, Carolina Mendez Valdez, Jamile dos Santos Picetti, et al., "Characteristics of fetuses evaluated due to suspected anencephaly: A population based cohort study in southern Brazil," *São Paulo Medical Journal* 133 (2015): 101–8.

50. For the latter argument see, e.g., comments on the article by Lyndsay Werking-Yip, "I had a late-term abortion. I am not a monster," in *New York Times*, October 19, 2019. For similar testimonies of Vietnamese women see Tine Gammeltoft, *Haunting Images: A Cultural Account of Selective Reproduction in Vietnam* (Berkeley: University of California Press, 2014).

51. Iulia Bicu Fernandes, "Interromper ou não interromper a gestação: Vivencias de gestantes de fetos com Anenefalia" (dissertation, Instituto Fernandes Figueia, Fiocruz, 2017).

52. Fernandes, "Interromper ou não interromper a gestação," 85, 95–96.

53. Fernandes, "Interromper ou não interromper a gestação," 97– 98. Since Fendandes recorded only the women's impressions, it is possible that some women might have misinterpreted the health providers' reactions. Nevertheless, even if that was the case, the women's testimonies reflect problematic interactions with professionals and a mutual lack of trust. Some women who lost an anencephalic fetus were offered psychological counseling, but only after the abortion or death of their child.

54. Fernandes, "Interromper ou não interromper a gestação," 96–97.

55. Fernandes, "Interromper ou não interromper a gestação," 92–93.

56. Fernandes, "Interromper ou não interromper a gestação," 69. It is possible that this woman was obliged to secure permission before the implementation of the 2012 law.

57. The document that provided the legal basis for "humanized" abortion in Brazil, *Atenção humanisada au abortamento: Norma technica de aborto*, does not mention mifepristone, banned in Brazil. It does not mention either peridural anesthesia or any other kind of pain relief, even when pregnancy is terminated following the death of the fetus in the womb. See Maria Isabel do Nascimento, Alfredo de Almeida Cunha, Sandra Regina dos Santos Muri Oliveira, et al., "Misoprostol use under routine conditions for termination of pregnancies with intrauterine fetal death," *Revista da Associação Médica Brasileira* 59, no. 4 (2013): 354–59.

58. Fernandes, "Interromper ou não interromper a gestação," 87–88.

59. L. Mandelbrot and G. Girard, "Aspects techniques des interruptions médicales de grossesse," *Mises à Jour en Gynecologie et Obstétrique* 32 (2008): 7–39; A. Agostini, C. Vayssiere, A. Gaudinau, et al., "Recommandations pour la pratique clinique: L'interruption volontaire de grossesse élaborées par le Collège national des gynécologues et obstétriciens français," CNGOF, 2016, https://ansfl.org/document/cngof-2016-livg-medicamenteuse/; J. M. Pelligrinelli, ed., *Interuption thérapeutique/médicale de la grosesse* (Geneva: Hopitaux Universitaires, 2014).

60. The combination of mefipristone and misoprostol is credited with shortening the time of abortion. On the other hand, according to some reports, abortions with misoprostol alone, combined with the administration of laminaria and performed by experienced practitioners generally lasted approximatively the same amount of time (4.8 to 5 hours from the beginning of the procedure) as abortions with misoprostol and mefipristone. The key reason might have been the skill and experience of the medical staff rather than the precise method employed. Erin Wingo, Sarah Raifman, Carmen Landau, Shelley Sella, and Daniel Grossman, "Mifepristone-misoprostol versus misoprostol-alone regimen for medication abortion at more than 24 weeks' gestation," *Contraception* 102 (2020): 99–103.

61. See, e.g., *Fiche d'information patiente: Interruption médicale de la grossesse* (CHU Caen); *Livret d'information à l'usage des parents: Interruption médicale de la grossesse* (Hopital Femme, Mère, Enfant, Hospices Civils de Lyon); and *Livret d'information à l'usage des parents: Interruption médicale de la grossesse* (Hopitaux de la région Languedoc-Roussillon). Feticide— usually by injection of potassium chloride to the fetal heart—while difficult for the woman who undergoes a termination of pregnancy and the professional who performs it, is usually presented as less traumatic than its alternative, the birth of a live fetus/child. Society for Family Planning, "Clinical guidelines: Induction of fetal demise before abortion," *Contraception* 81 (2010): 462–73.

62. On the other hand, the "new normal" of mourning rites for aborted fetuses or stillborn infants can be oppressive for some women. Dominique Memmi, *La deuxième vie des bébés morts* (Paris: Editions EHESS, 2011); Ilana Löwy, *Tangled Diagnoses: Prenatal Testing, Women and Risk* (Chicago: University of Chicago Press, 2018), chap. 1.

63. Debora Diniz and Marilena Correa, eds., *Aborto e saúde pública: 20 anos de pesquisas no Brasil* (Brasilia: Ministério de Saúde, 2008).

64. Human Rights Watch, *Neglected and Unprotected: The Impact of the Zika Outbreak on Women and Girls in Northeastern Brazil,* 2017, https://www.hrw.org/report/2017/07/13/neglected-and-unprotected/impact-zika-outbreak-women-and-girls-northeastern, 58. While in the case of rape a simple declaration of the woman that her pregnancy was a result of a rape should be sufficient to have an abortion in public hospital, in practice these women had numerous difficulties terminating their pregnancies. Alberto Pereira Madeiro and Debora Diniz, "Legal abortion services in Brazil—A national study," *Ciência e Saúde Coletiva* 21, no. 2 (2016): 563–72.

65. On debates about the legal basis of juridical abortion in Brazil see Maria Cristina Guilam, "O discurso do risco na prática do aconselhamento genético pré-natal" (PhD thesis, Instituto de Medicina Social, Universidade do Estado do Rio de Janeiro, 2003), 121–29; and Debora Diniz, "Aborto e inviabilidad fetal: El debate brasileño," *Cadernos de Saúde Pública* 21 (2005): 634–39.

66. A woman who petitions a court for permission to terminate her pregnancy can obtain help from the Public Defender's Office (Defensoria Publica), independent institution akin to the French Defenseur des droits. However, only a fraction of Brazilian women have access to this resource. Costa Fonseca, Domingues, Leal, et al., "Aborto legal no Brasil."

67. Flavia Westphal, Edward Araujo Júnior, Suzete Maria Fustinoni, and Anelise Riedel Abrahão, "Maternal risks and predictor factors for the termination of pregnancy in fetuses with severe congenital anomaly: Experience from a single reference center in Brazil," *Journal of Maternal-Fetal and Neonatal Medicine* 29, no. 23 (2016): 3762–67.

68. Only one among the 14 pairs of conjoined twins born alive at the maternity hospital of Ribeiro Preto University in the state of São Paolo was successfully separated after birth; all the others died either immediately after birth or a few weeks later. Anderson Tadeu Berezoski, Geraldo Duarte, Reinaldo Rodriguez, et al., "Gêmeos conjugados: Experiência de um hospital terciário do sudeste do Brasil," *Revista Brasileira de Ginecologia e Obstetrícia* 32, no. 2 (2010): 61–65.

69. M. L. Brizot, A. W. Liao, L. M. Lopes, et al., "Conjoined twins pregnancies: Experience with 36 cases from a single center," *Prenatal Diagnosis* 31 (2011): 1120–25.

70. Rosalie Mieko Yamamoto Nomura, Maria de Lourdes Brizot, Adolfo Wenjaw Liao, and Wagner Rodriguez Hernandes, "Conjoined twins and legal authorization for abortion," *Revista da Associação Médica Brasileira* 57, no. 2 (2011): 205–10. Because of the shape of conjoined twins, the woman cannot have a vaginal birth or a standard C-section. When a termination of pregnancy with conjoined twins is made in the early or middle second trimester, the fetuses are still relatively small, and the risk for the pregnant women is much lower.

71. This story was exceptional because it became public. In Brazil there are 6 legal abortions per day of girls of less than 14 years who are victims of rape. Matheus Magenta and Laís Alegretti, "Brasil registra 6 abortos por dia em meninas entre 10 e 14 anos estupradas," *BBC News Brasil*, August 17, 2020, https://www.bbc.com/portuguese/brasil-53807076.

72. "Promotoria vai investigar se grupos tentaram pressionar avó de menina estuprada a não autorizar aborto," *O Globo*, August, 16, 2020. According to Brazilian law, a women who declares that her pregnancy is the result of a rape is entitled to an abortion without additional legal or administrative steps.

73. Mayhill J. Fowler, "Conservative Brazilian groups hinder the legal abortion of a 10-year-old girl raped by her uncle," *OfftheBus*, August 17, 2020, https://www.offthebus.net /author/mayhill-j-fowler/.

74. Curumim was founded in Recife, Pernambuco. It is committed to reproductive justice, with special emphasis on the problems of poor women, young women, and women of color. Joanna Suarez, "De corpo e alma na luta: A enfermeira que batalha pelo aborto seguro há 40 anos," *My News*, September 29, 2021, https://canalmynews.com.br/mais/corpo-e-alma-na -luta-enfermeira-batalha-aborto-seguro-ha-40-anos/.

75. Aliny Gama and Carlos Madeiro, "Criança de 10 anos grávida de estupro realiza curetagem em PE: Menina estaria sendo estuprada há 4 anos pelo tio," *UOL*, August 17, 2020, https://www.uol.com.br/universa/noticias/redacao/2020/08/17/crianca-de-10-anos-expulsa -feto-e-passa-por-avaliacao-para-finalizar-aborto.htm. Several similar cases were recorded later, e.g., in 2022. Ana Laura Queiroz, "Menina de 11 anos estuprada é mantida em abrigo para evitar aborto," *Estado de Minas*, June 20, 2022. In 2022, changes in abortion laws in the

United States led to similar problems for doctors who provide abortions to minors. See, e.g., Sheryl Gay Stolberg and Ave Sasani, "An Indiana doctor speaks out on abortion, and pays a price," *New York Times*, July 28, 2022.

76. *Manual technico pre-natal* (Technical directory of prenatal tests), published by the Brazilian Health Ministry in 2006, quoted in Ana Elisa Rodrigues Baião, "A decisão informada no rastramento prenatal das aneuploidias" (master's thesis, Instituto Fernandes Figueira, Fiocruz, 2009). The text does not mention serological tests for an increased risk of fetal anomalies.

77. Claudia Sampaio Rodrigues, "Sentidos, limited e potentialidades de medecine fetal: A visão dos especialistas" (master's thesis, Instituto Fernandes Figueira, Fiocruz, 2010).

78. Lilian Krakowsky Chazan, "O aparelho é como um automovel: A pista é a paciente," *Physis—Revista de Saúde Coletiva* 21, no. 2 (2011): 601–27.

79. Veronique Mirlesse, "Diagnostic prénatal et médecine fœtale: Du cadre des pratiques à l'anticipation du handicap; Comparaison France–Brésil" (PhD thesis, University of Paris XIII, 2014).

80. Olga Luiza Bomfim, Orlando Coser, and Maria Elisabeth Lopes Moreira, "Unexpected diagnosis of fetal malformations: Therapeutic itineraries," *Physis—Revista de Saúde Coletiva* 24, no. 2 (2014): 607–22.

81. Lilian Krakowsky Chazan, "'É . . . tá grávida mesmo! E ele é lindo!' A construção de 'verdades' na ultra-sonografia obstétrica," *Manguinhos* 15, no. 1 (2008): 99–116.

82. Olga Luiza Bomfim, "A antecipação ultra-sonográfica de malformação fetal sob a ótica da mulher" (master's thesis, Instituto Fernandes Figueira, Fiocruz, 2009); Bomfim, Coser, and Lopes Moreira, "Unexpected diagnosis."

83. Lilian Krakowsky Chazan, "Vérités, attentes, spectacles et consommations: A propos de l'échographie obstétriquedans les cliniques de Rio de Janeiro," *in Les technologies de l'espoir: La fabrique d'une historie à accomplir*, ed. Annette Leibing and Virginie Turnay (Quebec: Presses Universitaires de Laval, 2010); Bomfim, "A antecipação ultra-sonográfica," 33–37; Bomfim, Coser, and Lopes Moreira, "Unexpected diagnosis."

84. Paradoxically, Brazilian advocates of liberalization of abortion also share this view. They too do not attempt to historicize or nuance the term *eugenic*, nor do they question the identification of eugenics with an absolute evil. I am grateful to Robert Wegner and Alessandra Barroso for this precision.

85. The 12 in-depth interviews with women who asked for permission to have an abortion for fetal anomaly between 2011 and 2016 were part of research on juridical abortions coordinated by Claudia Bonan, of the Instituto Fernandes Figueira, Fiocruz, together with Luiz Antionio Teixeira, of Casa Oswaldo Cruz, Fiocruz. The project, entitled "Malformações no Brasil: Patologia, genética e quadro legal," was approved by the IFF Ethics Committee on May 6, 2015. The women were selected from a registry of a major Brazilian maternal-and-child-health hospital that has a genetic counseling service; all the participants signed consent forms. Contact with many of the women in this registry was lost, and many among those who were successfully contacted did not wish to speak about their pregnancies. As in the case of Wendell Ferrera's interviews with adolescents who had undergone an illegal abortion and Iulia Bicu Fernandes's interviews with women diagnosed with fetal anencephaly, the sample comprised women willing to discuss the sensitive topic with a researcher and therefore probably was not entirely representative.

86. Fernandes, "Interromper ou não interromper a gestação."

87. On the difficulty of reconciling the language of human rights with the religious worldview see, e.g., Zvika Orr, Shifra Unger, and Adi Finkelstein, "Localization of human rights of people with disabilities: The case of Jewish ultra-orthodox people in Israel," *Human Rights Quarterly* 43 (2021): 93–116. The rejection of the language of individual rights in favor

of the language of responsibility and mutual obligations is shared by ultraorthodox Jews and Brazilian religious women, but the religious Jews studied by Orr and his colleagues did not mention a direct communication with God; such communication was always mediated by religious authorities.

88. A conservative Catholic may resist the principle that if the fetus is not viable, a woman should be allowed to end the pregnancy. Thus in 2016 the president of the Polish conservative ruling party, PiS, explained that his party aspired to ban abortion even in cases of a severely deformed, nonviable fetus, to make possible the baptism of the child. Krystyna Opozda, "Nic sie nie stalo" [Nothing had happened], Wprost.pl, November 2, 2021, https://www.wprost.pl /kraj/10535665/nic-sie-nie-stalo-zakazu-aborcji-nie-ma-tragedia-z-pszczyny-przeczy-narracji -pis.html. In 2021 the PiS-led government successfully banned all abortions for fetal indication in Poland.

89. No woman "choses" to learn that she is carrying a fetus with a severe anomaly. Nevertheless, Frenchwomen who were informed that they have to obtain the approval of an ethics committee for a late abortion for fetal anomaly were shocked to learn that other people, and not only they and their partners, were involved in what they saw as a decision that affected them, and them alone. Marie Gaille, "On prenatal diagnosis and the decision to continue or terminate a pregnancy in France: A clinical ethics study of unknown moral territories," *Medicine, Health Care and Philosophy* 19, no. 3 (2016): 381–91.

90. Löwy, *Tangled Diagnoses*, 125.

91. In situations of conflict patients are expected to fight for their "right to health" either individually, by suing the state, or collectively, through health activism. See, e.g., João Biehl, "Patient-citizen-consumer: Judicialization of health and metamorphoses of biopolitics," *Lua Nova* (São Paulo) 98 (2016): 77–105.

92. See Emilia Sanabria, *Plastic Bodies: Sex Hormones and Menstrual Suppression in Brazil* (Durham, NC: Duke University Press, 2016).

93. Tests like noninvasive prenatal testing (NIPT), coupled with chronic villous sampling (CVS), can detect genetic anomalies of the fetus early in pregnancy, but in Brazil such testing is available only to affluent women. Ilana Löwy, "Non-invasive prenatal testing: A diagnostic innovation shaped by commercial interests and the regulation conundrum," *Social Science and Medicine* 304 (2022), https://pubmed.ncbi.nlm.nih.gov/32534823/.

94. Ferrari, *Entre o segredo e a solidão*, 186–87.

95. Moran, *How to Be a Woman*, 240–41. Moran added that she had later discovered that her response was far from unusual; the main reaction of many women who terminated a pregnancy was relief.

96. Tom Phillips and Caio Baretto Briso, "Brazil: Outcry as religious extremists harass child seeking abortion," *Guardian*, June 18, 2020.

Chapter 3 · Surprises

1. Quoted in Sarah Boseley, "On the frontline of Brazil's war on Zika," *Guardian*, April 12, 2016.

2. On hypotheses about the origins of AIDS see, e.g., Jacques Papin, *The Origins of AIDS* (Cambridge: Cambridge University Press, 2011). The COVID-19 epidemic led to heated, still unresolved debates on the precise origins of the SARS-CoV-2 virus. Most experts believe that the virus had natural origins, but in 2022 some did not exclude a laboratory accident in Wuhan, China.

3. A. J. Haddow, M. C. Williams, J. P. Woodall, et al., "Twelve isolations of Zika virus from Aedes (Stegomyia) africanus (Theobald) taken in and above Uganda Forest," *Bulletin of the World Health Organization* 31 (1964): 57–69.

4. Brian Foy, Kevin Kobylinski, Joy Chilson, et al., "Probable non-vector-borne transmission of Zika virus, Colorado, USA," *Emerging Infectious Diseases* 17, no. 5 (2011): 880–82.

5. *Zika: The untold story*, 2016, https://www.youtube.com/watch?v=_yFPgaFJtRM.

6. A. H. Fagbami, "Zika virus infections in Nigeria: Virological and seroepidemiological investigations in Oyo State," *Journal of Hygiene* (Cambridge) 83 (1979): 213–19.

7. Duane J. Gubler, Nikos Vasilakis, and Didier Musso, "History and emergence of Zika virus," *Journal of Infectious Diseases* 216, suppl. 10 (2017): S860–66.

8. Mark Duffy, Tai-Ho Chen, W. Thane Hancock, et al., "Zika virus outbreak on Yap Island, Federated States of Micronesia," *New England Journal of Medicine* 360, no. 24 (2009): 2536–43.

9. Didier Musso, Hervé Bossin, Henri Pierre Mallet, et al., "Zika virus in French Polynesia, 2013–14: Anatomy of a completed outbreak," *Lancet Infectious Diseases* 18, no. 5 (2018): e172–e182, https://doi.org/10.1016/S1473-3099(17)30446-2.

10. John Pettersson, Vegard Eldholm, Stephen Seligman, et al., "How did Zika virus emerge in the Pacific Islands and Latin America?," *mBio* 7, no. 5 (2016) : e01239-16, https://doi.org/10.1128/mBio.01239-16.

11. Didier Musso, Claudine Roche, Emilie Robin, et al., "Potential sexual transmission of Zika virus," *Emerging Infectious Diseases* 21, no. 2 (2015): 259–61.

12. Recent studies favor the hypothesis of an early introduction of ZIKV to Brazil, probably in 2013. Larissa Catharina Costa, Rafael Valente Veiga, Juliane Fonseca Oliveira, et al., "New insights on the Zika virus arrival in the Americas and spatiotemporal reconstruction of the epidemic dynamics in Brazil," *Viruses* 13, no. 12 (2021), https://doi.org/10.3390/v13010012.

13. Nuno Rodrigues Faria, Raimunda do Socorro da Silva Azevedo, Moritz U. G. Kraemer, et al., "Zika virus in the Americas: Early epidemiological and genetic findings," *Science* 352, no. 6283 (2016): 345–49.

14. Gubio Campos, Antonio Bandeira, and Silvia Sardi, "Zika virus outbreak, Bahia, Brazil," *Emerging Infectious Diseases* 21, no. 10 (2015): 1885–86.

15. Camila Zanluca, Vanessa Campos Andrade de Melo, Ana Luiza Pamplona Mosimann, et al., "First report of autochthonous transmission of Zika virus in Brazil," *Memorias do Instituto Oswaldo Cruz, Rio de Janeiro* 110, no. 4 (2015): 569–72.

16. Ravi Mehta, Cristiane Nascimento Soares, Raquel Medialdea-Carrera, et al., "The spectrum of neurological disease associated with Zika and chikungunya viruses in adults in Rio de Janeiro, Brazil: A case series," *PLOS Neglected Tropical Diseases*, February 18, 2018, https://doi.org/10.1371/journal.pntd.0006212.

17. Michel Foucault, *La naissance de la clinique: Une archeologie du regard médical* (Paris: PUF, 1963), translated into English by A. M. Sheridan Smith as *The Birth of the Clinics: An Archeology of Medical Perception* (New York: Vintage Books, 1973).

18. Carlo Ginzburg, "Clues: Roots of a scientific paradigm," *Theory and Society* 7, no. 3 (1979): 273–88.

19. Celina Turchi upon being named the personality of the year by the journal *O Globo* in 2016, http://eventos.oglobo.globo.com/faz-diferenca/2016/vencedores/personalidade-2016-nome-do-vencedor/.

20. Laura Rodrigues, "Microcephaly and Zika virus infection," *Lancet* 387 (2016): 2070–71.

21. ANIS, *Zika, the film*, 2016, produced by Debora Diniz and her colleagues from the Institute of Bioethics, Human Rights and Gender (ANIS), affiliated with the University of Brasília, https://www.youtube.com/watch?v=j9tqtojaoGo.

22. Boseley, "On the frontline of Brazil's war on Zika."

23. Debora Diniz, *Zika: Do sertão nordestino à ameaça global* (Rio de Janeiro: Editora de Civilização Brasileira, 2016), translated into English by Diane Grosklaus Whitty as *Zika: From the Brazilian Backlands to Global Threat* (Chicago: University of Chicago Press, 2017).

24. Maria de Fatima Pessoa Militão de Albuquerque, Wayner Vieira de Souza, Thalia Velho Barreto Araújo, et al., "The microcephaly epidemic and Zika virus: Building knowledge in epidemiology," *Cadernos de Saúde Pública* 34, no. 10 (2018): e00069018.

25. Vivian Avelino–Silva and Esper Kallas, "Untold stories of the Zika virus epidemic in Brazil," *Review of Medical Virology* 28, no. 6 (2018): e2000, https://doi.org/10.1002/rmv.2000.

26. Quoted in Simon Schaffer, "Scientific discoveries and the end of natural philosophy," *Social Studies of Science* 16 (1986): 387.

27. Boseley, "On the frontline of Brazil's war on Zika."

28. Camila Costa, "Infectologista relata choque e desespero ao se deparar com início de epidemia de microcefalia," *BBC Brazil*, November 30, 2015, http://www.bbc.com/portuguese/noticias/2015/11/151127_depoimento_medica_microcefalia_cc.

29. Ana Lucia Azevedo, "'Estamos com os pés e mãos atados,' diz medico sobre zika," *O Globo*, December 5, 2015.

30. Rodrigues, "Microcephaly and Zika virus infection."

31. Carlos Brito, "Zika virus: A new chapter in the history of medicine," *Acta Medicina Portuguesa* 28, no. 6 (2015): 679–80.

32. Rivaldo Venâncio da Cunha, "Ao que tudo indica, problema do zika está só começando; temos muita dor pela frente," *Agencia Fiocruz de Noticias* (blog), Centro des Estudos Estratégicos, Fiocruz, February 26, 2016, http://www.cee.fiocruz.br/?q=node%2F116.

33. Jaime Larry Benchimol, ed., *Febre amarela: A doença e a vacina, uma história inacabada* (Rio de Janeiro: Editora Fiocruz, 2001).

34. Gustavo Corrêa Matta, Carolina de Oliveira Nogueira, Elaine Teixeira Rabello, and Lenir da Nascimento Silva, "Zika outbreak in Brazil: In times of political and scientific uncertainties mosquitoes can be stronger than a country," in *Framing Animals as Villains: Histories of Non-Human Disease Vectors*, ed. Christos Lynteris (London: Palgrave Macmillan, 2019), 211–26.

35. Eduardo Gómez, Fernanda Aguilar Perez, and Deisy Ventura, "What explains the lacklustre response to Zika in Brazil? Exploring institutional, economic and health system context," *BMJ Global Health* 3, no. 5 (2018): e000862, https://doi.org/10.1136/bmjgh-2018-000862; Gabriel Lopez and Luisa Reis Castro, "A vector in the (re)making: A history of *Aedes aegypti* as mosquitoes that transmit diseases in Brazil," in Lynteris, *Framing Animals as Villains*, 147–75.

36. Gloria Nazario-Pietri, "The role of research in policy and practice: The Zika phenomena in Puerto Rico," *Puerto Rico Health Sciences Journal* 37, suppl. 1 (2018): S33–S40.

37. The "Protocolo Atenção à Saúde em resposta à ocorrência de microcefalia relacionada à infecção pelo vírus Zika" is discussed in Gustavo Corrêa Matta, Carolina de Oliveira Nogueira, and Lenir da Silva Nascimento, "A literary history of Zika: Following Brazilian state responses through documents of emergency," in *Zika Frontiers: Social Change and Governance in the Age of Mosquito Pandemics*, ed. Kevin Bardosh (London: Routledge, 2020), 55–77.

38. Gómez, Perez, and Ventura, "What explains the lacklustre response to Zika?"

39. Guilherme Calvet, Renato S Aguiar, Adriana S. O. Melo, et al., "Detection and sequencing of Zika virus from amniotic fluid of fetuses with microcephaly in Brazil: A case study," *Lancet Infectious Diseases* 16, no. 6 (2016): 653–60.

40. Raimunda S. S. Azevedo, Marialva Araujo, Consuelo S. Oliveira, et al., "Zika virus epidemic in Brazil: II. Post-mortem analyses of neonates with microcephaly, stillbirths, and miscarriage," *Journal of Clinical Medicine* 7, no. 12 (2018): 496, https://doi.org/10.3390/jcm7120496.

41. Jernej Mlakar, Misa Korva, Nataša Tul, et al., "Zika virus associated with microcephaly," *New England Journal of Medicine* 374 (2016): 951–58.

42. "Epidemiological update: Complications potentially linked to the Zika virus outbreak, Brazil and French Polynesia," European Centre for Disease Prevention and Control, November 26, 2015, https://www.ecdc.europa.eu/en/news-events/epidemiological-update-complications -potentially-linked-zika-virus-outbreak-brazil-and.

43. Abortion for a fetal indication is legal in French Polynesia, as it is in France.

44. Marcia Turcato, ed., *Zika Virus in Brazil: The SUS Response* (Brasilia: Ministry of Health of Brazil, Secretariat of Health Surveillance, 2017), 38, http://portalarquivos.saude.gov .br/images/pdf/2017/setembro/21/zika-virus-in-brazil-2017.pdf.

45. Pan American Health Organization, "Epidemiological alert: Increase in microcephaly in the northeast of Brazil," November 17, 2015, https://www.paho.org/hq/dmdocuments/2015 /2015-nov-17-cha-microcephaly-epi-alert.pdf.

46. Marcia Trufinol, "A new mosquito-borne threat to pregnant women in Brazil," *Lancet Infectious Diseases* 16, no. 2 (2016): 156–57.

47. Lavinia Schuler-Faccini, Erlane M. Ribeiro, Ian M. L. Feitosa, et al., "Possible asso- ciation between Zika virus infection and microcephaly, Brazil 2015," *Morbidity and Mortality Weekly Reports* 65, no. 3 (2016): 59–62.

48. Team Reduas, "Report from physicians in the Crop-Sprayed Villages regarding Dengue-Zika, microcephaly, and mass-spraying with chemical poisons," February 6, 2016, http://reduas.com.ar/report-from-physicians-in-the-crop-sprayed-town-regarding-dengue -zika-microcephaly-and-massive-spraying-with-chemical-poisons/.

49. ABRASCO, "Nota técnica sobre microcefalia e doenças vetoriais relacionadas ao Aedes aegypti: Os perigos das abordagens com larvicidas e nebulizações químicas—fumacê," February 2, 2016, https://www.abrasco.org.br/site/noticias/institucional/nota-tecnica-sobre -microcefalia-e-doencas-vetoriais-relacionadas-ao-aedes-aegypti-os-perigos-das-abordagens -com-larvicidas-e-nebulizacoes-quimicas-fumace/15929/.

50. Comissão de Epidemiologia da Abrasco, "Zika virus: Challenges of public health in Brazil," *Revista Brasileira de Epidemiologia* 19, no. 2 (2016): 225–28, https://doiorg/10.1590/1980 -5497201600020001.

51. Thália Velho Barreto de Araújo, Ricardo Arraes de Alencar Ximenes, Demócrito de Barros Miranda-Filho, et al., "Association between microcephaly, Zika virus infection, and other risk factors in Brazil: Final report of a case-control study," *Lancet Infectious Diseases* 18, no. 3 (2018): 328–36.

52. Raphael Parens, Frederik Nijhout, Alfredo Morales, et al., "A possible link between pyriproxyfen and microcephaly," *PLOS Current Outbreaks* 9 (November 2017), https://doi .org/10.1371/currents.outbreaks.5afb0bfb8cf31d9a4baba7b19b4edbac.

53. Jorge Lopez-Camelo and Iêda Maria Orioli, eds., "ECLAMC, Final document," De- cember 30, 2015, http://www.eclamc.org/descargas/6.DocumentoECLAMCFinalV3.docx.

54. Eduardo Castilla and Iêda Orioli, "ECLAMC: The Latin-America Collaborative Study of Congenital Malformations," *Community Genetics* 7 (2004): 76–94.

55. Declan Butler, "Microcephaly surge in doubt," *Nature* 530 (February 3, 2016): 14–15; Cesar Gomes Victora, Lavinia Schuler-Faccini, Alicia Matijasevich, et al., "Microcephaly in Brazil: How to interpret reported numbers?," *Lancet* 387 (2016): 621–24.

56. Michel de Pracontal, "Adriana Melo: Zika provoque 'quelque chose de jamais vu,'" *Mediapart*, February 16, 2016.

57. See, e.g., Fernando Antônio Ramos Guerra, Juan Clinton Llerena Jr., et al., "Confiabili- dade das informações das declarações de nascido vivo com registro de defeitos congênitos no Município do Rio de Janeiro, Brasil, 2004," *Cadernos de Saúde Pública* 24, no. 2 (2008): 438–46; and Schuler-Faccini, Ribeiro, Feitosa, et al., "Possible association between Zika virus infection and microcephaly."

58. Zilton Farias Meira de Vasconcelos, Renata Campos Azevedo, Nathália Thompson, et al., "Challenges for molecular and serological ZIKV infection confirmation," *Child's Nervous System* 34, no. 1 (2018): 79–84.

59. Mariana Kikuti, Cristiane Cardoso, Ana Prates, et al., "Congenital brain abnormalities during a Zika virus epidemic in Salvador, Brazil, April 2015 to July 2016," *Eurosurveillance* 23, no. 45 (November 8, 2018), https://www.ncbi.nlm.nih.gov/pmc/articles/PMC6234531/.

60. Cristina Possas, Partricia Brasil, Mauro Marzochi, et al., "Zika puzzle in Brazil: Peculiar conditions of viral introduction and dissemination—A review," *Memorias do Instituto Oswaldo Cruz, Rio de Janeiro* 112, no. 5 (2017): 319–27.

61. Secretaria de Vigilância em Saúde, Ministério da Saúde, "Monitoramento integrado de alterações no crescimento e desenvolvimento relacionadas à infecção pelo vírus Zika e outrasetiologias infecciosas, até a Semana Epidemiológica 30 de 2018," *Boletim Epidemiológico* 49, no. 39 (2018), https://repositorio.observatoriodocuidado.org/bitstream/handle/handle/1671/2018-047.pdf?sequence=1&isAllowed=y.

62. Simon Romero, "After living Brazil's dream, family confronts microcephaly and economic crisis," *New York Times*, March 6, 2016.

Chapter 4 · *Zika in Brazil*

1. See, e.g., David M. Morens and Antony S. Fauci, "Pandemic Zika: A formidable challenge to medicine and public health," *Journal of Infectious Diseases* 216, suppl. 10 (2017): S857–S859.

2. Donald McNeil Jr., *Zika: The Emerging Epidemic* (New York: Norton, 2016).

3. Donald McNeil Jr., "How the response to Zika failed millions," *New York Times*, January 16, 2017.

4. Declan Butler, "Microcephaly surge in doubt," *Nature* 530 (February 3, 2016): 14–15; Daniel Lucey, "Editorial: Time for global action on Zika virus epidemic," *British Medical Journal* 352 (2016): 781. *Microcephaly epidemic* was shorthand for a cluster of anomalies of the fetus and the newborn.

5. Isaac Bogoh, Oliver Brady, Moritz Kraemer, et al., "Anticipating the international spread of Zika virus from Brazil," *Lancet* 377 (2016): 335–36.

6. David Heyman, Abraham Hodgson, Amadou Alpha Sall, et al., "Zika virus and microcephaly: Why is this situation a PHEIC?," *Lancet* 387 (2016): 719–21.

7. Heyman, Hodgson, Sall, et al., "Zika virus and microcephaly."

8. Steven Hatch, *Inferno: A Doctor's Ebola Story* (New York: St. Martin's Press, 2017).

9. Secretaria de Vigilância em Saúde, Ministério da Saúde, "Monitoramento integrado de alterações no crescimento e desenvolvimento relacionadas à infecção pelo vírus Zika e outras etiologias infecciosas, até a Semana Epidemiológica 28/2017," *Boletim Epidemiológico* 48, no. 24 (2017), https://www.gov.br/saude/pt-br/assuntos/boletins-epidemiologicos/por-assunto.

10. Patricia Brasil, Jose Pereira, Claudia Raja Gabaglia, et al., "Zika virus infection in pregnant women in Rio de Janeiro: Preliminary report," *New England Journal of Medicine* 375, no. 24 (2016): 2321–34.

11. Rivaldo Venâncio da Cunha, "Ao que tudo indica, problema do zika está só começando; temos muita dor pela frente," *Agencia Fiocruz de Noticias* (blog), Centro des Estudos Estratégicos da Fiocruz, February 26, 2016, https://cee.fiocruz.br/?q=node/116.

12. Anthony Fauci and David Morens, "Zika virus in the Americas—yet another arbovirus threat," *New England Journal of Medicine* 374, no. 7 (2016): 601–4.

13. Maria Teixeira, Maria da Conceição Costa, Wanderson de Oliveira, et al., "The epidemic of Zika virus–related microcephaly in Brazil: Detection, control, etiology, and future scenarios," *American Journal of Public Health* 106, no. 4 (2016): 601–5.

14. Gretchen Vogel, "Experts fear Zika's effects may be even worse than thought," *Science* 352 (2016): 1375–76.

15. Adriana Oliveira-Melo, Gustavo Malinger, Renato Ximenes, et al., "Zika virus intra-uterine infection causes fetal brain abnormality and microcephaly: Tip of the iceberg?," *Ultrasound in Obstetrics and Gynecology* 47 (2016): 6–7.

16. Sarah Boseley, "On the frontline of Brazil's war on Zika," *Guardian*, April 12, 2016.

17. Enny Paixao and Laura Rodrigues, "Editorial: What we need to know about Zika virus," *British Journal of Hospital Medicine* 77, no. 3 (2016): 124–25.

18. Maria de Fatima Pessoa Militão de Albuquerque, Wayner Vieira de Souza, Thália Velho Barreto Araújo, et al., "The microcephaly epidemic and Zika virus: Building knowledge in epidemiology, "*Cadernos de Saúde Pública* 34, no. 10 (2018): e00069018.

19. Cristina Possas, Patricia Brasil, Mauro Marzochi, et al., "Zika puzzle in Brazil: Peculiar conditions of viral introduction and dissemination—A review, "*Memorias de Instituto Oswaldo Cruz, Rio de Janeiro* 112, no. 5 (2017): 319–27.

20. Carlos Brito, "Zika virus: A new chapter in the history of medicine," *Acta Medicina Portuguesa* 28, no. 6 (2015): 679–80.

21. Debora Diniz, *Zika: De sertão nordestino á ameaça global* (Rio de Janeiro: Editora de Civilização Brasileira, 2016), translated into English by Diane Grosklaus Whitty as *Zika: From the Brazilian Backlands to Global Threat* (Chicago: University of Chicago Press, 2017).

22. Declan Butler, "Brazil's birth defects puzzle," *Nature* 435 (July 28, 2016): 475–76.

23. Claudia Collucci, "Brazil to investigate if other factors act with Zika to cause congenital defects," *British Medical Journal* 354 (2016): 4439.

24. Collucci, "Brazil to investigate if other factors act"; Marilia Sá Carvalho, Laís Freitas, Oswaldo Gonçalves Cruz, et al., "Association of past dengue fever epidemics with the risk of Zika microcephaly at the population level in Brazil," *Scientific Reports* 10 (2020): 1752, https://doi.org/10.1038/s41598-020-58407-7; Stephanie Petzold, Nisreen Agbaria, Andreas Deckert, et al., "Congenital abnormalities associated with Zika virus infection—Dengue as potential co-factor? A systematic review," *PLOS Neglected Diseases* 15, no. 1 (2020): e0008984, https://doi.org/10.1371/journal.pntd.0008984.

25. Dom Phillips and Nick Miroff, "Scientists are bewildered by Zika's path across Latin America," *Washington Post*, October 26, 2016.

26. On the difficulty of distinguishing between Zika, chikungunya, and dengue see, e.g., Juliane Oliveira Moreno Rodrigues, Lacita M. Skalinski, Aline Santos, et al., "Interdependence between confirmed and discarded cases of dengue, chikungunya and Zika viruses in Brazil: A multivariate time series analysis," *PLOS One* 5, no. 2 (2020): e0228347, https://doi.org/10.1371/journal.pone.0228347.

27. Wanderson Kleber de Oliveira, Claudio Henriques, Giovanini Coelho, et al., "Zika virus infection and associated neurologic disorders in Brazil," *New England Journal of Medicine* 376 (2017): 1591–93.

28. Marcia Turcato, ed., *Zika Virus in Brazil: The SUS Response* (Brasilia: Ministry of Health of Brazil, Health Surveillance Department, 2017), 6, http://portalarquivos.saude.gov.br/images/pdf/2017/setembro/21/zika-virus-in-brazil-2017.pdf.

29. Duschinka Guedes, Marcelo Paiva, Mariana Donato, et al., "Zika virus replication in the mosquito *Culex quinquefasciatus*," *Emerging Microbes & Infections* 6, no. 8 (August 9, 2017): e69, https://doi.org/10.1038/emi.2017.59.

30. Ricardo Lourenço-de-Oliveira and Anna-Bella Failoux, "Lessons learned on Zika virus vectors," *PLOS Neglected Tropical Diseases* 11, no. 6 (June 15, 2017): e0005511:2546.

31. Jayme Souza-Neto, Jeffrey Powell, and Mariangela Bonizzoni, "*Aedes aegypti* vector competence studies: A review," *Infection, Genetics and Evolution* 67 (2019): 191–207; Tereza

Magalhaes, Karlos Diogo Chalegre, Cynthia Braga, and Brian Foy, "The endless challenges of arboviral diseases in Brazil," *Tropical Medicine and Infectious Diseases* 5 (2020): 75, https://doi .org/10.3390/tropicalmed5020075.

32. Brian Foy, Kevin Kobylinski, Joy Chilson, et al., "Probable non-vector-borne transmission of Zika virus, Colorado, USA," *Emerging Infectious Diseases* 17, no. 5 (2011): 880–82; Didier Musso, Claudine Roche, Emilie Robin, et al., "Potential sexual transmission of Zika virus," *Emerging Infectious Diseases* 21, no. 2 (2015): 259–61.

33. See, e.g., Luisa Reis Castro and Carolina Nogeira, "Who should be concerned? Zika as an epidemic about mosquitoes and women (and some reflections on COVID-19)," Somatosphere, April 6, 2020, http://somatosphere.net/2020/zika-epidemic-mosquitos-women.html/. I was concerned about the low visibility of sexual transmission of Zika in Brazil and I discussed the risk of sexual propagation of Zika in several setting, e.g., at a public conference at Fiocruz in April 2017. https://www.youtube.com/watch?v=62wbnZWEDus. At that time, however, the Zika outbreak was already on the wane.

34. Inda Clancy, Robert Jones, Grace Power, et al., "Public health messages on arboviruses transmitted by *Aedes aegypti* in Brazil," *BMC Public Health* 21 (2021): 1362, https://doi.org /10.1186/s12889-021-11339. Only one poster among 37 analyzed mentioned that Zika could be transmitted through sexual contact. Human Rights Watch, *Neglected and Unprotected: The Impact of the Zika Outbreak on Women and Girls in Northeastern Brazil*, 2017, https:// www.hrw.org/report/2017/07/13/neglected-and-unprotected/impact-zika-outbreak-women -and-girls-northeastern, 67, 89.

35. Debora Diniz, Ali Moazzam, Ilana Ambrogi, and Luciana Brito, "Understanding sexual and reproductive health needs of young women living in Zika affected regions: A qualitative study in northeastern Brazil," *Reproductive Health* 17 (2020): 22, https://doi.org /10.1186/s12978-020-0869-4; Elizabeth Anderson, Kacey Ernst, Francisco Fernando Martins, et al., "Women's health perceptions and beliefs related to Zika virus exposure during the 2016 outbreak in northern Brazil," *American. Journal of Tropical Medicine and Hygiene* 102, no. 3 (2020): 629–33; Letícia Marteleto, Abigail Weitzman, Raquel Zanata Coutinho, and Sandra Valongueiro Alvez, "Women's reproductive intentions and behaviors during the Zika epidemic in Brazil," *Population and Development Review* 43, no. 2 (2017): 199–227.

36. Evaristo Medina-Cucurella, Jorge Acevedo-Canabal, Jeidiel De León-Arbucias, et al., "Zika-prevention knowledge among Hispanic women living in Puerto Rico: A cross-sectional study," in "Special issue on Zika," *Puerto Rico Health Sciences Journal* 37 (2018): S51–S56.

37. Amy Nunn, *The Politics and History of AIDS Treatment in Brazil* (New York: Springer, 2009).

38. Monica Malta, "Human rights and political crisis in Brazil: Public health impacts and challenges," *Global Public Health* 13, no. 11 (2018): 1577–84; Marcos Cueto and Gabriel Lopes, "Backlash in global health and the end of AIDS' exceptionalism in Brazil, 2007–2019," *Global Public Health* 17, no. 2 (2022): 815–22.

39. In her study of cervical cancer in Brazil, *Virtually Virgins: Sexual Strategies and Cervical Cancer in Recife, Brazil* (Stanford: Stanford University Press, 2003), Jessica Gregg observed an exclusive focus on women's sexuality no mention of men's role in infecting their partners with the human papillomavirus (HPV).

40. Flavio Codeco Coelho, Betina Durovni, Valeria Saraceni, et al., "Higher incidence of Zika in adult women than adult men in Rio de Janeiro suggests a significant contribution of sexual transmission from men to women," *Journal of Infectious Diseases* 51 (2016): 128–32.

41. Beatriz Macedo Coimbra dos Santos, Flavio Codeço Coelho, and Margaret Armstrong, "Zika: An ongoing threat to women and infants," *Cadernos de Saúde Pública* 34, no. 11 (2018): e00038218.

42. Juan Aguilar Ticona, Huma Baig, Nivison Nery, et al., "Risk of sexually transmitted

Zika virus in a cohort of economically disadvantaged urban residents," *Journal of Infectious Diseases* 224, no. 5 (2021): 860–64.

43. Eli Rosenberg, Kate Doyle, Jorge Munoz-Jordan, et al., "Prevalence and incidence of Zika virus infection among household contacts of patients with Zika virus disease, Puerto Rico, 2016–2017," *Journal of Infectious Diseases* 220 (2019): 932–39.

44. Tereza Magalhaes, Clarice Morais, Iracema Jacques, et al., "Follow-up household serosurvey in northeast Brazil for Zika virus: Sexual contacts of index patients have the highest risk for seropositivity," *Journal of Infectious Diseases* 223, no. 4 (2021): 673–85.

45. Magalhaes, Morais, Jacques, et al., "Follow-up household serosurvey in northeast Brazil," 680.

46. Taís da Cruz, Raquel Souza, Sandra Pelloso, et al., "Case report: Prolonged detection of Zika virus RNA in vaginal and endocervical samples from a Brazilian woman, 2018," *American Journal of Tropical Medicine and Hygiene* 100, no. 1 (2018): 183–86; Fabrício Morelli, Raquel Pantarotto Souza, Taís Elisângela da Cruz, et al., "Zika virus infection in the genital tract of non-pregnant females: A systematic review," *Journal of the São Paolo Institute of Tropical Medicine* 62 (2019), http://doi.org/10.1590/S1678-9946202062016; Raquel das Neves Almeida, Heloisa Antoniella Braz-de-Melo, Igor de Oliveira Santos, et al., "The cellular impact of the ZIKA virus on male reproductive tract immunology and physiology," *Cells* 9 (2020): 1006, https://doi.org/10.3390/cells9041006.

47. Andrew Haddow, Aysegul Nalca, Franco D. Rossi, et al., "High infection rates for adult macaques after intravaginal or intrarectal inoculation with Zika virus," *Emerging Infectious Diseases* 23, no. 8 (2017): 1274–81; Nisha Duggal, Erin McDonald, Jana Ritter, and Aaron Brault, "Sexual transmission of Zika virus enhances in utero transmission in a mouse model," *Scientific Reports* 8 (2018): 4510, https://doi.org/10.1038/s41598-018-22840-6.

48. Brasil, Pereira, Raja Gabaglia, et al., "Zika virus infection in pregnant women."

49. Keila Guimaraes, "The real infectious disease problem in Brazil isn't actually Zika, it's syphilis," *Quartz*, August 22, 2016, https://qz.com/763105/brazil-zika-syphilis-infant-mortality/.

50. *Boletim Epidemiológico Sífilis*, 2019, fig. 1, p. 13, http://www.aids.gov.br/pt-br/pub/2019/boletim-epidemiologico-sifilis-2019. Data on stillbirths and inborn anomalies attributed to syphilis recorded in the Brazilian Live Birth Information System, SINASC, are not considered very reliable.

51. *Boletim Epidemiológico Sífilis*, 2020, http://www.aids.gov.br/pt-br/pub/2020/boletim-sifilis-2020.

52. Cristiane Bomfim, "Por que os casos de sífilis não param de crescer no Brasil," *Veja*, November 8, 2019; Carlos Brito, "Brasil tem 18 casos de sífilis por hora, diz Ministério da Saúde," *Veja*, February 8, 2020; Jacielma de Oliveira Freire, Jaqueline Bohrer Schuch, Mariana Freire de Miranda, et al., "Prevalência de HIV, sífilis, hepatites B e C em gestantes de uma maternidade de Salvador," *Revista Brasileira de Saúde Materna e Infantil* (Recife) 21, no. 3 (2021): 955–63.

53. Cristiana Bastos, "From global to local and back to global: The articulation of politics, knowledge and assistance in Brazilian responses to AIDS," in *The Politics of AIDS: Globalization, the State and Civil Society*, ed. M. J. Follér and H. Thörn (London: Palgrave Macmillan, 2008), 225–54.

54. ABIA (Brazilian Interdisciplinary AIDS Association), "Understanding of the dismantlement of the AIDS response in Brazil," *Sexual Policy Watch*, May 27, 2019, https://sxpolitics.org/understanding-the-dismantling-of-the-aids-response-in-brazil/19855; Marcos Cueto and Gabriel Lopes, "AIDS, antiretrovirals and the international politics of global health, 1996–2008," *Social History of Medicine* 34, no. 1 (2021): 1–22; Cueto and Lopes, "Backlash in global health."

55. Adele Schwartz Benzaken, Gerson Fernando Mendes Pereira, Alessandro Ricardo, et al., "Adequacy of prenatal care, diagnosis and treatment of syphilis in pregnancy: A study with open data from Brazilian state capitals," *Cadernos de Saúde Pública* 36, no. 1 (2020): e00057219.

56. See, e.g., Rafael Garcia Torres, Ana Laura Neves Mendonça, Grazielle Cezarine Montes, et al., "Syphilis in pregnancy: The reality in a public hospital," *Revista Brasileira de Ginecologia e Obstetrícia* 41 (2019): 90–96; Samara Isabela Maia de Oliveira, Cecília Olívia Paraguai de Oliveira Saraiva, Débora Feitosa de França, et al., "Syphilis notifications and the triggering processes or vertical transmission: A cross-sectional study," *International Journal of Environmental Research in Public Health* 17 (2020): 984, https://doi.org/10.3390/ijerph17030984; and Carmen Lucia Muricy and Vitor Laerte Pinto Júnior, "Congenital and maternal syphilis in the capital of Brazil," *Revista da Sociedade Brasileira de Medicina Tropical* 48, no. 2 (2015): 216–19.

57. Anita Rita Paulo Cardoso, Maria Alix Leite Arauajo, Roumayne Fernandes, et al., "Underreporting of congenital syphilis as a cause of fetal and infant deaths in northeastern Brazil," *PLOS One* 11, no. 12 (2016): e0167255; Marquiony Marques dos Santos, Ana Karla Bezerra Lopes, Angelo Giuseppe Roncalli, and Kenio Costa de Lima, "Trends of syphilis in Brazil: A growth portrait of the treponemic epidemic," *PLOS One* 15, no. 4 (2020): e0231029.

58. Ana Paula Lopes de Melo, Tereza Lyra, Thália Velho Barreto de Araújo, et al., " 'Life is taking me where I need to go': Biographical disruption and new arrangements in the lives of female family carers of children with congenital Zika syndrome in Pernambuco, Brazil," *Viruses* 12, no. 12 (2020): 1410, https://doi.org/10.3390/v12121410.

59. Mark Seidner, Edward Ryan, and Isaac Bogach, "Gone or forgotten? The rise and fall of Zika virus," *Lancet Public Health* 3, no. 3 (2018): e109–e110.

60. Charles Rosenberg, "The tyranny of diagnosis: Specific entities and individual experience," *Milbank Quarterly* 80, no. 2 (2002): 245.

61. Pedro Vasconcelos, interview by Ana Lucia Azevedo, " 'Estamos com os pés e mãos atados,' diz médico sobre zika," *O Globo*, December 5, 2015.

62. Koichi Kameda, "Testing the Nation: Healthcare Policy and Innovation in Diagnostics for Infectious Diseases in Brazil" (PhD thesis, École des Hautes Études en Sciences Sociales, Paris, 2019).

63. Kameda, "Testing the Nation."

64. Alvina Clara Felix, Nathalia Santiago Sousa, Walter Figueiro, et al., "Cross reactivity of commercial anti-dengue immunoassays in patients with acute Zika virus infection," *Journal of Medical Virology* 89, no. 8 (2017):1477–79; Mariana Kikuti, Laura Tauro, Patrícia Moreira, et al., "Diagnostic performance of commercial IgM and IgG enzyme-linked immunoassays (ELISAs) for diagnosis of Zika virus infection," *Virology Journal* 15, no. 1 (2018): 108, https://doi.org/10.1186/s12985-018-1015-1016.

65. Kameda, "Testing the Nation."

66. Zilton Farias Meira de Vasconcelos, Renata Campos Azevedo, Nathália Thompson, et al., "Challenges for molecular and serological ZIKV infection confirmation," *Child's Nervous System* 34, no. 1 (2018): 79–84; Mirna Burciaga-Flores, Marissa Reyes-Galeana, Tanya Camacho-Villegas, et al., "Updating Zika diagnostic methods: The point-of-care approach," *Revista de Investigación Clínica* 76, no. 6 (2020): 344–52.

67. Vivian Iida Avelino-Silva, "Zika: The grim reality from a clinical researcher perspective" (paper presented at the International Symposium on Zika Virus Research, Marseille, June 4–6, 2018). Avelino-Silva discussed, among other things, the case of a pregnant woman who suspected she might have contracted Zika early in pregnancy and considered the possibility of an abortion.

68. Possas, Brasil, Marzochi, et al., "Zika puzzle in Brazil."

69. Wanderson Kleber Oliveira, Giovanny Vinícius Araújo de França, Eduardo Hage Carmo, et al., "Infection-related microcephaly after the 2015 and 2016 Zika virus outbreaks in Brazil: A surveillance-based analysis," *Lancet* 26, no. 390 (2017): 861–70; Oliver Brady, Aaron Osgood-Zimmerman, Nicholas Kassebaum, et al., "The association between Zika virus infection and microcephaly in Brazil, 2015–2017: An observational analysis of over 4 million births," *PLOS Medicine* 16, no. 3 2019): e1002755, https://doi.org/10.1371/journal.pmed.1002755.

70. Marion Koopmans, Xavier de Lamballerie, and Thomas Jaenisch, on behalf of ZIKAlliance Consortium, "Familiar barriers still unresolved—a perspective on the Zika virus outbreak research response," *Lancet Infectious Diseases* 19, no. 2 (2019): e59–e62, https://doi .org/10.1016/S1473-3099(18)30497-3.

71. Elisabeth Lopes Moreira, Karin Nielsen-Saines, Patricia Brasil, et al., "Neurodevelopment in infants exposed to Zika virus in utero," *New England Journal of Medicine* 379, no. 24 (2018): 2377–79.

72. Giovanny Vinícius Araújo de França, Vaneide Daciane Pedi, Márcio Henrique de Oliveira Garcia, et al., "Congenital syndrome associated with Zika virus infection among live births in Brazil: A description of the distribution of reported and confirmed cases in 2015–2016," *Epidemiologia e Serviços de Saúde* 27, no. 2 (2018): e2017473.

73. "Monitoramento integrado de alterações no crescimento e desenvolvimento relacionadas à infecção pelo vírus Zika e outras etiologias infecciosas, até a Semana Epidemiológica 30 de 2018," *Boletim Epidemiológico* 49, no. 39 (2018), https://repositorio.observatoriodocuidado .org/bitstream/handle/handle/1671/2018-047.pdf?sequence=1&isAllowed=y.

74. Ludwik Fleck, "On the crisis of 'reality,'" in *Cognition and Fact: Materials on Ludwik Fleck*, ed. Robert Cohen and Thomas Schnelle (1929; reprint, Dordrecht: Reidel, 1986), 59–78.

75. On the disastrous effect of the political and economic crisis on public health in Brazil at the time of Zika outbreak, see, e.g., Malta, "Human rights and political crisis in Brazil."

76. "Monitoramento integrado de alterações no crescimento e desenvolvimento relacionadas à infecção pelo vírus Zika e outras etiologias infecciosas, até a Semana Epidemiológica 30 de 2018."

77. Iêda Orioli, Helen Dolk, Jorge S. Lopez-Camelo, et al., "Prevalence and clinical profile of microcephaly in South America pre-Zika, 2005–14: Prevalence and case-control study," *British Medical Journal* 359 (November 21, 2017): j5018, https://doi.org/10.1136/bmj.j5018.

78. Antonio Silva, Marco A. Barbieri, Maria T. Alves, et al., "Prevalence and risk factors for microcephaly at birth in Brazil in 2010," *Pediatrics* 141, no. 2 (2018): e20170589. The authors of this study collected their data independently. The SINASC registry of inborn anomalies, they stressed, was often unreliable.

79. The proportion of "discarded" children was higher in the poor state of Alagoas than in the more affluent state of Bahia. ANIS, "Zika in Brazil: Women and children at the center of the epidemic," 2017, http://anis.org.br/wp-content/uploads/2017/06/Zika-in-Brazil_Anis _2017.pdf.

80. Charles Rosenberg, "Explaining epidemics," in *Explaining Epidemics, and Other Studies in the History of Medicine* (Cambridge: Cambridge University Press, 1992), 293–304.

81. Butler, "Brazil's birth defects puzzle."

Chapter 5 · Stratified Reproduction

1. Barbara Ribeiro, Sarah Hartley, Brigitte Nerlich, and Rusi Jaspal, "Media coverage of the Zika crisis in Brazil: The construction of a 'war' frame that masked social and gender inequalities," *Social Science and Medicine* 200 (2018): 137–44; Gustavo Corrêa Matta, Carolina de Oliveira Nogueira, and Lenir da Silva Nascimento, "A literary history of Zika: Following Brazilian state responses through documents of emergency," in *Zika Frontiers: Social Change and Governance in the Age of Mosquito Pandemics*, ed. Kevin Bardosh (London: Routledge,

2020); Clare Wenham, *Feminist Global Health Security* (Oxford: Oxford University Press, 2021).

2. This was the case in the first documented sexual transmission of Zika. Brian Foy, Kevin Kobylinski, Joy Chilson, et al., "Probable non-vector-borne transmission of Zika virus, Colorado, USA," *Emerging Infectious Diseases* 17, no. 5 (2011): 880–82.

3. Deisy Ventura, Danielle Rached, Jameson Martins, et al., "A rights-based approach to public health emergencies: The case of the 'More Rights, Less Zika' campaign in Brazil," *Global Public Health* 16, no. 10 (2021): 1–14.

4. I thank the UNFPA for permission to reproduce the song's lyrics. English translation quoted in Ventura, Rached, Martins, et al., "Rights-based approach to public health emergencies."

5. Germana Soares, cofounder and president of the association of mothers of children with CZS, the União de Mães de Anjos (UMA), called the fathers' desertion of impaired children "male abortion." Silvana Sobreira de Matosa, Luciana Campelo de Lira, and Fernanda Meira, "Deficiência, ativismo, gênero e cuidado na síndrome congênita do Zika vírus: Entrevista com Germana Soares," *Revista Antropológicas* 29, no. 2 (2018): 142–53.

6. Some researchers question the claim that susceptibility to diseases spread by mosquitoes, such as dengue fever, is associated with social status. Kate Mulligan, Jenna Dixon, Chi-Ling Joanna Sinn, and Susan J. Elliott, "Is dengue a disease of poverty? A systematic review," *Pathogens and Global Health* 109, no. 1 (2015): 10–18.

7. Finn Diderichsen, Lia Giraldo da Silva Augusto, and Bernadete Perez, "Understanding social inequalities in Zika infection and its consequences: A model of pathways and policy entry-points," *Global Public Health* 14, no. 5 (2019): 675–83.

8. Partial data published in 2016 indicate that 63.5% of the pregnant women diagnosed with Zika during the 2015–16 epidemic were either Black or Brown (*parda*). "Zika vírus: Perfil epidemiológico em mulheres," *Boletim Epidemiológico* 47, no. 37 (2016), http://combateaedes .saude.gov.br/images/pdf/Virus_Zika_perfil_epidemiologico_em_mulheres.pdf.

9. Marcia Trufinol, "A new mosquito-borne threat to pregnant women in Brazil," *Lancet Infectious Diseases* 16, no. 2 (2016): 156–57.

10. Camila Pimentel, Ana Paula Lopes de Melo, Sandra Valongueiro Alves, et al., "Zika in everyday life: Gender, motherhood and reproductive rights in Pernambuco State, northeast Brazil," in Bardosh, *Zika Frontiers*, 83.

11. BBC Brazil, "Como vive a 1ª geração de bebês com microcefalia por zika," December 12, 2018, https://www.youtube.com/watch?v=1nbe8kTLCP8&t=121s.

12. Wayner Vieira de Souza, Maria de Fatima Pessoa Militao de Albuquerque, Enrique Vaquez, et al., "Microcephaly epidemic related to the Zika virus and living conditions in Recife, northeast Brazil," *BMC Public Health* 18, no. 1 (2018): 130, https://doi.org/10.1186 /s12889-018-5039-z; Jimena Barbeito-Andrés, Lavinia Schuler-Faccini, and Patricia Pestana Garcez, "Why is congenital Zika syndrome asymmetrically distributed among human populations?," *PLOS Biology* 18, no. 8 (2018): https://doi.org/10.1371/journal.pbio.2006592.

13. De Souza, de Albuquerque, Vaquez, et al., "Microcephaly epidemic related to the Zika virus." It is reasonable to assume that when the Brazilian government announced that Zika was linked with inborn anomalies, some women from more affluent parts of Recife were already pregnant. The reportedly few children born with CZS in these parts of the city after November 2015 may have been partly the result of selective abortion.

14. Luísa Reis-Castro and Carolina de Oliveira Nogueira, "Uma antropologia da transmissão: Mosquitos, mulheres e a epidemia de Zika no Brasil," *Ilha* 22, no. 2 (2020): 21–63.

15. V. A. Dantas Melo, J. R. Santos Silva, and R. La Corte, "Use of mosquito repellents to protect against Zika virus infection among pregnant women in Brazil," *Public Health* 171 (2019): 89–96.

16. Helena Prado, "Ce que l'épidémie du virus Zika dévoile des droits reproductifs et sexuels au Brésil," *Cahiers des Ameriques Latines* 88–89 (2018): 90.

17. Eduardo Gómez, Fernanda Aguilar Perez, and Deisy Ventura, "What explains the lacklustre response to Zika in Brazil? Exploring institutional, economic and health system context," *BMJ Global Health* 3, no. 5 (2018): e000862, https://doi.org/10.1136/bmjgh-2018 -000862.

18. Talk by the pioneer of Zika studies, Claudio Maierovitch, at the ABRASCO meeting, December 7, 2019, "A epidemia zika e o devir nas emergências sanitárias," https://www.you tube.com/watch?v=1-eSfQJ8bnI.

19. Jeffrey Lesser and Uriel Kitron, "The social geography of Zika in Brazil," *NACLA Report on the Americas* 48, no. 2 (2016): 123–29.

20. Paulo Andrade Lotufo, "Zika epidemic and social inequalities: Brazil and its fate," *São Paulo Medical Journal* 134, no. 2 (2016): 95–96.

21. Debora Diniz and Ilana Ambrogi, "Research ethics and the Zika legacy in Brazil," *Developing World Bioethics* 17, no. 3 (2017): 142–43; Elizabeth Anderson, Kacey Ernst, Francisco Fernando Martins, et al., "Women's health perceptions and beliefs related to Zika virus exposure during the 2016 outbreak in northern Brazil," *American Journal of Tropical Medicine and Hygiene* 102, no. 3 (2020): 629–33.

22. Morgana Martins Krieger, Clare Wenham, Denise Nacif Pimenta, et al., "How do community health workers institutionalise: An analysis of Brazil's CHW programme," *Global Public Health* 8 (2021): 1507–24. The popular name of the *agentes de combate de endemias* was, and sometimes still is, "mosquito killers" (*mata mosquitos*).

23. Alfonsina Faya Robles, "Las agentes comunitarias de salud en el Brasil contemporaneo: La 'policia amiga' de las madres pobres," *Sexualidade Salud e Sociedade* 12 (2012): 92–126; João Nunes, "The everyday political economy of health: Community health workers and the response to the 2015 Zika outbreak in Brazil," *Review of International Political Economy* 27, no. 1 (2019): 146–66. See also Alex Nading, "'Love isn't there in your stomach': A moral economy of medical citizenship among Nicaraguan community health workers," *Medical Anthropology Quarterly* 27, no. 1 (2013): 84–102.

24. Clare Wenham, João Nunes, Gustavo Correa Matta, et al., "Gender mainstreaming as a pathway for sustainable arbovirus control in Latin America," *PLOS Neglected Tropical Diseases* 14, no. 2 (2020): e0007954, https://doi.org/10.1371/journal.pntd.0007954.

25. André Novais Oliveira, dir., *Temporada* (film), 2018.

26. Faye Ginsburg and Rayna Rapp, eds., *Conceiving the New World Order: The Global Politics of Reproduction* (Berkeley: University of California Press, 1995).

27. See, e.g., Wenham, *Feminist Global Health Security*.

28. Declaration of minister Marcelo Castro, November 18, 2015, http://www1.folha.uol .com.br/cotidiano/2015/11/1707967-microcefalia-pode-atingir-outrosestados- se-elo-com -zika-for-confirmado.shtml., quoted in Prado, "Ce que l'épidémie du virus Zika dévoile," 82; Marcelo Castro, "'Sexo é para amador, gravidez é para professional,' diz ministro sobre microcefalia," *Extra* (Rio de Janeiro), November 18, 2015, quoted in Reis-Castro and de Oliveira Nogueira, "Uma antropologia da transmissão."

29. Ana Luiza Vilela Borges, Caroline Moreau, Anne Burket, et al., "Women's reproductive health knowledge, attitudes and practices in relation to the Zika virus outbreak in northeast Brazil," *PLOS One* 13, no. 1 (2018): e0190024, https://doi.org/10.1371/journal .pone.0190024; Ann H. Kelly, Javier Lezaun, Ilana Löwy, et al., "Uncertainty in times of medical emergency: Knowledge gaps and structural ignorance during the Brazilian Zika crisis," *Social Science and Medicine* 246 (2020): 112787, https://doi.org/10.1016/j.socscimed .2020.112787.

30. Raquel Zanatta Coutinho, Aida Villanueva Montalvo, Abigail Weitzman, and Letícia

Junqueira Marteleto, "Zika virus public health crisis and the perpetuation of gender inequality in Brazil," *Reproductive Health* 18 (2021), https://doi.org/10.1186/s12978-021-01067-1.

31. Debora Diniz, "Vírus Zika e mulheres," *Cadernos de Saúde Pública* 32 (2016): e00046316, https://www.scielo.br/j/csp/a/4wsWG3TkLXVMqNNTdW3JmcK/?format=pdf&lang=pt. According to the study "Nascer no Brasil," 55% of all pregnancies in Brazil, and 70% of pregnancies among teenaged girls, are unplanned. Maria de Carmo Leal, ed., *Nascer no Brasil: Inquérito nacional sobre parto e nascimento* (Rio de Janeiro: ENSP, Fiocruz, 2014).

32. Paige Baum, Anna Fiastro, Shane Kunselman, et al., "Ensuring a rights-based health sector response to women affected by Zika," *Cadernos de Saúde Pública* 32, no. 5 (2016): e00064416, http://doi.org/10.1590/0102-311X00064416; Human Rights Watch interviews with activists in Pernambuco, Paula Viana, Ediclea Santos, Maria Santiago, and Vera Barone, in Human Rights Watch, *Neglected and Unprotected: The Impact of the Zika Outbreak on Women and Girls in Northeastern Brazil*, 2017, https://www.hrw.org/report/2017/07/13/neglected-and-unprotected/impact-zika-outbreak-women-and-girls-northeastern, 53.

33. Human Rights Watch interviews with activists revealed the difficulties lower-class Brazilian women faced in trying to access reliable contraception during the Zika epidemic. Human Rights Watch, Neglected and Unprotected, 55–57, 63–64.

34. Fredi Alexander Diaz-Quijano, Daniele Maria Pelissari, and Alexandre Dias Porto Chiavegatto Filho, "Zika-associated microcephaly epidemic and birth rate reduction in Brazilian cities," *American Journal of Public Health* 108, no. 4 (2018): 514–16; Marcia Castro, Qiuyi Han, Lucas Carvalho, Cesar Victora, and Giovanny França, "Implications of Zika virus and congenital Zika syndrome for the number of live births in Brazil," *PNAS* 115, no. 24 (2018): 6177–82.

35. Debora Diniz, Marcelo Medeiros, and Alberto Madeiro, "Brazilian women avoiding pregnancy during Zika epidemic," *Journal of Family Planning and Reproductive Health Care* 43, no. 1 (2017): 80–81; Borges, Moreau, Burket, et al., "Women's reproductive health knowledge."

36. Susan Mayor, "Abortion requests increase in Latin America after Zika warning, figures show," *British Medical Journal* 353 (2016): 3492, https://doi.org/10.1136/bmj.i3492; Abigail Aiken, James Scott, Rebecca Gomperts, et al., "Requests for abortion in Latin America related to concern about Zika virus exposure," *New England Journal of Medicine* 375, no. 4 (2016): 396–98. Only a small fraction of Brazilian women who wish to terminate a pregnancy use Women on the Web services.

37. Rozeli Maria Porto and Patricia Rosalba Salvador Moura, "O corpo marcado: A construção do discurso midiático sobre Zika vírus e microcefalia," *Cadernos de Gênero e Diversidade* 3, no. 2 (2017): 158–91. Emilia Sanabria described the disparaging attitude of SUS doctors toward women seeking contraceptive advice. Emilia Sanabria, "From sub- to super-citizenship: Sex hormones and the body politic in Brazil," *Ethnos* 75, no. 4 (2010): 377–401.

38. Letícia Marteleto, Abigail Weitzman, Raquel Zanata Coutinho, and Sandra Valongueiro Alvez, "Women's reproductive intentions and behaviors during the Zika epidemic in Brazil," *Population and Development Review* 43, no. 2 (2017): 215. Women from Recife who participated in a focus group organized by Marteleto and her colleagues said that they would consider abortion for CZS, while according to Carneiro and Fleischer, the Recife women they interrogated did not see abortion for CZS as an option. Rosamaria Carneiro and Soraya Resende Fleischer, "'I never expected this, it was a big shock': Conception, pregnancy and birth in times of Zika through the eyes of women in Recife," *Interface* (Botucatu) 22, no. 66 (2018): 709–23. The reason for divergent reports on views of women interrogated in these two studies may be that Marteleto and her colleagues asked women about their intentions

in a hypothetical case of pregnancy with ZIKV infection, while Carneiro and Fleischer interviewed mothers of children with CZS.

39. Paula Freitas, Gabriella Soares, Helaine Mocelin, et al., "How do mothers feel? Life with children with congenital Zika syndrome," *International Journal of Gynecology and Obstetrics* 148, suppl. 2 (2020): 20–28. The quotations are from interviews with mothers of children with CZS in the state of Espírito Santo.

40. Layla Pedreira Caravalho, "Vírus Zika e direitos reprodutivos entre as políticas transnacionais, as nacionais e as ações locais," *Cadernos de Gênero e Diversidade* 3, no. 2 (2017): 134–57.

41. Marteleto, Weitzman, Coutinho, and Alvez, "Women's reproductive intentions and behaviors," 213–14.

42. Ventura, Rached, Martins, et al., "Rights-based approach to public health emergencies." On the role of the small but very active Recife-based feminist group Curumim see, e.g., Mara Régian, "Grupo Curumim de Recife faz campanha para conscientizar mulheres sobre Zika," *Radio EBC-Brasil*, May 2, 2016, https://radios.ebc.com.br/viva-maria/edicao/2016-05 /grupo-curumim-de-recife-faz-campanha-para-concientizar-mulheres-sobre-zika; and Shena Cavalho, "It's not just about a mosquito: Changing the conversation on Zika," *New Humanitarism*, October 27, 2016, https://www.newsdeeply.com/womenandgirls/community/2016/10/27 /not-just-mosquito-changing-conversation-zika.

43. Ventura, Rached, Martins, et al., "Rights-based approach to public health emergencies."

44. See, e.g., Régian, "Grupo Curumim de Recife faz campanha para conscientizar mulheres sobre Zika"; and Cavalho, "It's not just about a mosquito."

45. Shena Cavallo, "Brazil declares Zika crisis over, but is it?," International Women's Health Coalition, May 19, 2017, https://iwhc.org/2017/05/brazil-declares-zika-crisis/.

46. Julia Carneiro, "The Brazilian doctor who connected Zika to birth defects," *BBC Brazil*, March 10, 2016, https://www.bbc.com/news/world-latin-america-35763232.

47. Pan American Health Organization, *Zika Ethics Consultation: Ethics Guidance on Key Issues Raised by the Outbreak* (Washington, DC, 2016), 7. On the problematic position of international organizations on abortion rights see Florencia Luna, "Public health agencies' obligations and the case of Zika," *Bioethics* 31, no. 8 (2017): 575–81.

48. Human Rights Watch, *Neglected and Unprotected*, 71. Some women reported being tested for Zika in a SUS facility and then never receiving the results.

49. World Health Organization, "Pregnancy management in the context of Zika virus infection: Interim guidance update 13 May 2016," .https://apps.who.int/iris/bitstream/handle /10665/204520/WHO_ZIKV_MOC_16.2_eng.pdf?sequence=1; Olufemi Oladapo, João Paulo Souza, Bremen De Mucio, et al., "WHO interim guidance on pregnancy management in the context of Zika virus infection," *Lancet Infectious Diseases* 4 (August 2016): e510–e11, https:// www.thelancet.com/journals/langlo/article/PIIS2214-109X(16)30098-5/fulltext.

50. Ascom Cosems, Ministerio da Saude, "Saúde amplia acesso a diagnóstico e cuidado das gestantes e bebês," November 18, 2016, https://www.cosemsrn.org.br/noticia/saude-amplia -acesso-a-diagnostico-e-cuidado-das-gestantes-e-bebes/.

51. Interviews with Thereza de Lamar, Ministry of Health official, in Brasília, April 19, 2017; Eliane Germano, head of the Healthcare Department, Recife Secretariat of Health, April 6, 2017; and Leticia Katz, head of the Women's Healthcare Department, Pernambuco Secretariat of Health, Recife, October 21, 2016, quoted in Human Rights Watch, *Neglected and Unprotected*, 71.

52. Ana Paula Lopes de Melo, Tereza Lyra, Thália Velho Barreto de Araújo, et al., " 'Life is taking me where I need to go': Biographical disruption and new arrangements in the lives of

female family carers of children with congenital Zika syndrome in Pernambuco, Brazil" *Viruses* 12, no. 12 (2020): 1410, https://doi.org/10.3390/v12121410.

53. Vivian Avelino–Silva and Esper Kallas, "Untold stories of the Zika virus epidemic in Brazil," *Review of Medical Virology* 28, no. 6 (2018): e2000, https://doi.org/10.1002/rmv.2000. On the rise in internet searches for information about abortive drugs during the Zika epidemic see Alexandra Wollum, Sara Larrea, Caitlin Gerdts, and Kinga Jelinska, "Requests for medication abortion support in Brazil during and after the Zika epidemic," *Global Public Health* 16, no. 3 (2020): 366–77.

54. Marilia Sá Carvalho, ed., "Zika," special issue, *Cadernos de Saúde Pública* 32, no. 5 (2016), http://doi.org/10.1590/0102-311X00046316.

55. Drauzio Varella, "'Aborto já é livre no Brasil. Proibir é punir quem não tem dinheiro,' diz Drauzio Varella," interview by Ricardo Senra, *BBC Brazil*, February 2, 2016, https://www.bbc.com/portuguese/noticias/2016/02/160201_drauzio_aborto_rs.

56. Norman MacAlister Gregg, "Congenital cataract following German measles in the mother," *Transactions of the Ophthalmological Society of Australia* 3 (1941): 35–46. On the history of rubella epidemics and their role in the abortion debate see Leslie Reagan, *Dangerous Pregnancies: Mothers, Disabilities and Abortion in Modern America* (Berkeley: University of California Press, 2012).

57. D. P. Murphy, *Congenital Malformations: A Study of Parental Characteristics, with Specific Reference to the Reproductive Process*, 2nd ed. (Philadelphia: J. B. Lippincott, 1947), 106.

58. M. Sheridan, "Final report of a prospective study of children whose mothers had rubella in early pregnancy," *British Medical Journal* 2, no. 5408 (1964): 536–39; F. Neva, C. Alford, and T. Weller, "Emerging perspectives on rubella," *Bacteriological Review* 28, no. 4 (1964): 444–51.

59. Julia Bell, "On rubella in pregnancy," *British Medical Journal* 1, no. 5123 (1959): 686–88, quotation on 686.

60. Julia Bell, "Correspondance," *British Medical Journal* 1, no. 5132 (1959): 1302.

61. Bell "On rubella in pregnancy," 686.

62. Bevis Brock, "Rubella in pregnancy," *British Medical Journal* 1, no. 5129 (1959): 1117.

63. Ilana Löwy, "Zika and microcephaly: Can we learn from history?," *Physis—Revista de Saúde Coletiva* 26, no. 1 (2016), https://doi.org/10.1590/S0103-73312016000100002.

64. On the use of misoprostol as abortifacient in Brazil see Ilana Löwy and Marilena Correa, "The 'abortion pill' misoprostol in Brazil: Women's empowerment in a conservative and repressive political environment," *American Journal of Public Health* 110, no. 5 (2020): 677–84. On the widespread use of risky abortion methods by Brazilian women see, e.g., Debora Diniz, "Aborto no Brasil: Uma pesquisa domiciliar com técnica de urna," *Ciência e Saúde Coletiva* 15, suppl. 1 (2010): 2105–12. Diniz's survey was published in 2010, but more recent investigation did not indicate an amelioration of the conditions in which Brazilian women from the lower classes ended unwanted pregnancies.

65. Marteleto, Weitzman, Coutinho, and Alvez, "Women's reproductive intentions and behaviors," 218.

66. One Brazilian study at that time indicated that up to one-third of women infected with ZIKV might give birth to children with CZS. Patricia Brasil, Jose Pereira, Claudia Raja Gabaglia, et al., "Zika virus infection in pregnant women in Rio de Janeiro: Preliminary report," *New England Journal of Medicine* 375, no. 24 (2016): 2321–34.

67. ANIS, ADI 5581, "Protocoal ação no Supremo Tribunal Federal: Proteçao de diretos violados na emergencia de saúde pública do virus Zika," petition to the Supreme Court supported by ANIS and ANADEP, ANIS press release of August, 24, 2016. I was among the scholars—together with Rebecca Cook, University of Toronto; Eva Kittay, Stony Brook

University; Laura Rodrigues, London School of Hygiene and Tropical Medicine; and two Brazilian scholars, the jurist Alberto Silva Franco and the economist Fernando Gaiger Silveira—who wrote expert opinions in support of ADI 5581; these opinions were annexed to the petition submitted to the Supreme Court.

68. Projeto de Lei, no. 4396, "Para prever aumento de pena no caso de aborto cometido em razão da microcefalia ou anomalia do feto," https://www.camara.leg.br/proposicoesWeb /prop_mostrarintegra;jsessionid=8DFB38FDDD490B5E9E0C07214F8A4C39.proposicoesWeb Externo1?codteor=1433470&filename=Tramitacao-PL+4396/2016. The bill did not pass.

69. Answer to the demand of ANADEP of September 5, 2016, Procuratoria Geral da República, document no. 207.857/2016-AsJConst/SAJ/PGR, September 16, 2016.

70. Bruna Gonçalves, "Gestantes com zika vírus sofrem com falta de informações," *Jornal do USP*, July 20, 2019.

71. Agencia Senado, "Possível liberação do aborto de fetos com microcefalia pelo STF é criticada na CAS," April 25, 2019, https://www12.senado.leg.br/noticias/materias/2019/04/25 /possivel-liberacao-do-aborto-de-fetos-com-microcefalia-pelo-stf-e-criticada-na-cas.

72. G1 Rio, "Polícia fecha clínica de aborto e prende 10 durante ação em Caxias, RJ," *O Globo*, March 15, 2013. This taking of a bleeding woman from an operating table in an abortion clinic was not an isolated case; it happened again during a raid on an "upscale" abortion clinic in Rio de Janeiro in April 2016. Elisa Clavery, "Médico de hospital público no Rio e assessor parlamentar são presos em clínica de aborto," *O Globo*, April 6, 2016.

73. Supremo Tribunal Federal Brasil, Habeas Corpus 124.306, August 9, 2016, 2.

74. Amanda Greenberg, "Will the Zika virus enable a transplant of Roe v. Wade to Brazil?," *University of Miami Inter-American Law Review* 49, no. 1 (2017): 51–87.

75. Naara Luna, "The debate on abortion in the chamber of deputies in Brazil between 2015 and 2017: Conservative agenda and resistance," *Sexualidad, Saúde y Sociedad* 33 (2019): 240–72.

76. Partido Socialismo e Liberdade, "Arguição de Descumprimento de Preceito Fundamental," Brasília, March 6, 2017.

77. Paula Guimarães and Sonia Corrêa, "Brazil: Abortion rights at the Supreme Court," *Sexuality Policy Watch*, April 11, 2017, https://sxpolitics.org/abortion-rights-at-the-brazilian -supreme-court/16796.

78. Natacha Cortez, "ADPF 442: Tudo que você precisa saber sobre a audiência deaborto no STF," *Marie Claire*, August 3, 2018; Manuela Andreoni and Ernesto Londono, "Brazil's Supreme Court considers decriminalizing abortion," *New York Times*, August 3, 2018.

79. Renata Teixeira Jardim, "Aborto no STF: O debate sobre a ADPF 442," *Themis*, August 6, 2018, http://themis.org.br/wp-content/uploads/2018/08/20180804-stf.jpg.

80. Sonia Correa, "Brazilian Supreme Court public hearing on the decriminalization of abortion: Antecedents, contents and effects," *Sexual Policy Watch*, September 2018, https:// www.sxpolitics.org/wp-content/uploads/2018/09/Brazilian-Supreme-Court-Public-Hearing -on-the-Decriminalization-of-Abortion-2018.pdf; Jonatan Sacramento and Maria Conceição da Costa, "Zika vírus, expertises e moralidades: A ADPF 442 e as controvérsias em torno da descriminalização do aborto," *Ilha* 22, no. 2 (2020): 200–228.

81. Advocacia Geral da União, "AGU defende no Supremo a inconstitucionalidade do aborto em casos de Zika vírus," April 24, 2020, https://www.gov.br/agu/pt-br/comunicacao /noticias/agu-defende-no-supremo-a-inconstitucionalidade-do-aborto-em-casos-de-zika -virus-924639; *Noticias Supremo Tribunal Federal Brasil*, Portal STF, May 1, 2020, http:// www.stf.jus.br/portal/cms/verNoticiaDetalhe.asp?idConte.

82. Catholic News Agency, "Brazil's Supreme Court rejects effort to legalize abortion in Zika cases," *CNA*, April 27, 2020, https://www.catholicnewsagency.com/news/brazils-supreme -court-rejects-effort-to-legalize-abortion-in-zika-cases-17289.

83. Lucila Szwarc, "Les services d'accueil et de conseils en avortement sûr à Buenos Aires et en banlieue : De la réduction des risques à l'avortement populaire" (MSc thesis, EHESS, Paris, 2013).

84. Simon Cauchemez, Marianne Besnard, Priscilla Bompard, et al., "Association between Zika virus and microcephaly in French Polynesia, 2013–15: A retrospective study," *Lancet* 387 (2016): 2125–32.

85. Carneiro and Fleischer, " 'I never expected this, it was a big shock,' " 720–21.

86. Iulia Bicu Fernandes, "Interromper ou não interromper a gestação: Vivencias de gestantes de fetos com Anenefalia" (dissertation, Instituto Fernandes Figueira, Fiocruz, 2017).

87. Several women who participated in focus groups conducted by Mateleto and her colleagues declared that they believed an abortion should be legal in cases of microcephaly. Marteleto, Weitzman, Coutinho, and Alvez, "Women's reproductive intentions and behaviors," 211.

88. Heron Werner, Daniele Sordé, Celso Hygino, et al., "First-trimester intrauterine Zika virus infection and brain pathology: Prenatal and postnatal neuroimaging findings," *Prenatal Diagnosis* 36, no. 8 (2016): 785–89; Brasil, Pereira, Raja Gablia, et al., "Zika virus infection in pregnant women."

89. Clare Wenham, Amaral Arevalo, Ernestina Coast, et al., "Zika, abortion and health emergencies: A review of contemporary debates," *Globalization and Health* 15, no. 49 (2019): 49, https://doi.org/10.1186/s12992-019-0489-3.

90. Wenham, Arevalo, Coast, et al., "Zika, abortion and health emergencies."

91. Pan American Health Organization, *Zika Ethics Consultation.*

92. Abigail Aiken, Catherine Aiken, and James Trussell, "In the midst of Zika pregnancy advisories, termination of pregnancy is the elephant in the room," *BJOG* 124 (2017): 546–48.

93. "Carta de recomendação para o enfrentamento das consequências da epidemia de Zika virus no Brasil. Fiocruz, 2019," http://expozika.fiocruz.br/site/wp-content/uploads/2020/10/05-carta-de-recomendacao.pdf.

94. Quoted in Ann Kelly, Javier Lezaun, Ilana Löwy, and Koichi Kameda, "Imperfect diagnosis: The truncated legacy of Zika testing," *Social Studies of Science* 51, no. 5 (2021): 683–706.

95. Debora Diniz, "Comment: The protection of women's fundamental rights violated by Zika epidemics," *American Journal of Public Health* 106, no. 8 (2016): e9, https://doi.org/10.2105/AJPH.2016.303246.

96. Pablo Valente, "Zika and reproductive rights in Brazil: Challenge to the right to health," *American Journal of Public Health* 107, no. 9 (2017): 1376–80. Valente's argument about the existence of "legal instrument that allow abortion only in case of fetal malformation" is a fiction: no country has legalized abortion only in such cases.

97. Diane Paul and Ilana Löwy, "On objectivity in prenatal genetic care," *OBM Genetics* 2, no. 2 (2018), https://doi.org/10.21926/obm.genet.1802022.

98. ANIS, *Zika, the film,* https://www.youtube.com/watch?v=j9tqtojaoGo; the exchange between Melo and Loizy takes place in the first four minutes of the film.

99. Anahí Guedes de Mello and Gabriela Rondon, "Feminism, disability, and reproductive autonomy: Abortion in times of Zika in Brazil," Somatosphere, February 17, 2020, http://somatosphere.net/2020/abortion-zika.html/.

100. De Mello and Rondon, "Feminism, disability, and reproductive autonomy." De Mello, who is disabled herself, is a disability rights activist; Rondon represented Brazil on the executive committee of the Consorcio Latinoamericano contra el Aborto Inseguro (CLACAL, Latin American Consortium against Unsafe Abortion).

101. Debora Diniz, *Zika: From the Brazilian Backlands to Global Threat,* trans. Diane Grosklaus Whitty (Chicago: University of Chicago Press, 2017).

102. In France the great majority of abortions for a fetal indication are for anomalies classified as severe by experts. Marc Dommergues, Laurent Mandelbrot, Dominique Mahieu-Caputon, et al., "Termination of pregnancy following prenatal diagnosis in France: How severe are the foetal anomalies?," *Prenatal Diagnosis* 30 (2010): 531–39.

103. Marcia Turcato, ed., *Zika Virus in Brazil: The SUS Response* (Brasilia: Ministry of Health of Brazil, Health Surveillance Department, 2017), http://portalarquivos.saude.gov.br/images/pdf/2017/setembro/21/zika-virus-in-brazil-2017.pdf.

104. A Frenchwoman who decides to terminate a pregnancy after 14 weeks needs the approval of an interdisciplinary ethics committee. However, such committees rarely reject women's demands. Ilana Löwy, *Tangled Diagnosis: Prenatal Testing, Women and Risk* (Chicago: University of Chicago Press, 2018), chap. 3.

105. "Nos queremos o conhecimento de vôces." Debora Diniz and Luciana Brito, "Epidemia provocada pelo vírus Zika: Informação e conhecimento," *RECIIS, Revista Eletrônica de Comunicação, Informação e Inovação em Saúde* 10, no. 2 (April–June 2016), "notas de conjunctura," | https://www.reciis.icict.fiocruz.br. Joselito and Maria Carolina probably suspected that because severe microcephaly was visible in the second-trimester ultrasound, it had been diagnosed by the ultrasound expert at the public hospital, who had then elected to hide this information from the couple.

106. Anthony Cousien, Sylvie Abel, Alice Monthieux, et al., "Assessing Zika virus transmission within households during an outbreak in Martinique, 2015–2016," *American Journal of Epidemiology* 188, no. 7 (2019): 1389–96.

107. National Institute of Statistics and Economic Studies (INSEE), France, data from 2018 census, https://www.insee.fr/fr/statistiques/2011101?geo=DEP-972#chiffre-cle-2.

108. The majority of the inhabitants of Martinique are Catholic, but there is a growing presence of evangelicals, mainly Adventists. In 2020 there were 49 Catholic parishes in Martinique and 70 relatively smaller, evangelical churches. https://fr.wikipedia.org/wiki/Martinique.

109. Institut de Veille Sanitaire, France, "Infection par le Zika chez la femme enceinte," March, 11, 2016, https://solidarites-sante.gouv.fr/IMG/pd f/zika_femme_enceinte-reperes-110316.pdf; Haut Conseil de Sante, "Surveillance des femmes enceintes dans le cadre de l'épidémie de Zika," May 4, 2016, https://www.hcsp.fr/explore.cgi/avisrapportsdomaine?clefr=532.

110. Mehdi Mejdoubi, Alice Monthieux, Tiphaine Cassan, et al., "Brain MRI in infants after maternal Zika virus infection during pregnancy," *New England Journal of Medicine* 377, no. 14 (2017): 1399–1400; Bruno Schaub, Michèle Gueneret, Eugénie Jolivet, et al., "Ultrasound imaging for identification of cerebral damage in congenital Zika virus syndrome: A case series," *Lancet Child and Adolescent Health* 1 (2017): 45–55.

111. Karen Sohan and Cathy Cyrus, "Ultrasonographic observations of the fetal brain in the first 100 pregnant women with Zika virus infection in Trinidad and Tobago," *Gynecology and Obstetrics* 139, no. 3 (2017): 278–83.

112. Schaub, Gueneret, Jolivet, et al., "Ultrasound imaging for identification of cerebral damage," 51, 54.

113. Claudia Sampaio Rodrigues, "Sentidos, limited e potentialidades de medecine fetal: A visão de especialistas" (master's thesis, Instituto Fernandes Figuiera, Fiocruz, 2010).

114. Lilian Krakowsky Chazan, "'É . . . tá grávida mesmo! E ele é lindo!' A construção de 'verdades' na ultra-sonografia obstétrica," *Manguinhos* 15 (2008): 99–116; Veronique Mirlesse, "Diagnostic prénatal et médecine fœtale: Du cadre des pratiques à l'anticipation du handicap; Comparaison France–Brésil" (PhD thesis, University of Paris XIII, 2014).

115. Human Rights Watch, *Neglected and Unprotected*, 71.

116. Veronique Mirlesse and Isabelle Ville described the reluctance of some Brazilian

experts in the public sector to provide precise information about the consequences of an observed fetal malformation. They quote a pediatrician who explained to parents: "First of all, we don't know the exact situation. . . . An ultrasound scan provides an image, like a portrait. If you take my portrait home with you today, to introduce me to your family, you'll say 'Here is the paediatrician we met.' From the image you show them, they'll be able to tell I have problems with my sight, because of my glasses, but will they know that I speak French? So an ultrasound scan shows a structure, not a function. We only see the function when the challenge is there and we have to meet it." Mirlesse and Ville, "The uses of ultrasonography in relation to foetal malformations in Rio de Janeiro, Brazil," *Social Science and Medicine* 87 (2013): 173. The prenatal blurring of prognoses of fetuses with severe CZS—in many cases pregnant women were told that it was impossible to know what the future of the child would be even though the experts were aware of the high probability that the child would have a severe handicap— reflected a similar trend.

117. Schaub, Gueneret, Jolivet, et al., "Ultrasound imaging for identification of cerebral damage," 48. Brazilian doctors often note that lower-class Brazilian women who use SUS services are very religious and would have categorically rejected terminating a pregnancy for a fetal anomaly. It is possible that this view that poor women's beliefs and attitudes are radically different from those of middle-class women makes a very difficult situation bearable.

Chapter 6 · *Mães de Micro*

1. ANIS, *Zika, the film*, 2016, https://www.youtube.com/watch?v=j9tqtojaoGo.

2. Debora Diniz and Ilana Ambrogi, "Research ethics and the Zika legacy in Brazil," *Developing World Bioethics* 17, no. 3 (2017): 142–43.

3. Eleomar Vilela Moraes, Olegário Rosa Toledo, Flávia Lúcia David, et al., "Implications of the clinical gestational diagnosis of ZIKV infection in the manifestation of symptoms of postpartum depression: A case-control study," *BMC Psychiatry* 19, no. 1 (2019): 199, https://doi.org/10.1186/s12888-019-2157-9.

4. Paula Freitas, Gabriella Soares, Helaine Mocelin, et al., "How do mothers feel? Life with children with congenital Zika syndrome," *International Journal of Gynecology and Obstetrics* 148, suppl. 2 (2020): 20–28. This study was based on detailed interviews with 14 mothers of children with CZS in the state of Espírito Santo. Some mothers reported extremely brutal statements made by doctors, but such statements appear to have been exceptional.

5. Ana Paula Lopes de Melo, Tereza Lyra, Thália Velho Barreto de Araújo, et al., "'Life is taking me where I need to go': Biographical disruption and new arrangements in the lives of female family carers of children with congenital Zika syndrome in Pernambuco, Brazil," *Viruses* 12, no. 12 (2020): 1410, https://doi.org/10.3390/v12121410.

6. Rosamaria Carneiro and Soraya Resende Fleischer, "'I never expected this, it was a big shock': Conception, pregnancy and birth in times of Zika through the eyes of women in Recife," *Interface* (Botucatu) 22, no. 66 (2018): 713–15 . Carneiro and Fleischer asked mothers of children with CZS to keep diaries and record their daily experiences.

7. Ministério da Saúde, Agência Nacional de Vigilância Sanitária, Brasília, *Nota técnica sobre critérios técnicos para gerenciamento do risco sanitário no uso de hemocomponentes em procedimentos transfusionais frente à situação de Emergência em Saúde Pública de Importância nacional por casos de infecção por vírus Zika no Brasil,* Publication no. 001 (December 2015); "Estratégia de ação rápida para o fortalecimento da atenção à saúde e da proteção social de crianças com microcefalia," ordinance no. 405 (February 2016). See also Gustavo Corrêa Matta, Carolina de Oliveira Nogueira, and Lenir da Silva Nascimento, "A literary history of Zika: Following Brazilian state responses through documents of emergency," in *Zika Frontiers: Social Change and Governance in the Age of Mosquito Pandemics,* ed. Kevin Bardosh (London: Routledge, 2020), 55–77.

8. ANIS, "Zika in Brazil: Women and children at the center of the epidemic," 2017, http://anis.org.br/wp-content/uploads/2017/06/Zika-in-Brazil_Anis_2017.pdf.

9. Maria Conceição N. Costa, Luciana Lobato Cardim, Maria Gloria Teixeira, et al., "Case fatality rate related to microcephaly: Congenital Zika Syndrome and associated factors; a nationwide retrospective study in Brazil," *Viruses* 12 (2020): 1228, https://doi.org/10.3390/v12111228; Maria Gloria Teixeira, "A epidemia zika e o devir nas emergências sanitárias," at the ABRASCO meeting, December 7, 2021, https://www.youtube.com/watch?v=1-eSfQJ8bnI.

10. "Monitoramento integrado de alterações no crescimento e desenvolvimento relacionadas à infecção pelo vírus Zika e outras etiologias infecciosas, até a Semana Epidemiológica 30 de 2018," *Boletim Epidemiológico* 48, no. 39 (2018), https://repositorio.observatoriodocuidado.org/handle/handle/1671.

11. Adeilson Cavalcante, introduction to *Zika Virus in Brazil: The SUS Response*, ed. Marcia Turcato (Brasilia: Ministry of Health of Brazil, Health Surveillance Department, 2017), 6, http://portalarquivos.saude.gov.br/images/pdf/2017/setembro/21/zika-virus-in-brazil-2017.pdf. The title of Graciliano Ramos's book, *Vidas secas* (Dry lives), is a reference to the severe droughts frequent in northeastern Brazil and to their effects on the inhabitants of that region.

12. Alessandra Gomes Mendes, Daniel de Suza Campos, Letícia Batista Silva, et al., "Facing a new reality from the Zika Virus Congenital Syndrome: The families' perspective," *Ciência e Saúde Coletiva* 5, no. 10 (2020): 3785–94.

13. Diniz and Ambrogi, "Research ethics and the Zika legacy in Brazil"; C-News, "A rotina de sacrifícios de mulheres para criar filhos portadores do zika vírus," January 16, 2019, http://g1.globo.com/globo-news/jornal-globo-news/videos/v/a-rotina-de-sacrificios-de-mulheres-para-criar-filhos-portadores-do-zika-virus/7298901/Y6PBGUUna9P6meglReAM7e7Ky GAoronU9LWShphCMIA5fXco.

14. Carneiro and Fleischer, "'I never expected this, it was a big shock,'" 716.

15. The parable of going to Florence and landing in the Netherlands was written by the Down syndrome activist Emily Pearl Kingsley in 1987. It is reproduced in Andrew Salomon, *Far from the Tree: Parents, Children and the Search for Identity* (New York: Scribner, 2012), chap. 4.

16. Russell Parry Scott, Luciana Campelo de Lira, Silvana Sobreira de Matos, et al., "Therapeutic paths, care and assistance in the construction of ideas about maternity and childhood in the context of the Zika virus," *Interface* (Botucatu) 22, no. 66 (2018): 673–84.

17. Barbara Marques, Raquel Lustosa, Thais Valim, and Soraya Fleischer, eds., *Micro-histórias para pensar macropolíticas* (São Carlos: Áporo Editorial, 2021).

18. Diniz and Ambrogi, "Research ethics and the Zika legacy in Brazil."

19. Lopes de Melo, Lyra, Barreto de Araújo, et al., "'Life is taking me where I need to go.'"

20. Carneiro and Fleischer, "I never expected this, it was a big shock," 721.

21. Ilana Löwy and Marilena Correa, "The 'abortion pill' misoprostol in Brazil: Women's empowerment in a conservative and repressive political environment," *American Journal of Public Health* 110, no. 5 (2020): 677–84.

22. Russell Parry Scott, Marion Teodósio Quadros, Ana Cláudia Rodriguez, et al., "A epidemia de Zika e as articulações das mães num campo tensionado entre feminismo, deficiência e cuidados," *Cadernos de Gênero e Diversidade* 3, no. 2 (2017), https://doi.org/10.9771/cgd.v3i2.22013. On the importance for mães de micro of labeling children with CZS as "special children" and "angels" see, e.g., Marion Teodosio de Quadros, Russell Parry Scott, and Alfonsina Faya Robles, "'Enfants spéciaux,' 'bébés-micro,' 'bébés anges' . . . objectivation, et subjectivations du corps des enfants atteints du syndrome congénital, du virus Zika à Pernambouc, Brésil," in *Socialisation familiale des jeunes enfants*, ed. Anne Dupuy (Paris: Eres, 2021), 221–40.

23. UMA, founded in Pernambuco in November 2015, was probably the first association

of mothers of children with CZS; it remained numerically the most important among them. Many other such associations were founded later, such as the Associação das Mães Escolhidas (AME), of Juazeiro do Norte, Ceará, founded in February 2016; MED-RN de Rio Grande do Norte, founded in March 2016; Abraço a Microcefalia de Salvador, Bahia, founded in April 2016; the Associação Mães Unidas pelo Amor de pessoas com microcefalia, of Mato Grosso, founded in January 2017; the Associação de Mães de Anjos de Minas (AMAM), of Belo Horizonte, Minas Gerais, founded in April 2017; the Associação Mães de Anjos da Paraíba (AMAP), of Campina Grande, Paraíba, founded in May 2017; the Associação Macro Amor de Mossoró, of Rio Grande do Norte, founded in June 2017; the Associação Lótus de Famílias Vítimas da Síndrome Congênita do Zika Vírus e outras Neuropatias, of Rio de Janeiro, founded in July 2017; Pais de Anjos da Bahia (APAB), of Salvador Bahia, founded in August 2017; the Associação das Famílias de Anjos do Estado de Alagoas (AFAEAL), of Maceió, Algoas, founded in September 2017; the Associação Mais de Fé—Microcefalia não é o fim (AMF), of Manaus, Amazonas, founded in October 2017; the Associação Filhos da Benção (AFB), of Fortaleza, founded in January 2018; the Associação de Mães de Microcéfalos (AMMI), of Piauí, founded in 2018; the Associação de famílias com crianças com microcefalia por Zika e microcefalia por outras patologias em Goiás (AMIZ-Goiás), of Goiás, founded in February 2019; and the Associação Maranhense de Apoio às Crianças com Microcefalia (AMACRIM), of São Luís, Maranhão, founded in June 2020. Many of these associations have strong links with Catholic or evangelical churches.

24. Declaration of UMA, quoted in Camila Pimentel, Ana Paula Lopes de Melo, Sandra Valongueiro Alves, et al., "Zika in everyday life: Gender, motherhood and reproductive rights in Pernambuco State, northeast Brazil," in Bardosh, *Zika Frontiers*, 86.

25. Luciana Campello de Lira, Russel Parry Scott, and Fernanda Meira, "Trocas, gênero, assimetrias e alinhamentos: Experiência etnográfica com mães e crianças com síndrome congênita do Zika," *Revista Antropológicas* 28, no. 2 (2017): 231.

26. Soraya Fleischer and Flavia Lima, eds., *Micro: Contribuições da Antropologia* (Brasilia: Editora Athalia, 2020); Marques, Lustosa, Valim, and Fleischer, *Micro-histórias para pensar macropolíticas*.

27. Silvana Sobreira de Matos, Marion Teodósio de Quadros, and Ana Cláudia Rodrigues da Silva, "A negociação do acesso ao benefício de prestação continuada por crianças com Síndrome Congênita do Zika Vírus em Pernambuco," *Anuário Antropológico* 44, no. 2 (2019): 229–60.

28. On the status and difficulties of care professions in Brazil see, e.g., Helena Hirata, *Le care, théories et pratiques* (Paris: La Dispute, 2021).

29. Soraya Fleischer, "Me chama de mamae," in Marques, Lustosa, Valim, and Fleischer, *Micro-histórias para pensar macropolíticas*, 221–26. On narratives of mothers of children with multiple handicaps see, e.g., Myriam Winance, "Histoires de normes: Articuler récits biographiques et analyses des processus de normalisation par les sciences sociales," in *Repenser la normalité: Perspectives critiques sur le handicap*, ed. J.-P. Tabin, M. Piecek, C. Perrin, and I. Probst (Lormont: Editions Le Bord de l'eau, 2019), 35–57.

30. Aissa Simmas Petronilho, "Quantidade, qualidade, temporalidade: Microcefalia e políticas de desenvolvimento," in Marques, Lustosa, Valim, and Fleischer, *Micro-histórias para pensar macropolíticas*, 87–91.

31. Maya Mayblin, "The madness of mothers: Agape love and the maternal myth in northeast Brazil," *American Anthropologist* 114, no. 2 (2012): 240–52.

32. Lopes de Melo, Lyra, Barreto de Araújo, et al., "'Life is taking me where I need to go.'"

33. Rozeli Maria Porto, "Zika vírus e itinerários terapêuticos: Os impactos da pós-epidemia no Estado do Rio Grande do Norte," *Ilha* 22, no. 2 (2020): 169–99.

34. Anna Guiland, "Our babies are 'little warriors': How love is transforming tragedy in

the wake of Brazil's Zika outbreak," *Telegraph*, September 18, 2018, https://www.telegraph.co
.uk/news/0/babies-little-warriors-love-transforming-tragedy-wake-brazils/.

35. On the parallel between the spread of epidemics and infodemics see Adam Kucharski, *The Rules of Contagion: Why Things Spread—and Why They Stop* (London: Wellcome Collection, 2020).

36. Debora Diniz, *Zika: From the Brazilian Backlands to Global Threat*, trans. Diane Grosklaus Whitty (Chicago: University of Chicago Press, 2017), 121.

37. Andrew Jacobs, "Conspiracy theories about Zika spread through Brazil with the virus," *New York Times*, February 16, 2016.

38. Naomi Smith and Tim Graham, "Mapping the anti-vaccination movement on Facebook," *Information, Communication and Society* 22, no. 9 (2019): 1310–27.

39. Such rumors might also have been one of the reasons Debora Diniz received death threats and was obliged to leave Brazil. Dom Phillips, "Professor forced into hiding by death threats over Brazil abortion hearing," *Guardian*, August 2, 2018.

40. Shawn Smallman, "Conspiracy theories and the Zika epidemic," *Journal of International and Global Studies* 9, no. 2 (2018): 1–13.

41. Meg Stalcup, "The invention of infodemics: On the outbreak of Zika and rumors," *Somatosphere*, March 16, 2020, http://somatosphere.net/2020/infodemics-zika.html/.

42. Mathew Connelley, *Fatal Misconception: The Struggle to Control World Population* (Cambridge, MA: Harvard University Press, 2008).

43. Rockefeller Foundation, "Background on The Rockefeller Foundation and Zika," 2016, https://www.rockefellerfoundation.org/zika-statement/.Websites that spread the rumor about links between the RF and the deliberate spread of ZIKV displayed images of invoices for mailing ZIKV samples from the RF's virology laboratory to other laboratories. Indeed, the RF's virology laboratory became a reference laboratory for ZIKV, and samples of this virus were sent to other laboratories to facilitate a correct diagnosis.

44. On the rapid spread of rumors linking Zika to vaccines see Heidi Larson, *Stuck: How Vaccine Rumors Start—And Why They Don't Go Away* (Oxford: Oxford University Press, 2020), 8–9.

45. Amanda Taub and Max Fisher, "The Interpreter: How YouTube misinformation resolved a WhatsApp mystery in Brazil," *New York Times*, August 15, 2019.

46. Clarissa Simas, Loveday Penn-Kekana, Hannah Kuper, et al., "Hope and trust in times of Zika: The views of caregivers and healthcare workers at the forefront of the epidemic in Brazil," *Health Policy and Planning* 35, no. 8 (2020): 953–62.

47. See, e.g., Paul Farmer, "From Haiti to Rwanda: AIDS and accusations," in *Partner to the Poor: A Paul Farmer Reader*, ed. H. Saussy (Berkeley: University of California Press, 2010); and Eugene Richardson, Timothy McGinnis, and Raphael Frankfurter, "Ebola and the narrative of mistrust," *BMJ Global Health* 4 (2019): e001932, https://doi.org/10.1136/bmjgh-2019 -001932.

48. John Carey, Victoria Chi, D. J. Flynn, Brendan Nyhan, and Thomas Zeitzoff, "The effects of corrective information about disease epidemics and outbreaks: Evidence from Zika and yellow fever in Brazil," *Science Advances* 6, no. 5 (January 29, 2020): https://doi.org/10 .1126/sciadv.aaw7449.

49. Carneiro and Fleischer, " 'I never expected this, it was a big shock,' " 718. Eva's conviction that her doctor blamed vaccines for microcephaly—a conviction linked with a rumor that pregnant women were immunized with banned or unauthorized vaccines—does not necessarily mean that this was a faithful reconstitution of what her doctor had said. Brazilian health professionals usually support vaccination, and it is somewhat difficult to imagine a physician, even less a specialist, telling a patient to distrust vaccines. Nevertheless, this testimony shows poor communication between health providers and mothers of CZS children.

As several women attested, "We did not know what was normal. They did not explain anything to us." Carneiro and Fleischer, "'I never expected this, it was a big shock,'" 715.

50. Wanderson Kleber de Oliveira, Daniela Buosi Rohlfs, Eduardo Marquez Macario, et al., *Síndrome congênita associada a infecção pelo virus Zika: Situação epidemiologica, acoes desinvolvidase desafios de 2015 a 2019* (Brasilia: Secretaria de Vigiliancia em Saúde, Ministério da Saúde, 2019).

51. Antony Duttine, Tracey Smythe, Míriam Ribiero Calheiro de Sá, et al., "Congenital Zika syndrome—assessing the need for a family support programme in Brazil," *International Journal of Environmental Research in Public Health* 17 (2020): 3559, https://doi.org/10.3390/ijerph17103559.

52. Tracy Smythe, Monica Matos, Julia Reis Antony Duttine, Silvia Ferrite, and Hanna Kupfer, "Mothers as facilitators for a parent group intervention for children with congenital zika syndrome: Qualitative findings from a feasibility study in Brazil," *PLOS One* 15, no. 9 (2020): e0238850, https://doi.org/10.1371/journal. pone.0238850.

53. Cora Coralina dos Santos Junqueira, Alane Barreto de Almeida Leôncio, Elenice Maria Cecchetti Vaz, et al., "Stimulation of children with congenital Zika syndrome at home: Challenges for the caregivers," *Revista Gaúcha de Enfermagem* 41 (2020): e20190247, https://doi.org/10.1590/1983-1447.2020.20190247.

54. Luciana Lira and Helena Prado, "Les effets collatéraux de la recherche sur l'épidémie de Zika au Brésil," *Anthropologie et Santé* 21 (2020), https://doi.org/10.4000/anthropologiesante.7972.

55. Diniz and Ambrogi, "Research ethics and the Zika legacy in Brazil."

56. Soraya Fleischer and Thais Valim, "Meu filho foi quem me ensinou a falar," in Marques, Lustosa, Valim, and Fleischer, *Micro-histórias para pensar macropolíticas*, 63–67; Thais Valim, "Ciência para quem?," in Marques, Lustosa, Valim, and Fleischer, *Micro-histórias para pensar macropolíticas*, 145–48; Soraya Fleischer, "'Mas vai ter resultado essa pesquisa, né?': Zika, mães e ciência no Brasil," in Marques, Lustosa, Valim, and Fleischer, *Micro-histórias para pensar macropolíticas*, 149–52.

57. Ana Claudia Knihs de Carvalho, "Sobre fé, santos e remédios," in Marques, Lustosa, Valim, and Fleischer, *Micro-histórias para pensar macropolíticas*, 74–77.

58. Silvana Sobreira de Matos, Luciana Campelo de Lira, and Fernanda Meira, "Deficiência, ativismo, gênero e cuidado na síndrome congênita do Zika vírus: Entrevista com Germana Soares," *Revista Antropológicas* 29, no. 2 (2018): 150.

59. Diniz and Ambrogi, "Research ethics and the Zika legacy in Brazil."

60. On the difficulties of integrating the knowledge of users of science and experts see, e.g., Bruno Strasser, Jerome Baudry, Dana Mahr, Gabriela Sanchez, and Elise Tancoigne, "'Citizen science'? Rethinking science and public participation," *Science and Technology Studies* 32, no. 2 (2019): 52–76.

61. Lira and Prado, "Les effets collatéraux de la recherche sur l'épidémie de Zika au Brésil."

62. Luciana Lira and Helena Prado, "'Nossos filhos não são cobaias': Objetificação dos sujeitos de pesquisa e saturação do campo durante a epidemia de Zika," *Ilha* 22, no. 2 (December 2020): 96–131; Lira and Prado, "Les effets collatéraux de la recherche sur l'épidémie de Zika au Brésil."

63. Soraya Fleischer, ed., "Field report, Zika" (University of Brasília, January 2019), 7–8, https://opendocs.ids.ac.uk/opendocs/bitstream/handle/20.500.12413/14407/FIELD%20 REPORT_Fleischer_2019_1%2 02.pdf?sequence=1&isAllowed=y.

64. Maria Joana Passos, Gustavo Matta, Tereza Maciel Lyra, et al., "The promise and pitfalls of social science research in an emergency: Lessons from studying the Zika epidemic in Brazil, 2015–2016," *BMJ Global Health* 5, no. 4 (2020): e002307, https://gh.bmj.com/content/5/4/e002307.

65. Lira, Scott, and Meira, "Trocas, gênero, assimetrias e alinhamentos," 206–37.

66. Lira and Prado, "Les effets collatéraux de la recherche sur l'épidémie de Zika"; Lira and Prado, "'Nossos filhos não são cobaias.'"

67. Lira, Scott, and Meira, "Trocas, gênero, assimetrias e alinhamentos," 218.

68. Simas, Penn-Kekana, Kuper, et al., "Hope and trust in times of Zika."

69. Simas, Penn-Kekana, Kuper, et al., "Hope and trust in times of Zika."

70. Mendes, Campos, Silva, et al., "Facing a new reality from the Zika Virus Congenital Syndrome," 3792. Anthropologists who documented tensions between mothers of CZS children and scientists who studied them and researchers who emphasized the mothers' (in this case, one mother's) gratitude observed small groups of mães de micro. I am not aware of studies that investigated larger groups of mothers of children with CZS.

71. Lira, Scott, and Meira, "Trocas, gênero, assimetrias e alinhamentos," 218.

72. See https://portal.fiocruz.br/noticia/fiocruz-aprova-tres-mocoes-na-conferencia -nacional-de-saude.

73. João Biehl, Mariana P. Socal, Varun Gauri, et al., "Judicialization 2.0: Understanding right-to-health litigation in real time," *Global Public Health* 14, no. 2 (2019): 190–99.

74. Lira and Prado, "'Nossos filhos não são cobaias.'"

75. Jessica S. Cranston, Sophia Finn Tiene, Karin Nielsen-Saines, et al., "Association between antenatal exposure to Zika virus and anatomical and neurodevelopmental abnormalities in children," *JAMA Network Open* 3, no. 7 (2020): e209303. The opposite is true too. About half the children born to mothers infected with ZIKV during pregnancy and declared symptom free at birth developed some degree of neurological impairment, mainly delays in cognition and the acquisition of language, in the first two years of life. Massaroni Pecanha, Saint Clair Gomes Junior, Sheila Moura Pone, et al., "Neurodevelopment of children exposed intrauterus by Zika virus: A case series," *PLOS One* 15, no. 2 (2020): e0229434, https://doi.org /10.1371/journal.pone.0229434.

76. Thais Masetti, Dafne Herrero, Julliana Alencar, et al., "Clinical characteristics of children with congenital Zika syndrome: A case series," *Arquivio Neuropsychiatria* 78, no. 7 (2020): 403–11.

77. Anne Wheeler, Danielle Toth, Ty Ridenour, et al., "Developmental outcomes among young children with congenital Zika syndrome in Brazil," *JAMA Network Open* 3, no. 5 (2020): e204096, https://doi.org/10.1001/jamanetworkopen.2020.4096. This study was conducted with CZS children in Recife, an especially closely observed group.

78. Heloisa Viscaino Fernandes Souza Pereira, Stella Pinto dos Santos, Ana Paula Rodriguez Lazzari Amancio, et al., "Neurological outcomes of congenital Zika syndrome in toddlers and preschoolers: A case series," *Lancet Child and Adolescent Health* 4 (2020): 378–87.

79. https://www.bbc.com/news/av/world-latin-america-35643345/the-story-of-the-brazil -s-zika-bucket-baby. The short film was made in February, 2016. (accessed January 13, 2022).

80. The Associated Press photographer Felipe Dana, who took photos of José Wesley Campos at the age of 3 months, told a somewhat different story. See https://globalnews.ca /news/2497368/in-photos-photographer-reflects-on-bucket-baby-brazil-child-born-with-zika -virus-linked-microcephaly/.

81. Mauricio Savarese, "From shrieks in bucket to laughs, Brazil Zika baby improves," *Associated Press*, June 6, 2018, https://apnews.com/0686869cf5294b3aab134ce11386cc23.

82. Thais Valim, "Sintomas e tratamentos: Fases de cuidado dos bebês nascidos com a Síndrome Congênita do Zika Vírus," in Marques, Lustosa, Valim, and Fleischer, *Micro-histórias para pensar macropolíticas*, 96–100; Flavia Lima and Soraya Fleischer, "Dilemas alimentares: A complexa ciência de cuidar de crianças com a Síndrome Congênita do Zika Vírus," in Marques, Lustosa, Valim, and Fleischer, *Micro-histórias para pensar macropolíticas*,

78–86. As a rule, children with moderate CZS have less distressing trajectories, as do those born without visible brain anomalies.

83. Carneiro and Fleischer, "'I never expected this, it was a big shock,'" 713–15.

84. Stephanie Nolen, "The forgotten virus: Zika families and researchers struggle for support," *New York Times*, August 16, 2022.

85. Alessandra Santana Soares Barros, "Deficiência, sindrome congênita do zika e produção de conhecimento pela antropologia," *Revista Scientia* (Salvador) 6, no. 1 (2021): 142–63.

86. Barros, "Deficiência, sindrome congênita do zika e produção de conhecimento," 157.

87. Eliza Williamson, "Care in the time of Zika: Notes on the 'afterlife' of the epidemic in Salvador (Bahia), Brazil," *Interface* (Botucatu) 22, no. 66 (2018): 685–96.

88. Williamson, "Care in the time of Zika," 689.

89. Freitas, Soarez, Mocelin, et al., "How do mother feel?" This study was based on detailed interviews with 25 "Zika mothers" from the state of Espírito Santo in southeastern Brazil. See also Deisiane Amorim da Silva and Érica Quinaglia Silva, "Saúde mental no enfoque das mulheres afetadas pelo Zika vírus: Um estudo etnográfico no Estado do Pará, Brasil," *Cadernos de Saúde Pública* 36, no. 8 (2020): e00100019, https://www.scielo.br/j/csp/a/cBkXygT4rmmybRyHnwkmjwt/?lang=pt.

90. Carlo Caduff, "Hot chocolate," *Critical Inquiry* 45, no. 3 (2019): 787–803. Other anthropologists, among them Clara Han, Lisa Stevenson, Angela Gracia, Julie Livingston, and Veena Das, similarly documented the difficulty of caring. They questioned an automatic association of care with good intentions, good feelings, and good outcomes and proposed a more nuanced descriptions of care's ambivalence.

91. Aryn Martin, Natasha Myers, and Ana Viseu, "The politics of care in technoscience," *Social Studies of Science* 45 (2015): 1–17.

92. Anne Marie Mol, *The Logic of Care: Health and the Problem of Patient Choice* (London: Routledge, 2011), 10.

93. Freitas, Soarez, Mocelin, et al., "How do mother feel?," 27.

94. Ilana Ambrogi, Luciana Brito, and Debora Diniz, "The vulnerabilities of lives: Zika, women and children in Alagoas State, Brazil," *Cadernos de Saúde Pública* 36, no. 12 (2020): e00032020, https://doi.org/10.1590/0102-311X00032020.

95. Congresso Nacional, "Projeto de lei de conversão n° 26 de 2019 (proviente de Medida Provisoria n° 894 de 2019)," September 4, 2019, https://www.in.gov.br/en/web/dou/-/medida-provisoria-n-894-de-4-de-setembro-de-2019-214566522. The demand for a minimum pension for each child with CZS had been included in the petition ADI 5581, supported by ANIS and ANADEP, the National Association of Public Defenders, and submitted to the Supreme Court in August 2016. Press release, ANIS, August 24, 2016.

96. A transcription of the parliamentary debates of September–October 2019 can be found at https://www.congressonacional.leg.br/materias/medidas-provisorias/-/mpv/138553.

97. Rodrigo Baptista, "Familiares criticam MP que prevê pensão para crianças com microcefalia por Zika," Senadonotícias, October 10, 2019, materias/2020/04/08/sancionada-lei-que-garante-pensao-vitalicia-a-criancas-atingidas-por-zika-virus.

98. "Senado confirma pensão vitalícia para crianças atingida pelo Zika vírus," February 5, 2020, Agência Senado, https://www12.senado.leg.br/noticias/materias/2020/02/05/senado-confirma-pensao-vitalicia-para-criancas-atingidas-pelo-zika-virus.

99. Senadonotícias, "Sancionada lei que garante pensão vitalícia a crianças atingida por Zika vírus," April 8, 2020, Agência Senado, https://www12.senado.leg.br/noticias/materias/2020/04/08/sancionada-lei-que-garante-pensao-vitalicia-a-criancas-atingidas-por-zika-virus.

100. The participation of Zika activists in the elaboration of this law is described in

Silvana Sobreira de Matos and Ana Cláudia Rodrigues da Silva, "'Nada sobre nós sem nós': Associativismo, deficiência e pesquisa científica na Síndrome Congênita do Zika Vírus," *Ilha* 22, no. 2 (December 2020): 132–67.

101. See http://expozika.fiocruz.br/en/ (accessed January 13, 2022). The main mothers' and parents' association linked with the exhibition was the Associação Lótus, from the state of Rio de Janeiro, which has had long-standing links with Fiocruz.

102. The first version of the document "Epidemia de zika no Brasil: Lições aprendidas e recomendações" was drafted in August 2018, and its definitive version was published in 2019. See http://expozika.fiocruz.br/site/wp-content/uploads/2020/10/05-carta-de-recomendacao.pdf.

103. Lenir Silva, Mariana Albuquerque, and Marta Fabíola Mayrink, "Exhibition 'Zika Affecting Lives': An experience report," *Saúde Debate* 45, no. 130 (2021): 861–70. The authors do not list the activist groups that participated in the organization of the Fiocruz exhibition or discuss their contributions.

104. UMA's leader, Germana Soares, discussed the abandonment of CZS children by their fathers in her TED talk "Como transformar a superação em uma missão?," March 6, 2018, https://www.youtube.com/watch?v=u-iOwWGs8gA.

105. Silva, Albuquerque, and Mayrink, "Exhibition 'Zika Affecting Lives,'" 866–67.

106. Silva, Albuquerque, and Mayrink, "Exhibition 'Zika Affecting Lives,'" 864.

107. The last chapter of this book discusses the difference between a call to "reduce inequalities," a relatively consensual slogan, and a striving to put an end to social injustice.

Chapter 7 · After Zika

1. Jeremy Greene and Dora Vargha, "How epidemics end," *Boston Review*, June 30, 2020, https://www.bostonreview.net/special_project/thinking-pandemic-project-page/.

2. Erica Charters and Kristin Heitman, "How epidemics end: Introduction," University of Oxford University, How Epidemics End, A multidisciplinary project, accessed January 14, 2022, https://epidemics.web.ox.ac.uk/how-epidemics-end-introduction#/.

3. On the rules that govern the declaration of a disease as a public health emergency of international concern see Marc Eccleston-Turner and Clare Wenham, *Declaring a Public Health Emergency of International Concern: Between International Law and Politics* (Bristol: Bristol University Press, 2021).

4. Jenny Lei Ravelo, "Peter Sands: HIV and TB needs even greater post-pandemic," *Devex,* September 9, 2021, https://www.devex.com/news/peter-sands-hiv-tb-and-malaria -needs-even-greater-post-pandemic-101574. On the colonial root of defining a disease as "endemic" see Jacob Steere-Williams, "Rethinking 'herd' mentalities and rethinking the value of the history of public health," *American Journal of Public Health*, November 10, 2022, https:// ajph.aphapublications.org/doi/abs/10.2105/AJPH.2022.307148.

5. On "neglected diseases" and silenced populations see, e.g., João Nunes and Denise Nacif Pimenta, "A epidemia de Zika e os limites de saúde global," *Lua Nova* (São Paulo) 98 (2016): 21–46.

6. *Boletim Epidemiológico Zika*, 2020, https://www.gov.br/saude/pt-br/assuntos/media /pdf/2020/dezembro/11/boletim_epidemiologico_svs_47.pdf.

7. Gretchen Vogel, "One year later, Zika scientists prepare for a long war," *Science* 354 (December 2, 2016): 1088–89; Kate Wighton, "Zika epidemics likely to end within three years," Imperial College London, July 14, 2016, https://www.imperial.ac.uk/news/173474/zika -epidemic-likely-within-three-years/.

8. Jose Ueleres Braga, Clarisse Bressan, Ana Paula Razal Dalvi, et al., "Accuracy of Zika virus disease case definition during simultaneous dengue and chikungunya epidemics," *PLOS One* 12, no. 6 (2017): e0179725, https://doi.org/10.1371/journal.pone.0179725.

9. Jon Cohen, "Where has all the Zika gone?," *Science* 357 (August 18, 2017): 631–32.

10. Monica Malta, "Human rights and political crisis in Brazil: Public health impacts and challenges," *Global Public Health* 13, no. 11 (2018): 1577–84.

11. David Heymann, Joanne Liu, and Louis Lillywhite, "Partnerships, not parachutists, for Zika research," *New England Journal of Medicine* 374, no. 16 (2016): 1504–5.

12. Marcia Turcato, ed., *Zika Virus in Brazil: The SUS Response* (Brasilia: Ministry of Health of Brasil, Health Surveillance Department, 2017), 19, http://portalarquivos.saude.gov .br/images/pdf/2017/setembro/21/zika-virus-in-brazil-2017.pdf.

13. International cooperation did not play an important role in Brazil's public health authorities' response to Zika, criticized as being lackluster. Eduardo Gómez, Fernanda Aguilar Perez, and Deisy Ventura, "What explains the lacklustre response to Zika in Brazil? Exploring institutional, economic and health system context," *BMJ Global Health* 3, no. 5 (2018): e000862, https://pubmed.ncbi.nlm.nih.gov/30397514/.

14. Donald McNeil Jr., "How the response to Zika failed millions," *New York Times*, January 16, 2017.

15. Clare Wenham, Amaral Arevalo, Ernestina Coast, et al., "Zika, abortion and health emergencies: A review of contemporary debates," *Globalization and Health* 15, no. 49 (2019), https://doi.org/10.1186/s12992-019-0489-3.

16. Nunes and Pimenta, "A epidemia de Zika e os limites de saúde global." For a critique of global health as a Western enterprise see, e.g., Seye Abimbola and Madhukar Pai, "Will global health survive its decolonisation?," *Lancet* 396 (2020): 1628–29; and Clare Herrick and Kirsten Bell, "Epidemic confusions: On irony and decolonisation in global health," *Global Public Health* 17, no. 8 (2022): 1467–78, https://doi.org/10.1080/17441692.2021.1955400. On the trend to replace the striving for health justice with the sanitized framework of "social determinants of health" see Thomas Cousins, Michelle Pentecost, Alexandra Alvergne, et al., "The changing climates of global health," *BMJ Global Health* 6 (2021): e005442, https://doi.org/10 .1136/ bmjgh-2021-005442.

17. Deisy Ventura, "Infectious diseases served as an excuse to change the global health agenda," *Bulletin of the Brazilian Society of Tropical Medicine*, October 14, 2017, http://www .sbmt.org.br/portal/doencas-infectocontagiosas-tem-servido-como-pretexto-para-mudanca -na-agenda-da-saude-global/?lang=en.

18. Laura Rodriges, "Zika: The tragedy and the opportunities," *American Journal of Public Health* 106, no. 4 (2016): 582.

19. Deisy Ventura, "From Ebola to Zika: International emergencies and the securitization of global health," *Cadernos de Saúde Pública* 32, no. 4 (2016): e00033316, https://doi.org/10 .1590/0102-311X00033316.

20. Barbara Ribeiro, Sarah Hartley, Brigitte Nerlich, and Rusi Jaspald, "Media coverage of the Zika crisis in Brazil: The construction of a 'war' frame that masked social and gender inequalities," *Social Science and Medicine* 200 (2018): 137–44.

21. John Maurice, "The Zika virus public health emergency: 6 months on," *Lancet* 388 (2016): 450.

22. Maria Joana Passos, Gustavo Matta, Tereza Maciel Lyra, et al., "The promise and pitfalls of social science research in an emergency: Lessons from studying the Zika epidemic in Brazil, 2015–2016," *BMJ Global Health* 5, no. 4 (2020): e002307, https://doi.org/10.1136 /bmjgh-2020-002307. The practical outcome of the massive investment in fundamental research on Zika was modest. A similar focus on fundamental research during the Ebola epidemic had led to an efficient treatment and a vaccine.

23. WHO, "Zika strategic response plan—revised for July 2016–December 2017," June 2016, https://www.who.int/publications-detail-redirect/zika-strategic-response-plan---revised-for -july-2016-december-2017.

24. Passos, Matta, Lyra, et al., "Promise and pitfalls of social science research in an emergency," 3.

25. Passos, Matta, Lyra, et al., "Promise and pitfalls of social science research in an emergency." "Abraço a microcefalia" is a smaller and less well known group of activists than the Pernambuco-based União de Mães de Anjos.

26. Nunes and Pimenta, "A epidemia de Zika e os limites de saúde global."

27. Ventura, "From Ebola to Zika."

28. David M. Morens and Anthony S. Fauci, "Pandemic Zika: A formidable challenge to medicine and public health," *Journal of Infectious Diseases* 216, suppl. 10 (2017): S857–S859.

29. Marion Koopmans, Xavier de Lamballerie, and Thomas Jaenisch, on behalf of ZIKAlliance Consortium, "Familiar barriers still unresolved—a perspective on the Zika virus outbreak research response," *Lancet Infectious Diseases* 19, no. 2 (2019): e59–e62, https://doi .org/10.1016/S1473-3099(18)30497-3.

30. George Weisz and Noémi Tousignant, "International health research and the emergence of global health in the late twentieth century," *Bulletin of the History of Medicine* 93, no. 3 (2019): 365–400.

31. Severino Jefferson Ribeiro da Silva, Jurandy Júnior Ferraz de Magalhaes, and Lindomar Pena, "Simultaneous Circulation of DENV, CHIKV, ZIKV and SARS-CoV-2 in Brazil: An inconvenient truth," *One Health* 12 (December 16, 2020): 100205, https://doi .org/10.1016/j.onehlt.2020.100205; Creuza Rachel Vicente, Theresa Cristina Cardoso da Silva, Larissa Dell'Antonio Pereira, and Angelica E. Miranda, "Impact of concurrent epidemics of dengue, chikungunya, zika, and COVID-19," *Journal of the Brazilian Society of Tropical Medicine* 54 (2021): e0837-2020, https://doi.org/10.1590/0037-8682-0837-2020.

32. Tereza Magalhaes, Karlos Diogo Chalegre, Cynthia Braga, and Brian Foy, "The endless challenges of arboviral diseases in Brazil," *Tropical Medicine and Infectious Diseases* 5 (June 2020): 75, https://doi.org/10.3390/tropicalmed5020075.

33. Malta, "Human rights and political crisis in Brazil."

34. Isabel Rodriguez-Barraquer, Marli Cordeiro, Cynthia Braga, et al., "From re-emergence to hyperendemicity: The natural history of the dengue epidemic in Brazil," *PLOS Neglected Tropical Diseases* 5, no. 1 (2011): e935, https://www.ncbi.nlm.nih.gov/pmc/articles/PMC3014978/.

35. Magalhaes, Chalegre, Braga, and Foy, "Endless challenges of arboviral diseases in Brazil."

36. GBD 2017, DALYs, and HALE Collaborators, "Global, regional, and national disability-adjusted life-years (DALYs) for 359 diseases and injuries and healthy life expectancy (HALE) for 195 countries and territories, 1990–2017: A systematic analysis for the Global Burden of Disease Study 2017," *Lancet* 392 (2018): 1859–1922.

37. Carol Isoux, "Dengue: Sanofi au cœur d'une affaire de vaccin mortel aux Philippines," *Le Nouvel Observateur*, November 27, 2018.

38. Euzebiusz Jamrozik and Michael Selgelid, "Ethics, health policy, and Zika: From emergency to global epidemic?," *Journal of Medical Ethics* 44, no. 5 (2017): 343–48.

39. The official recommendation of the Brazilian Health Ministry was to offer "morphological ultrasound" for risk of Zika-induced brain malformations at 30 to 35 weeks of pregnancy, while the WHO recommended such a test at 18 to 20 weeks of pregnancy. Human Rights Watch, *Neglected and Unprotected: The Impact of the Zika Outbreak on Women and Girls in Northeastern Brazil*, 2017, https://www.hrw.org/report/2017/07/13/neglected-and -unprotected/impact-zika-outbreak-women-and-girls-northeastern, 69–71.

40. Elisabeth Lopes Moreira, Karin Nielsen-Saines, Patricia Brasil, et al., "Neurodevelopment in infants exposed to Zika virus in utero," *New England Journal of Medicine* 379, no. 24 (2018): 2377–79; Vinicius de Melo Marques, Camilla Sousa Santos, Isabella Godinho Santiago, et al., "Neurological complications of congenital Zika virus infection," *Pediatric Neurology* 91 (2019): 3–10.

41. A. E. Ades, Claire Thorne, Antoni Soriano-Arandes, et al., "Researching Zika in pregnancy: Lessons for global preparedness," *Lancet Infectious Diseases* 20 (2020): e61–e68, https://doi.org/10.1016/S1473-3099(20)30021-9; Margaret Honein, Kate Woodworth, and Christopher Gregory, "Neurodevelopmental abnormalities associated with in utero Zika virus infection in infants and children," *JAMA Pediatrics* 174, no. 3 (2020): 269–76.

42. Alan Brown, Patricia Cohen, Jill Harkavy-Friedman, et al., "Prenatal rubella, premorbid abnormalities, and adult schizophrenia," *Biological Psychiatry* 49 (2001): 473–86.

43. Maria Alice Rosa Ribeiro, *História sem fim: Inventário da saúde pública, São Paolo, 1880–1930* (São Paolo: Editora UNESP, 1993), 270.

44. Mauricio Barreto, Gloria Teixeira, Francisco Bastos, et al., "Successes and failures in the control of infectious diseases in Brazil: Social and environmental context, policies, interventions, and research needs," *Lancet* 377 (2011): 1877–89; Malta, "Human rights and political crisis in Brazil."

45. Dominichi Miranda de Sá, "A voz do Brasil: Miguel Pereira e o discurso sobre o 'imenso hospital,'" *História, Ciências, Saúde—Manguinhos* 16, no. 1 (2009): 333–48.

46. Alfrânio Peixoto, *A defesa sanitaria do Brasil* (Rio de Janeiro, 1922), quoted in Gilberto Hochman, *A era de saneamento* (Rio de Janeiro: Editora Hucitec, 1998), 70.

47. Rosamaria Carneiro, introduction to *Micro: Contribuições de antropologia*, ed. Soraya Fleischer and Flavia Lima (Brasilia: Editora Athalia, 2020), 15.

48. Michelle Murphy, "Unsettling care: Troubling transnational itineraries of care in feminist health practices," *Social Studies of Science* 45 (2015): 717–37. Murphy's message resonates with Peter Burke's affirmation that historians' task is to remind people of what they would like to forget. Peter Burke, "History as social memory," in *Varieties of Cultural History* (Ithaca, NY: Cornell University Press, 1997), 59.

Conclusion

1. See Paula Treichler, *How to Have Theory in an Epidemic: Cultural Chronicles of AIDS* (Durham, NC: Duke University Press, 1999).

2. Paul Wendel Giessler, "Public secrets in public health: Knowing not to know while making scientific knowledge," *American Ethnologist* 40, no. 1 (2013): 13–34.

3. Charles Rosenberg, "Explaining epidemics," in *Explaining Epidemics, and Other Studies in the History of Medicine* (Cambridge: Cambridge University Press, 1992), 293–304.

4. Didier Fassin, *Life: A Critical User's Manual* (Cambridge: Polity Press, 2018), 123–24.

5. Thomas Cousins, Michelle Pentecost, Alexandra Alvergne, et al., "The changing climates of global health," *BMJ Global Health* 6, no. 3 (2021): e005442, https://doi.org/10.1136/bmjgh-2021-005442.

6. Nancy Fraser, "On justice: Lessons from Plato, Rawls, and Ishiguro," *New Left Review* 74 (2012): 41–51.

7. Emilia Sanabria, "From sub- to super-citizenship: Sex hormones and the body politic in Brazil," *Ethnos* 75, no. 4 (2010): 377–401.

8. Sanabria, "From sub- to super-citizenship," 394, 396.

9. Fraser, "On justice," 48.

10. On the judicialization of the "right to health" in Brazil see, e.g., João Biehl, "The judicialization of biopolitics: Claiming the right to pharmaceuticals in Brazilian courts," *American Ethnologist* 40, no. 3 (2013): 419–36.

11. See http://expozika.fiocruz.br/en/ (accessed January 15, 2022). Some Brazilian states provide important additional aid for families of children with CZS: medical and rehabilitation services, childcare in a public day care facility accompanied by a professional caregiver, subsidized lodging. Access to such advantages is uneven, however, even within a given state.

12. Poliana Cardoso Martins, Rosangela Minardi Mitre Cotta, Fabio Farias Mendes, et al.,

"Conselhos de saúde e a participação social no Brasil: Matizes da utopia," *Physis* 18, no. 1 (2008): 105–21.

13. Avishai Margalit, *The Decent Society* (Cambridge, MA: Harvard University Press, 1996).

14. This is a broad generalization. The relationships between the private and public health sectors varies among European countries, and some offer combinations of private and public health insurance. Moreover, in Western Europe too, affluent individuals who rely exclusively on private health facilities perceive the access to "better" health care as one of the privileges that come with their wealth. The US configuration is different because of the absence of a national health service.

15. One should add that when a treatment for a given pathology is very expensive, it is usually not covered even by a good private health insurance. In such cases, middle-class individuals too may sue the Brazilian state in order to oblige it to pay for their therapy, in the name of their "right to health." Such interventions may be likened to, for example, efforts of cancer patients in the United Kingdom to obtain the purchase of expensive experimental anti-cancer drugs by the National Health Service and their struggle with the National Institute for Clinical Excellence over the definition of the benefit-risk ratio of a drug, although in the United Kingdom their efforts usually are not mediated by courts.

16. The failures of policies that put the onus of avoiding births of children with CZS on women are summarized in Clare Wenham, *Feminist Global Health Security* (Oxford: Oxford University Press, 2021).

17. In mid-November 2015, when the Brazilian state declared the Zika outbreak an emergency (ESPIN), there was no way to know how far and wide the microcephaly epidemic would spread. At that point there was an urgent need to protect all pregnant women and those who might become pregnant from an infection with ZIKV. As it turned out, the microcephaly epidemic was concentrated mainly in northeastern Brazil and lasted a relatively short time. In November 2015 a significant number of the women who later gave birth to CZS children were already pregnant. Measures that might have reduced the number of children with severe Zika syndrome among low-income women might have been, in ascending order, easy access to quality contraception to allow women to delay pregnancy; protecting women in the first trimester of pregnancy from ZIKV infection through education about the Zika risk, distribution of effective insect repellents, and information on the danger of unprotected sex; making abortion available for pregnant women infected with ZIKV early in pregnancy; and offering a second-trimester diagnostic ultrasound, coupled with the possibility of terminating the pregnancy, to all pregnant women in epidemic areas. Taking into account the unique biological traits of the Zika outbreak in Brazil—a narrow epidemic peak and a belated warning about Zika risks—the possibility of ending a pregnancy following a diagnosis of a serious brain malformation of the fetus might have been the most effective way to reduce the number of children born with severe CZS. However, this measure was seen as especially problematic and did not receive much attention in public debates on Zika.

18. Alessandra Santana Soares Barros, "Deficiência, sindrome congênita do zika e produção de conhecimento pela antropologia," *Revista Scientia* (Salvador) 6, no. 1 (2021): 142–63.

19. ANIS, *Zika, the film*, 2016, https://www.youtube.com/watch?v=j9tqtojaoGo.

20. For a short interview with Loizy, who speaks about her financial difficulties, among others things, see https://www.youtube.com/watch?v=JndxTFExhRo. The interview is included in the ANIS document *Mujeres de Epidemia: Una campaña para promoción de derechos sexuales y reproductivos frente a la epidemia del virus Zika en Brasil* (Brasilia, 2016), https://clacaidigital.info/handle/123456789/910.

21. See, e.g., Marcella Alsan, Amitabh Chandra, and Kosali Simon, "The great unequalizer:

Initial health effects of Covid-19 in the United States," *Journal of Economic Perspectives* 35, no. 3 (2021): 25–46.

22. People affected by Ebola—with the exception of health care workers—belonged mainly to lower social strata, but until now the spread of Ebola has mainly been determined by geographic and not socioeconomic factors.

23. Soraya Fleischer, ed., "Field report, Zika" (University of Brasília, January 2019), 7–8, https://opendocs.ids.ac.uk/opendocs/bitstream/handle/20.500.12413/14407/FIELD%20 REPORT_Fleischer_2019_1%202.pdf?sequence=1&isAllowed=y.

24. For an exception see, e.g., Philip Blumenshine, Arthur Reingold, Susan Egerter, et al., "Pandemic influenza planning in the United States from a health disparities perspective," *Emerging Infectious Diseases* 14, no. 5 (2008): 709–14.

25. Reuters, "Brazil warns women to delay pregnancy amid Covid-19 surge," *Guardian*, April 17, 2021; Flavia Milhorance, "Calamity of maternal deaths: Covid concern grows for Brazil's pregnant," *Guardian*, May 3, 2021.

26. Letícia Marteleto, "Scarred by Zika and fearing new COVID-19 variants, Brazilian women say no to another pandemic pregnancy," *Conversation*, April 28, 2021; Letícia Marteleto and Molly Dondero, "Navigating women's reproductive health and childbearing during public health crises: Covid-19 and Zika in Brazil," *World Development* 139 (2021): 105305, https://search.bvsalud.org/global-literature-on-novel-coronavirus-2019-ncov/resource/pt /covidwho-957485.

27. Claudia Fonseca and Soraya Fleicher, "Vulnerabilities within and beyond the pandemic: Disability in Covid-19 Brazil," in *Viral Loads: Anthropologies of Urgency in the Time of COVID-19*, ed. Lenore Manderson, Nancy J. Burke, and Ayo Wahlberg (London: UCL Press, 2021), 243–60.

28. Silvana Sobreira de Matos, " 'Unidos pelo contágio?' Novas precarizações das famílias que têm filhos com a Síndrome Congênita do Zika Vírus em tempos de pandemia da COVID-19," *Boletim Cientistas Sociais* 53 (June 2020), http://anpocs.org/index.php/publicacoes-sp -2056165036/boletim-cientistas-sociais/2375-boletim-n-53-cientistas-sociais-e-o-coronavirus.

29. Thais Maria Moreira Valim, Barbara Marciano Marques, and Raquel Lustosa, " 'Parece que estamos voltando no tempo': Direitos das crianças com a Síndrome Congênita do Zika Vírus e de suas cuidadoras em face de duas epidemias," *Disability Studies Quarterly* 41, no. 3 (2021), https://dsq-sds.org/article/view/8390/6198.

30. Silvana Sobeira de Matos and Ana Claudia Rodriguez da Silva, "Quando duas epidemias se encontram: A vida das mulheres que têm filhos com a Síndrome Congênita do Zika Vírus na pandemia da COVID-19," *Cadernos de Campo* (São Paulo) 29, supplement (2020): 329–40.

31. Ed Yong, "We are already barreling toward the next epidemic," *Atlantic*, September 29, 2021.

32. Rosenberg, "Explaining epidemics."

ABRASCO (Brazilian Association for Collective Health), 9, 97, 98, 149, 174
AIDS, 80 ,117, 187, 188, 203
Alves, Damares, 65
Alves, Rodriguez, 22
AMAR (Union of Mothers and Families, Rare Diseases), 165
Amaral, Claudio, 40
Ambrogi, Ilana, 162
American Journal of Public Health, 107, 150, 192
amniocentesis, 71, 153, 154, 157
amniotic fluid, 94, 95
ANADEP (National Association of Public Defenders), 142
Andrade, Antonio José Farias de 28
anencephaly, 60–63, 68, 72, 75, 148
ANIS (Institute of Bioethics, Human Rights, and Gender, Brasilia), 48, 145, 149, 151, 152, 160, 167, 194, 210
Anopheles mosquito, 127
ANVISA (National Agency of Sanitary Vigilance), 119, 120
Araújo Thália Velho Barreto de, 60
Argentina, 146
Astra-Zeneca, 197
Atenas Project, Savador, Bahia, 54–60.
Avila, Medardo, 97
Aylward, Bruce, 193
Azevedo, Juvenal Siqueira Fliho, 48, 142

Barros, Alessandra Santana Soares, 179
Barroso, Luis Roberto, 144
Bauer, Johannes, 30
BBC, 1, 137

Bean William, 20
Beauvoir, Simone de, 52
Bell, Julia, 140, 141
Benchimol, Jaime, x
Biehl, Joaõ, 16
Big Pharma, 167
Bio-Manguinhos, Fiocruz, 45, 120, 175
Bispo, Ana de Filippis, 94
body stalk malformation, 73
Bolsa Familia, 42, 129, 208
Bolsonaro, Jair, xvii, 7, 188
Bonan, Claudia, xv
BPC (Permanent State Pension), 143, 184
Brasil, Patricia, 87, 191
Brazilian Federal Court of Accounts, 129
Brazilian Society of Infectious Diseases, 117
"Brazilionaires," 10
breast feeding, 79
Briggs, Laura, 6
Brito, Carlos, 91
Brito, Luciana, 154, 167
Brito, Maria Lucia, 89
Brock, Bevis, 141
Buarque, Chico, 56, 59

C-section, 58, 74
Cadernos de Saude Publica (journal), 139
Caduff, Carlo, 181
Calcavante, Adeilson, 161
Câmara, Raphael, 146
Camargo, Rosana, 117
Campos, José Wesley, 1, 177, 178
Canguilhem, George, xi
Cantrell pentalogy, 71

Cardoso, Fernando Henrique, 42

Caritas Diocesiana (Diocesian Charity Association), 40

Carneiro, Rosamaria, 147, 161, 168, 201

Carta, Mino, 10

Castro, Marcelo, 133

CDC (Centers for Disease Control and Prevention, [US]), 96, 103, 192

Center of Medical Virology, Fiocruz, Rio de Janeiro, 44

Chacham, Alexandra, 58

chikungunya, x, 4, 6, 84, 86, 87, 112, 115, 119, 197

Collor, Fernando, 42

community health workers, 130–132

Comte, Auguste, 22

CNS (National Conference on Health), 174

Confederations Cup soccer tournament, 85

conjoined twins, 65, 69

Correa, Marilena, xv

COVID-19, vii, xii, xiii, xvii, 185, 196, 197, 211–213

Crawford, Porter, 28

Cruz, Oswaldo, 5, 22, 23, 41

Cuba, ix, 18, 19

Culex mosquitoes, 113

Cunha, Rivaldo Venâcano da, 90, 107

Curumim (group), 66, 127, 136, 137

cytomegalovirus (CMV), 5, 84, 90, 156, 198, 199

Dana, Felipe, 1, 2

DDT, 38

dengue, x, 2, 4, 5, 6, 40–44, 84, 86, 87, 107, 112, 119, 197

DFID (UK Department for International Development) 193

Diniz, Debora, xv, 13, 89, 150, 151, 154, 162, 194, 212

Diniz, Simone, 58

DNERu (National Department of Rural Endemic Diseases), 39

DNSP (National Department of Public Health), 24, 39

Down syndrome, 161, 170

Dream Team do Passinho group, 126, 127

Ebola, 104, 105, 190, 197

ECDC (European Centre for Disease Prevention and Control), 95, 96

ECLAMC (Latin American Collaborative Study of Congenital Malformations), 98, 99, 100, 124

encephalitis, 34

endemic disease control agents, 131

epidural anesthesia, 58, 62, 63

episiotomy, 58

ESPIN (Public Health Emergency of National Importance), xi, 12, 92, 124, 188, 209

European Union's Horizon Program, 194

Evandro Chagas Hospital, Fiocruz, 87

Evandro Chagas Institute, Ananindeaua, 91

"eugenic" abortion, 68, 69, 146, 149, 151, 167

Exposis (insect repellent), 129

expressivist objection, 150, 151

Falwell, Jerry, 187

FAMERJ (Federation of Associations of Residents of the State of Rio de Janeiro), 40

Fassin, Didier, 204

Fauci, Anthony, 107, 195

Federal Court of Accounts, Brazil, 129

Fernandes Figuera Innstitute, Rio de Janeiro, 106

Fernandes, Iulia, xv, 60–63, 70

Ferrari, Wendell, xv, 50–53,

Ferreira, Solange, 1, 2, 178

fetal alcohol syndrome, 106

feticide, 63

Filippis, Ana Bispo de, 94

Findlay, George Marshall, 34, 35

Fiocruz: Archive Center (Rio de Janeiro), ix; Mato Grosso do Sul, 90; Museum of Life, 184; Recife, 89, 113 ; Rio de Janeiro, ix, 106, 174, 175

Fisher, Max, 166

Fleck, Ludwik, 3, 123

Fleischer, Soraya, 147, 161, 168

forceps, 58

Foy, Brian, 115

Fraga, Clementino, 25

Franco, Itamar, 42

Fraser, Nancy, 15, 205, 206, 207, 209, 211

Freitas, Paula, 182

French Polynesia, 12, 84, 85, 86, 95, 113, 147

fumigation, 5; 23, 25, 40, 41, 92, 93

FUNASA (National Foundation of Health), 39

Galton Laboratory, University College, London, 140

Gates Foundation, 166, 167

Geissler, Paul Wenzel, 5

GHSA (Global Health Security Agenda), 192

Ginzburg, Carlo, 87
Global Fund to Fight Tuberculosis, AIDS and
    Malaria, 187
Goethe, Johann van, 90
Gorgas, William, 20
Greene Jeremy, 187
Gregg, Norman, 140
Guardian (newspaper), 108
Guillain-Barré syndrome, 84, 85, 86, 105, 112
Guimarães, Aloisio Soarez, 48
Guiteras, Juan, 20

Haddow, Alexander, 81, 82
Haddow, Andrew, 82
Hatch, Steven, 105, 106
Heller, Leo, 9
Henriques, Cláudio Maierovitch, 133
hepatitis B, 34, 35
hepatitis outbreak, US army, 35
Heymann, David, 190
holoprosencephaly, 67
Hotez, Peter, 103
Horizon 2020 program, 194
Hudson, Paul, 30
hydrocephaly, 65, 72, 73
Hygiene Institute, Saõ Paolo, 27

Ishiguro, Kazuo, 205, 206, 207

Jenner Institute, Oxford University, 197

Kameda, Koichi, xvi
Kelly, Ann, xv
"key focus" theory, 24, 25
Ko, Albert, 104
Kypra (drug), 164

Lancet (journal), 96, 104, 128
Lechanal, Guillaume, 5
Lévi-Strauss, Claude, 202
Lezaun, Javier, xv
Lima, Angelo Moreira de Costa, 33
Lima, Henrique de Rocha, 29
Lima, Mariana, xv
Lima, Nisia Trindade, xv, 184
lissencephaly, 88
Ljubliana, Slovenia, 152
Lobato, Monteiro, 3

Loizy, Amanda, 151, 152, 210
Lovell, Anne, xvi
Lula (Luiz Inácio Lula da Silva), 7, 42
Lyra, Jorge, 14

MAB (Friends of Neighborhoods Association),
    40, 41
Magalhães Rodrigo, x
Manguinhos (favela) 175, 176
Manton, Paul, 5
Marchoux, Emile, ix, 20, 21
Margalit, Avishai, 15
Marteleto, Leticia, 142
Martin, Aryn, 181
Martinique, 155–157
Martins, Polyana Cardoso, 208
Matias, Maria da Conceiçao Alcantara Oliveira,
    153, 154
Matta, Gustavo, xv
Matta, Roberto de, 206, 209
McNeil, Donald, 103, 104
MED (Mothers Elected by God group), 166
Medida Provisoria 895(law), 182–184
Mello, Anahi Guedes de, 152
Melo, Adriana, 88, 89, 94, 95, 137, 151, 159, 177, 210
Mendes, Chico, 204
MERS (Middle East Respiratory Syndrome), 191,
    211
microcalcifications, 88, 148
mifepristone, 56, 59, 63
Minha Casa, Minha Vida program, 164
misoprostol (Cytotec), 52, 54, 56, 57, 59, 63, 163
Moebius syndrome, 163
Mol, Anne Marie, 181
Monsanto, 167
Moral Majority Report, 187
Moran, Caitlin, 53, 77
Morens, David, 107, 194
"More Rights, Less Zika" campaign, 126, 136
MRI (magnetic resonance imaging), 123, 149, 155
Murphy, Douglas, 140
Murphy, Michelle, 202
Myers, Natasha, 181

Nascer no Brasil project, 58
necrotorium, 17, 18
Never Let Me Go (novel), 205, 206, 207, 211
New York Times, viii, xiii, 101, 103, 166, 178, 179

NIAID (National Institute of Allergy and Infectious Diseases, USA) 107
Noguschi, Hideo, 29

Oliveira, Andre Novaes, 132
Olympic Games, Rio de Janeiro, 110, 116, 195
Operation Herold, 47, 144
Osterholm, Michael, 192
Oswaldo Cruz Institute, 23, 33, 44
oxytocine, 58

Pacific Islands, 2, 103
PAHO (Pan American Health Organization), 6, 25, 37, 39, 95, 96, 137, 149, 193
Paixao, Emily, 109
Pasteur Institute Archive, ix,
Pasteur Institute, ix, 20, 29
Pedro I Hospital, Campina Grande, 88
Penna, Henrique de Azevedo, 33
Pereira, Miguel, 23, 200
Perente, Raphael, 212
pesticides, 97, 167
PHEIC (Public Health Emergency of International Concern), 12, 104, 105, 119, 121, 124, 189, 190, 194
PHS (Public Health Service [US]), 38
Pimenta, Denise, xv
polyhydramniosis, 65
Population Council, 167
Prado, Helena, xvi,
private health insurance, 76
PSOL (Socialism and Freedom Party), 145
Puerto Rico, 93, 114, 115
pyriproxyfen, 97, 98

Ramos, Gracilliano, 161
Rawls, John, 205
Reed Mission, 18, 19
Reed, Walter, 19
Ribeiro, Maria Alice Rosa, 200
Rockefeller Institute Archive Center, ix
Rodrigues, Laura, 88, 109
Rodrigues, Weverton, 46
Roe vs. Wade, 145
Rondon, Gabriela, 152
Rosenberg, Charles, 3, 9, 118, 119
Roussef, Dilma, 110, 188
Roux, Emile, 20
rubella, 5, 81, 90, 140, 141, 199

Salimbeni, Alessandro Taurelli, ix, 20
Sanabria, Emilia, xvi, 76, 206, 207,
Sanitary Movement, Brazil, 23, 24; 200
Sanofi, 197
Santos, Géssica Eduardo dos, 153, 154
Santos, Verônica, 179
São Sebastião Isolation Hospital, 20
SARS (severe acute respiratory syndrome), xii, 211
SARS-CoV2, xii, 196, 197, 212
Sawyer, Wilbur, 31, 32, 35
scarlet fever, 123
Schatzmayr, Hermann, 44
Schikore, Jutta, 8
Sellards, Andrew, 29
Senegal, ix, 20
Serological Institute, Manguinhos, 23
Simond, Paul, ix, 20, 21
SINAN (National Notifiable Disease Information System), 119
SINASC (Brazilian Registry of Birth Anomalies), 96, 99
Smith, Hugh, 32, 33
Soares, Germana, 101, 128, 165, 170, 184, 186
Social Sciences and Zika Network, xi, 15
Soper, Fred Lowe, 25, 26, 28, 32, 36, 37
Souto, Lucia, 40, 41
Spanish Flu, vii
St. Bartholomew's Hospital, London, 141
Standard Oil, 167
STF (Brazilian Supreme Court), 142, 150
STF's abortion debate, 142–146,
stillborn children, 61, 67, 68
Stokes, Adrian, 30
SUCAM (Superintendence of Public Health Campaigns), 39, 40,
syphilis, congenital, 4, 5, 117, 118

Taub, Amanda, 166
Team Redudas, 97, 98
Temer, Michel, 188
Temporada (film), 132
Theiller, Arnold, 34, 35
Theiller, Max, 29, 30, 32, 35
TORCH infections, 4, 198
Tousignant, Noémie, 195
toxoplasmosis, 4, 156
Treichel, Paula, 203

trisomy 13 (Patau syndrome), 71
trisomy 18 (Edwards syndrome), 61

Uganda, 81, 82, 167
UKAID, 194
ultrasound (obstetrical), 67, 137, 138, 141, 147, 148, 149, 154, 155–157
UMA (Union of Mothers of Angels), 163, 164, 165, 184, 186
UNFPA (United Nations Population Fund), 126, 127, 136
United Nations Development Programme, 185
USAID, 193
Ustra, Carlos Alberto Brilhante, 188

Va'a canoe event, 85
"vaccine revolt", 22
Valente, Pablo, 150
Van dee Linden, Vanessa, 89
Varella, Druzio, 50, 140
Vargas, Getulio, 26
Vargha Dora, 187
Vasconcelos, Pedro, 91, 94
Veja Magazine, 117
ventriculomegaly, 88
Ventura, Deisy, 192, 194
Verne, Jules, x
Viana, Paula, 66
Victa, Gabriela, xv
Vidas Secas (book), 161

Virchow, Rudolf, 6
visceroctomy, 17, 18, 31
Viseu, Ana, 181

Watson, Katie, 49,50
Weber, Rosa, 145
Weisz, George, 195
Wellcome Archive and Manuscript Collection, ix
Wellcome Trust, 194
Wenham, Clare, 192
WhatsApp, 164, 166, 168
WHO (World Health Organization), 12, 100, 104, 105, 121, 149, 189, 190, 192, 193
"wicked problem", 8
Williamson, Elisa, 180
Wolbachia (bacterium), 43
Women on the Web, 59, 134
World Cup soccer tournament, 85

Yap Island, 12, 81, 83, 84
Yellow fever vaccine 17 D, 32, 33 34, 44, 45
Yellow fever vaccine 17 E, 32
YouTube, 167

Zika Social Science Network, xvi, 194
Zika: From the Brazilian Backlands to Global Threat (book), 13, 212
Zika: The Film, 151, 158, 210
ZIKAlliance, 195